WOMEN IN MEDICINE IN THE LONG NINETEENTH CENTURY

Nineteenth Century Science, Technology and Medicine Sources
Series Editors: Piers J. Hale and Meegan Kennedy

Available:

Science and Sound in Nineteenth-Century Britain
Edited by Edward J. Gillin
4 volume set

Forthcoming:

Women in Medicine in the Long Nineteenth Century
Edited by Claire Brock
4 volume set

Scientific Methodology in Nineteenth-Century Britain
Edited by Charles H. Pence
4 volume set

Electric Power in Victorian Britain
Edited by Nathan Kapoor
4 volume set

Insects in Victorian Culture
Edited by John Clark
4 volume set

Evolution in Victorian Culture
Edited by Piers J. Hale
5 volume set

Nineteenth-Century British Microscopy
Edited by Meegan Kennedy
4 volume set

Meteorology in Nineteenth-Century Society
Edited by Aitor Anduaga
4 volume set

Women, Gender and Science in Victorian Culture
Edited by Leila McNeill & Anna N. Reser
4 volume set

WOMEN IN MEDICINE IN THE LONG NINETEENTH CENTURY

Edited by
Claire Brock

Volume I
Debates

Routledge
Taylor & Francis Group
LONDON AND NEW YORK

First published 2025
by Routledge
4 Park Square, Milton Park, Abingdon, Oxon OX14 4RN

and by Routledge
605 Third Avenue, New York, NY 10158

Routledge is an imprint of the Taylor & Francis Group, an informa business

British Library Cataloguing-in-Publication Data
A catalogue record for this book is available from the British Library

ISBN: 978-1-032-20788-9 (set)
ISBN: 978-1-032-20789-6 hbk (vol I)
ISBN: 978-1-003-26523-8 ebk (vol I)

DOI: 10.4324/9781003265238

Typeset in Times New Roman
by Apex CoVantage, LLC

For my nieces, Ella Giddings and Beatrice Dew, and my niece and goddaughter, Rose Dew. May they always enjoy learning, be inspired by their surroundings, and challenge expectations.

CONTENTS

NINETEENTH-CENTURY SCIENCE, TECHNOLOGY AND MEDICINE: SOURCES AND DOCUMENTS GENERAL EDITORS' INTRODUCTION

This volume is part of the Routledge Historical Resources primary source collection, "Nineteenth-Century Science, Technology and Medicine: Sources and Documents." This series offers a fresh look at the historical development of science, technology, and medicine through the eyes of subject experts and specialists from around the world. The series provides curated access to significant primary-source documents on these subjects, collating and contextualizing these valuable resources so that they may ground not just scholarly research but undergraduate and graduate research and teaching as well. As well as being published in print and ebook formats, the contents of this and all other volumes in this series will be available through the Routledge Historical Resources database, where they will be presented in a fully integrated and searchable format, together with supplemental secondary sources and images and newly-commissioned scholarly written and video essays.

Our editors have framed their volumes around themes they consider most pertinent to understanding nineteenth-century developments in their chosen field and its significance to broader changes in nineteenth-century British culture and society. Often the editors have chosen to provide short extracts to illustrate particular points or themes; in other cases, they have provided entire essays, book chapters, or periodical articles as appropriate. Each volume is prefaced by an introductory essay in which the editors review their topic and discuss the significance of their sources. They also frame each entry or collection of related entries with explanatory headnotes. Thus, each volume or set of volumes will provide a useful resource of easy-to-navigate, well-contextualized sources curated by an expert eye, which will serve as a useful introduction for those unfamiliar with the field. Since the editors build each volume to represent a unique, deeply-considered scholarly perspective on the foundational primary sources for a particular subject, the series should also prove valuable to established scholars, even those with deep experience in the field. Indeed, given the range of topics covered and sources collated in this series, we anticipate that this project will foster an exciting and insightful interdisciplinary perspective on the histories and cultures of nineteenth-century British science, technology, and medicine. We as general editors have learned a lot through our engagement with the editors who have contributed to this project, and we believe that wider audiences will do so too.

Throughout the project we have asked editors to comment on the state of the existing historiographical debate, and to specify where their own work fits in. Some editors have chosen to do this through the provision of recommendations for further reading; others do so through explicit commentary on this topic in their introductory essays, and in the headnotes and footnotes to each of the sources they have selected.

The histories of science, technology, and medicine are wide and often disparate fields, even though they are often encountered by students in the context of a single university department. Although they have much in common, scholars of science, technology, and medicine also propose field-specific questions and approaches; these are represented in the project through the disparate interests of the range of scholars contributing to the series. We have also worked to bring the insights of literary scholars as well as historians to the project.

We have made every effort to cover major nineteenth-century themes and topics in the scientific and technological disciplines as well as to give space to specialist topics. Of course, as is inevitably the case in a project of this nature, which must rely on the availability of expert scholars in particular fields, there will remain gaps. We have attempted to address these where we can in the form of introductory essays and video essays in the database. We do believe, though, that the reader and researcher will find that this project presents the major themes, as well as many specialist topics, in detail, and with scholarly rigour.

We are very grateful to Routledge for their invitation to take on this project, and we would especially like to thank the commissioning editor Rachel Douglas, her successor, Laura Pilsworth, and Simon Alexander. Most of all, however, we are grateful to the extensive list of scholars from around the world who have agreed to contribute, and who make this series what it is.

Meegan Kennedy and Piers J. Hale

ACKNOWLEDGMENTS

For commissioning this project, I would like to thank Piers Hale and Meegan Kennedy, and Rachel Douglas, followed by Simon Alexander, at Routledge. Marie Roberts at Apex CoVantage was exemplary: thank you. The brilliant Dr Lisa Coar put Sorabji on the curriculum and introduced me to her work. I am grateful to the University of Leicester for granting a term of study leave to complete this project in 2023.

Several organisations have very kindly made the reproduction of sources in these volumes possible. Many thanks to the following: The Dr Matilda A. Evans Collection of Archival Material, National Museum of African American History and Culture, Smithsonian Institution, Washington, DC for the image of the Taylor Lane Hospital Operating Theatre in Volume III; The Women's Library at the London School of Economics Library for extracts from *The Woman Worker* in Volume IV; The Royal Free NHS Foundation Trust for the *London (Royal Free Hospital) School of Medicine for Women Magazine* in Volumes III and IV; The *British Medical Journal* for May Thorne's 'The After Effects of Abdominal Section' in Volume IV.

With everlasting thanks to my family for all the loving support, and to Ben Dew, as always, for absolutely everything.

CHRONOLOGY: SELECTED KEY DATES

1848 Establishment of the Boston Female Medical Society, which became New England Female Medical College in 1852, the first institution devoted to the education of women in medicine, and in 1873, when merging with Boston University, the first co-educational medical school in America.

1849 Elizabeth Blackwell graduated in medicine from University of Geneva, New York, becoming the first woman to achieve this feat in modern times.

1858 Medical Act created General Medical Council in Britain and tighter regulation of profession.

1862 Marie Zakrzewska opened the New England Hospital for Women and Children.

1864 Rebecca Lee Crumpler became first African American woman to earn a M.D.

Mary Edwards Walker contracted as an assistant surgeon to the Union Army. Awarded Medal of Honor in 1865.

1865 Elizabeth Garrett gained Licentiate of Society of Apothecaries, the first woman to qualify as a doctor in Britain.

1867 The Russian Nadezhda Prokofyevna Suslova qualified as the first woman M.D. from Zurich and became Russia's first woman doctor.

1873 Elizabeth Garrett Anderson elected as member of British Medical Association.

1874 Opening of London School of Medicine for Women; from 1877 the Royal Free Hospital admitted women for clinical study.

1876 Britain permitted medical and university education for women.

1879 Association of Registered Medical Women founded in Britain; forerunner of Medical Women's Federation in 1917.

1886 Anandi Gopal Joshi graduated from the Woman's Medical College of Pennsylvania to become the first woman doctor in India.

1890 Emma Constance Stone became the first woman to be registered with the Medical Board of Victoria, and the first woman to practise in Australia.

1895 *London School of Medicine for Women Magazine* was first published.

1895 Louisa Aldrich-Blake became the first woman to achieve the Master of Surgery degree.

1907 Mabel St Clair Stobart set up the Women's Sick and Wounded Convoy Corps.

1911 Eleanor Davies-Colley became first female Fellow of Royal College of Surgeons.

1914 Louisa Garrett Anderson and Flora Murray led Women's Hospital Corps to France a month after the start of the Great War, where they create a woman-run hospital at the Hôtel Claridge, Paris.

1915 Establishment of the American Medical Women's Association.

GENERAL INTRODUCTION

In November 1924, former medical student turned journalist, Florence Fenwick Miller, wrote an article in the *Fortnightly Review* about 'Pioneer Medical Women'. Fenwick told a narrative of triumph and progress in recent British history:

> Others followed, and many more doors were opened as years went on; and the progress of medical women has been steadily successful, until the Great War came, and a final seal on their competence as proven. In Serbia first, in Malta, in France, and finally in England, large hospitals for wounded and sick men were entirely staffed by women surgeons; and if anybody wants testimony to their work – well, let them ask the brave patients!
>
> Little by little opposition was converted into favour. Hundreds of women have passed on to the medical register and engaged in practical work. School after school, qualification after qualification, has been opened. One after another of the men's established schools of medicine, forgetting that once mixed education in these matters shocked male feelings too terribly, have offered instruction to men and women together. At the present time women are taught with men at some of the great London hospitals' medical schools, at the universities of Scotland, and at English and Irish provincial schools, as well as alone at the London School for Women; they can take the M.D. degree of all the universities of Great Britain, or the Licentiate and Membership of the conjoint Boards of the Royal Colleges of Surgeons and Physicians (the qualification that most men practitioners hold), as well as many foreign and Colonial degrees. Surely in the history of the progress of mankind so extraordinary a change was never so quickly worked.[1]

Fenwick Miller, who had joined Sophia Jex-Blake in the fight to study at the University of Edinburgh, characterised herself as so devoted to the cause that she was akin to the underaged boy soldiers of the recent Great War; at 16, she had 'anticipate[d] the boys who "joined up" too young'.[2] The battle, Fenwick Miller concluded, had been won – the extraordinariness of the change had been unprecedented in its speed and absoluteness. Doors, which had been slammed in the faces of the pioneers, were readily opened for the post-war generation. Medical women were treated equally, accepted, desired, and praised for their professional skills, both by their male counterparts and by their patients.

This four-volume collection will tell the story, for the first time, of these momentous years through the eyes of the people who experienced them. Such participants ranged from prospective medical women, their supporters and their detractors, but also their potential and actual patients. I will also tell a global tale, focusing predominantly, but not exclusively, upon Anglophone contexts. Medical women were fundamentally international in their outlook from the outset, as they attempted to assist women across the world socially or religiously precluded from trained and professional care. By bringing all these sources together, a unique insight into a novel phenomenon can be explored. The period covered across these volumes – from the middle of the nineteenth century until the start of the Great War – allows a consideration of more than simply one generation of medical women. Unlike Fenwick Miller's focus, while the 'pioneers' are present, they are seen as representatives of a certain time, but also points of comparison, beneficial or otherwise, for those who came after. In making this choice to expand beyond the obvious, I want to show the opportunities as well as the setbacks for those women who entered the medical profession over these seven decades. This was in addition to the dialogues different generations and countries had internally and with each other. The range chosen is deliberate because it shows continuity and change in support and opposition; vitally, it must be recognised that debates moved, emerged, disappeared, but reappeared at later dates, even when questions and problems had supposedly been solved. There was as much discussion about female suitability for practise in the 1850s as there was in the midst of the Great War.

Fenwick Miller's optimistic trajectory was mirrored, in some ways, by the narratives of some of the contributions here. Yet it would be inaccurate to argue that the path was smooth and the way to the doors was not strewn with obstructions. The doors themselves to co-education in Britain, for example, would also be firmly, if temporarily, shut once more – again – after Fenwick Miller's assertions that the changes were completed.[3] If there was one consistent theme throughout this whole period, it was that medical women were constantly having to prove their worth to ensure they met the expectations of their professional colleagues and ever-expectant patients, but also, importantly against their own high standards. Narratives were created around medical women; they were, after all, a fascinating, if not new, phenomena, as many were keen to illustrate when they provided histories of women's participation in medicine dating back to ancient times. As the *Lancet* recognised, when the British-born, American-educated Elizabeth Blackwell graduated in 1849, she was only the 'first woman medical graduate in the modern meaning of the phrase'.[4] These nineteenth and early twentieth-century aspirants represented simply the most recent attempt to secure a foothold in the professional world. Yet, medical women established their own narratives, too. Such accounts led both to cross-cultural links and internal dissension over issues ranging from, for example, the benefits of co- or single-sex education and the questions over who to treat and why. As we will see, medical women wrote for the press, lay and professional, for men, women, and children, for their own institutions or places of learning, for their colleagues, male or female. They also aimed to record the movement of which they were a part and for actual or potential patients. The writings collected here show that female medical professionals wrote to convince others, as well as to reassure themselves and to consolidate their positions, skills, and institutions. Formats and genres by and about medical women included pamphlets, magazine, newspaper and periodical articles, and fictional texts. But, as recognised here anew, the visual and aural aspects of female medical students and practitioners were also important. Contemporaries could see depictions of this strange species and hear about them in drawing rooms and places of entertainment. They were far more than a textual phenomenon. What was most fascinating about medical women, however, and this has not been fully recognised by historians keen to explore the movement as a whole before, was their diversity. Even if they came from similar backgrounds, the same countries, or even the same continents, they were individuals. These volumes intend to bring out medical women from a mass in which others placed them and which they sometimes positioned themselves.

One fundamental example of this was ensuring that women were represented alongside each other regardless of colour and race. By doing so, it was possible to consider similarities as well as differences in outlook, ways of practising, and public perceptions. I was influenced, in this sense, by a contemporary comment made right at the end of the period considered here by S. Maria Steward, M.D. *In Woman in Medicine, read before the National Association of Colored Women's Clubs at Wilberforce, Ohio in August 1914*, Steward remarked that

> The list of earnest medical women might easily be augmented, matched up, and given colored tone, by the names of their sisters of a darker race in the profession, who too have taken advantage of stepping into the doors of medical opportunity [. . . .] These have made, and are making, records for themselves that will be handed down in history to the distinguished credit of our own race. These women have measured up with their sisters in white, and in some instances have, as students, carried off the highest honors of their classes.[5]

It was such new ways of thinking about medical women within and across a global context that provided inspiration for these volumes, 'augmenting', 'matching up', 'measuring up', and giving 'colored tone' to the usual picture. I want the conversations and the dialogues that span the four volumes to spark novel readings of female practitioners in their own contexts, but also in the wider questions surrounding women's right to practise medicine that were taking place between the mid-nineteenth and early twentieth century. As medical women, they were inherently engaged in and with issues which drove contemporary society, such as female and infant welfare, the appropriateness or otherwise of modern surgery, patient care, and women's employment and rights. Bringing together the source material here in all its variations can, therefore, illuminate and provide new perspectives on international debates surrounding key cultural, social, and political questions of the long nineteenth century in which medical women were deeply involved.

VOLUME I: DEBATES

The first volume will explore the range of reactions to medical women from the mid-nineteenth century up until the start of the Great War in 1914. By covering this period, readers will be introduced to ongoing debates surrounding women in medicine, via sources which explore the possibilities for – as well as the problems of – female professional practice. The perspectives of detractors and supporters, as well as medical women themselves, will be taken into account, and especial consideration given to opinions which were not neatly divided along gender lines. Conversations between the generations and across continents will be compared. Of key concern here will be a nuanced tracing through primary material of changes in the perception of medical women, as well as the ways in which lingering prejudices disappeared or remained well into the twentieth century. Ultimately, therefore, this volume will focus on two key areas: first, the debates and challenges surrounding the education of women as medical and surgical practitioners; and, second, women's physical and mental 'fitness' to practise. It will also, by extension, explore the areas in which it was felt by various groups constituted the 'natural' or 'appropriate' areas for women to display their expertise. By establishing the ongoing contextual, social, and political factors with which nineteenth and early twentieth-century medical women had to contend, this volume provides a foundation for the discussions within the other three volumes.

VOLUME II: MEDICAL WOMEN IN FICTION

As an exciting, demanding, and for some, repulsive, novelty and phenomenon, the medical woman was fictionalised swiftly in the second half of the nineteenth century. This volume will reproduce literary examples, which explore the many facets of women's entry into the medical profession, and their experiences once qualified. In keeping with other volumes in this series, 'Medical Women in Fiction' will broaden literary and cultural understanding of female doctors through the selection of sources which are less well-known or more difficult to find, as well as considering global examples or contexts. Short stories and magazine fiction will be paired with ephemeral songs or plays, for example, showing how the medical woman became a potential part of quotidian life. Victorian British works are paired with American novels from the 1900s to explore the medical woman's similarities and differences, based on geographical location. By choosing sources which reveal both supportive and derogatory assessments, and by male and female authors, a wide range of opinions regarding women's efficacy as medical practitioners will be considered. Moving into the Edwardian period will also permit reproduction of more unfamiliar works, and show that the medical woman, remained a continuing object of fascination into the early twentieth century, despite both critical assumptions to the contrary and the growth in her numbers.

VOLUME III: GLOBAL EXPERIENCES

This volume will explore medical women as a global phenomenon. Scholars working on the history of women in medicine tend to be geographically specific, so this is a topic yet to be thoroughly researched. I will focus on Anglophone sources, especially those from the Americas, Asia, and Australasia, but will also present African, Middle Eastern and Arabic examples. The volume will consider, firstly, how especially British and American medical women travelled internationally to treat patients who, for reasons of religious, cultural, or social beliefs, were reluctant to seek treatment from male doctors. In this instance, missionary zeal was balanced with concern for women's health and welfare. Secondly, the volume will include material written by those who qualified as medical women and practised either in their national context or those educated abroad, who then returned home to pursue their careers. The latter will make more widely available works by women of colour, including, for example, the African American woman doctor, Rebecca Lee Crumpler, and Indian female medical practitioner, Rukhmabai. It will also, importantly, allow their writings to be positioned in dialogue with others. The reproduction of previously unpublished student magazines will be a key part of this volume. This will illustrate the sheer range of destinations to which female practitioners were sent or chose to go, but shows also the attempts to replicate the sense of community wherever former students were, all over the world. Ultimately, it will place the medical woman of the nineteenth and early twentieth century, for the first time, in an international conversation about her professional expectations and responsibilities.

VOLUME IV: PATIENT PERSPECTIVES

Historians have argued that the patient disappeared from the clinical encounter at the end of the eighteenth century.[6] The selections for this volume, which focus on or are told from the patient's perspective, confirm that the patient was, indeed, very much a key part of this far from hierarchical relationship. Vital to the acceptance of medical women, indeed, was the willingness of patients – largely women and children initially – to be treated by them. By the end of 1914, this more usual patient base was expanded to include injured soldiers. To provide a full consideration of the medical and surgical world of this period, it is necessary to explore patients, both of male and female medical professionals, to complete this collection of sourcebooks. 'Patient Perspectives' will examine the contemporary fear that hospital patients, mostly of working-class origin, were being experimented upon by their overly eager, ambitious, and vivisecting doctors; something in which surgeons especially were seen to be complicit. Women too, however, carried out abdominal and gynaecological surgery, and performed clitoridectomies. How medical women justified their actions, as well as how their patients viewed them, will be the focus of this final volume. Additionally, the voice of those who experienced 'medical tyranny' will be considered to examine what happened when patients fought back publicly against the medical establishment. For the first time since the 1910s, the exceptionally rare writing of former nurse and non-consenting patient, Alice Beatty, a cause célèbre in the late nineteenth century, will be reproduced in full.

***

All four volumes are intended ultimately to encourage historians to rethink the medical woman and explore her varied impact upon the societies in which she operated. The narrative of the female practitioner's progress from a very few pioneers to the triumphs and developments of the Great War has inevitably tended to lend the story a Whiggish bent. Fractures and divisions were apparent amongst and between women in medicine, however, as in any profession. Before the doors opened, however (im)permanently, there were attitudes, opinions, and prejudices to negotiate and renegotiate both within and without the world of medicine. In 1884, the publisher and rights for women campaigner Emily Faithfull wrote about *Three Visits to America*, which involved a 'curious incident a propos of the assertion that a man always objects to the admission of women into his own profession'. Faithfull described an incident when Dr George Hoggan was travelling by train to identify the body of American practitioner, Dr Susan Dimock of Boston, who had been drowned in the shipwreck of the Schiller off the Isles of Scilly. He sat in a carriage where he found

> an old lady engaged in a vehement discussion on 'woman's sphere'. The opposition was maintained by two young ladies, who were evidently staunch champions of a woman's right to make use of her own talents for the good of others. As the veteran representative of the clinging-dependence-upon-man-theory found that the forces were against her, she turned to the new-comer for sympathy and assistance.
>
> 'I am sure', she said, 'that this gentleman does not approve of women who compete with men in trade and professions'.
>
> 'On the contrary, madam', Dr Hoggan replied, 'I am quite in favour of women undertaking any work for which they are fitted'.
>
> 'Surely', she exclaimed with horror, 'the idea of a woman doctor is thoroughly repulsive to you?'
>
> 'Certainly not', he answered quietly, 'though I am a medical man myself'.

> 'I am certain that you would never dream of marrying such a woman', she cried, thinking now at least she should obtain the convincing answer wherewith most to discomfit her young marriageable opponents'.
>
> 'Madam', replied Dr Hoggan placidly, 'that is just what I have done. My wife is a doctor in London, with an excellent practice'. *Tableaux.*[7]

In similar fashion to these train travellers, readers of these volumes are asked to put aside assumptions about beliefs and practices supposedly held by certain groups in the late nineteenth and early twentieth centuries. Women did not always support their own sex, and men, professionals included, were not inherently antagonistic to female practitioners of medicine and surgery. Different sides fed off and used the material and arguments of others. There was often more similarity in opposite corners of these ongoing conflicts than has previously been acknowledged. Opinions about women in medicine were divided, but fruitfully tracing those debates can reveal nuances even in moments of change and continuity, progression and stasis; Faithfull's *tableaux* was, in fact, perpetually in motion. To put it as Florence Fenwick Miller did when she looked back upon this momentous period, extraordinary developments were, indeed, swiftly worked. Those working within, however, experienced both the halts and the strains as well as the thrills and pleasures of becoming medical women. As a testament to their struggles, challenges, and successes, it is important that we recognise this.

Notes

1 F. Fenwick Miller, 'Pioneer Medical Women [A Record and A Remembrance]', *Fortnightly Review*, CXVI:695 (November 1924), pp. 692–706; on p. 706.
2 Fenwick Miller, 'Pioneer Medical Women', p. 700.
3 See, for example, C. Brock, "Women in Surgery after the Great War', in *The Palgrave Handbook of Women and Science: History, Cultures and Practice since 1660*, eds., Claire Jones and James Bainbridge (Cham: Palgrave Macmillan, 2022), pp. 593–610.
4 'Obituary; Elizabeth Blackwell', *Lancet*, 175:4528 (11 June 1910), pp. 1657–1658; on p. 1658.
5 S.M. Steward, M.D., *Woman in Medicine: A Paper Read Before the National Association of Colored Women's Clubs at Wilberforce, Ohio, August 6, 1914* (Wilberforce, Ohio: n.p., 1914), pp. 17–18.
6 For debates around the patient, see, for example, F. Condrau 'The Patient's View Meets the Clinical Gaze', *Social History of Medicine*, 20:3 (December 2007), pp. 525–540.
7 E. Faithfull, *Three Visits to America* (Edinburgh: David Douglas, 1884), p. 115.

INTRODUCTION

In an 1897 article for the *Ludgate Magazine*, reproduced in this volume, doctor and writer Arabella Kenealy described the initial reactions to women's mid-nineteenth-century desire to enter the medical profession formally. Contemporary responses were characterised, she suggested, by 'oppositions, disabilities and insults' on the one hand and 'chivalries, encouragements and generosities' on the other. Such polarity in the early days had been replaced at the end of the century by the question of numbers. Medical women were here to stay – now an accepted fact – but how many would there be, in what fields should they practise, and where and to whom would they take their hard-won medical knowledge?

Kenealy's succinct assessment of the past fifty years forms an ideal starting place to consider the debates surrounding medical women in the nineteenth and early twentieth centuries. Firstly, while there were clearly opposing sides, Kenealy did not gender these factions. Key, indeed, to the reams of newspaper, periodical, professional, fictional, and myriad other interventions, was that it was impossible to place male reactions in one corner, female in the other. Both could be found at either end, as well as places in between. Secondly, the antithesis of Kenealy's presentation of history, simplified here into containing supporters of and detractors from the cause, was rarely apparent. Debates were divisive, but they were often torn by their own contradictions. As Kenealy herself and as others excerpted in this volume would discover, support, as well as disdain, could wax and wane, but was perennially contingent on the specific behaviour and achievements of individuals. Medical women could and did find their own dual identities coming adrift from each other, despite the tightly bound hyphenation of Kenealy's choice of 'medical-women'. At times, the woman usurped the professional, and vice versa. Due to the smallness of their numbers, one may be used to represent the whole in an exemplary or a demonic light, and this affected perceptions of the individual, but reflected, ultimately, on the whole.

This introduction will be split into three parts, exploring the interwoven and overlapping themes of the sources chosen for this volume. The first section, 'Histories', will look at the ways in which debates about medical women from varied perspectives placed them against historical precedents in order to weigh up their contemporary right to practise. 'Suitabilities', the second area to be examined, will focus on the most prevalent concern which exorcised all combatants across the period covered here. Why were women peculiarly suited to the medical profession or why, alternatively, were they wholly unsuitable for training or developing a career in this field? For the concluding thread, 'Reputations', one of the women covered in this volume, American Civil War veteran Mary Edwards Walker, will be considered as a microhistorical case study. Walker was publicly debated across the medical and lay presses in relation to the reception of her character and writings, and she was tellingly used to debate the value – or otherwise – of 'medical-women'.

HISTORIES

Reflection on the past, whether ancient or recent, was a key concern for debates about medical women. There were so many attempts to do this, indeed, that it ultimately became a standard way of discussing the topic. Although by no means the first to write in such a manner, this was most famously to be seen in Sophia Jex-Blake's *Medical Women: Two Essays* (1872), later republished as *Medical Women: A Thesis and a History* in 1886, which drew links between ancient and modern treatments of female medical ambitions. A number of sources collected in this volume explored a similar theme, from the earliest, Samuel Gregory's *Letter to Ladies in Favor of Female Physicians* (first published in 1850), via Edwin A. Pratt's *Pioneer Women* of 1897, to Beatrice Harraden's 1915 *Windsor Magazine* investigation into 'Women Doctors in the War'. Contributors to the debates were keen to draw on either a long history of previous successes in the medical field or a Whiggish narrative of adversity to triumph in the more immediate past. Detractors, in a contradictory fashion, were equally keen to insist upon an historical trajectory that was mired only in continuity of failure by the early twentieth century. Stasis and lack of development, rather than onward movement and progression, characterised this particular brand of assessment.

Gregory's argument lamented recent changes that had led to female ignorance about their own bodies and the bodies of their sex more generally. Women had become 'such a profound mystery to themselves'. He put the blame squarely on the usurpation of midwifery by men, which, he suggested, was far more prevalent in America than in Europe. Despite the supposed enlightened times in which they lived, contemporaries were actually worse off than more distant, barbaric societies, as China or Russia were perceived to be. Such stark divisions were also apparent within America, however. Gregory admonished the Northern states' retrograde attitude in comparison to the Southern, where even the illiterate 'colored woman' acted as extremely valuable midwives. Although ostensibly *Letters to the Ladies*, Gregory does not often make an appeal to this particular audience beyond the preface and the conclusion, and evidently had a wider remit. Indeed, his focus on the backwardness of the present was used cunningly to show that attitudes in the past were more natural. For, he noted, if something had been carried out successfully for centuries then it was 'no new idea, no untried experiment, no innovation or revolution'. It was simply a restoration of what was right and proper. Throughout this treatise, Gregory played very effectively with any reader who might want to express horror at women's upstart demands to practise obstetrics by steadily convincing them of its historically-proven propriety.

Whereas today's attitudes to midwifery were less enlightened than those of the past, Gregory further utilised their opposite – a more scientific contemporary medicine – to link female practitioners to less harmless modes of obstetric intervention. By drawing on examples of disfiguring and disabling birth defects caused by unnecessary instrumental deliveries, *Letters to the Ladies* made a plea for older, safer practices which were less injurious both to women and to their children. Very recent experimental developments which had resulted in the pain-killing devices of ether and chloroform were condemned in additions to the second and third editions of *Letters*. While acknowledging their potential in serious surgical operations, Gregory could not condone their use for what should be a natural process. In this instance, he attacked the present (and by implication the future) for destroying history's more reliable modes of delivery. With both celebration of the past as more advanced than the present and denigration of the present as scientific and yet brutal, Gregory achieved his aim of placing female practitioners right in the centre of the debate and, by implication, women as the only feasible future of obstetrics.

Others sought to harness the most recent developments in the history of medical women's attempts to qualify as professionals to provide a more immediate and, often, still living, reminder of struggles and progress. In *Seven Lamps of Medicine*, Mary Scharlieb drew the attention of her London School of Medicine for Women (LSMW) audience to their privileged, full, and detailed education, which was in stark contrast to the piecemeal and interrupted learning of some of the first British women to attempt medical studies, such as Elizabeth Garrett Anderson, Sophia Jex-Blake, and Isabel Thorne. Nearly two decades later, at the start of the twentieth century, the latter began her narrative of the establishment of the LSMW with a reminder, in similar fashion to Scharlieb, that the present was a very different place for the aspiring female medical student. With what comes across as an admonishing tone, she advised those preparing for entry into the profession to consider her own recollections carefully. In doing so, they would be able to see both how her generation had negotiated a difficult, obstacle-strewn past to success, as well as appreciate that it had been the hard-won efforts of this cohort which would allow those tackling medical studies in the early 1900s to profit from such smooth and easy education. By providing exemplars, Thorne warned that the past was something from which current aspirants could learn, but which also would haunt with expectation. The long list of qualities concluding her work that were required for the ideal medical woman ensured that the weight of history would hang like a millstone around the necks of future generations. Correspondingly, Edwin A. Pratt's *Pioneer Women* utilised a rehashing of the recent histories of Sophia Jex-Blake and Elizabeth Garrett Anderson in combination with actually interviewing the *grande dame* of medical women, Elizabeth Blackwell, to show how the past was very much still present and keenly observing trends in education and practise from retirement in Hastings. Indeed, Blackwell's positioning herself as perpetually avant-garde in her attitudes ensured that she formed 'a sort of minority en permanence'; the trace of the past always there, and forever just ahead, in medical women's future trajectory.

William Dale presented a very different future for medicine, but one which was as intimidating. His frontispiece from 1860 offered a visual analysis of the present state of the medical profession, where the legitimate, properly qualified base of the professional tree branched off into illegitimate and poisonous fumes which were all-pervasive. Near the top of the tree, reaching off into the future, were 'lady dabblers in physic', a new, frighteningly modern and fashionable emanation inextricably linked to quackery, foreign qualifications, and 'specialism'. Dale's image was an odd one in many ways, which linked old-fashioned bone setting of the past with recent 'vulgar' trends, all unstoppably growing, upas-like and insidiously, into the minds of the undiscriminating general public. While the roots of the profession were steady and firm, it was both the newer and the older developments which projected out into an uncertain future. Although intending to picture women as part-time amateurs, the positioning of the 'lady dabblers' revealed the potential reach of their threat. Nearly half a century later, by 1907, as the *Observer* article on 'Lady Doctors' confirmed, considerable success had been achieved by women in the profession in terms of numbers and also regarding public perception: Dale's fears had been realised – the medical marketplace was polluted. What the *Observer* piece also noted, however, was that the growth was partial and restricted. Women had achieved a great deal, but careers were still curbed and prospects limited. The fume-like projections of Dale's upas tree 'lady dabblers', denied solidity and dispersed into the air, had potentially come to a less toxic pass.

In contrast, Beatrice Harraden emphasised the more positive aspects of continuity with the past in her discussion of 'Women Doctors in the War' from 1915. By describing Elizabeth Garrett Anderson's presence at the departure of her daughter, Louisa, to serve in France, Harraden brought together the generations, while simultaneously emphasising their differences. No matter how much she wished to accompany Louisa on her ambitious journey into the unknown, Elizabeth Garrett Anderson's time had passed. Unlike Thorne's perception that early twentieth-century medical women did not recognise the struggles of history, Harraden saw this challenge as simply another with which women had always fought and would contend anew. With such a 'spirit', they had done it before, and they could do it again. The Great War was a new opportunity: medical women were heading off towards a new battlefield with the force of the past and the possibilities of the future in front of them.

SUITABILITIES

Alongside medical women's place in history, their appropriateness to practise medicine was repeatedly invoked in debates. This argument developed into two related strands: physical and mental. For detractors, women were too weak in mind and body to be able to withstand the stresses and strains of everyday medicine. Supporters, on the other hand, drew attention to the fact that medicine did not need physical strength, especially as it developed more scientifically, and women were equally, if not superiorly, mentally agile. What one side saw as unnecessary, prurient curiosity about matters medical, the other saw as necessary to avoid female ignorance and suffering. Most fascinating about these debates, however, was that absolute focus on the strengths of body and mind grew into regular weaknesses of argument on both sides. Too often, strains showed.

Kenealy argued that doctors were born not made, rendering medicine available to all. In contrast, Mary Scharlieb connected women and medicine inextricably throughout her writings, belying the argument made by opponents of female medical education, such as William Dale, that deeper understanding 'unsexed'. *A Woman's Words to Women* was written by an author who presented herself both as doctor and mother, who had lived in India and in Britain. All these qualities and all this personal experience, Scharlieb argued, permitted her to address her readers – women from childhood, youth, motherhood, and beyond – with several layers of interrelated expertise. Indeed, *A Woman's Words to Women* was a no-nonsense, clearly expressed, but medically-inflected advice manual, which did not shy away from proving the moral rightness of all women knowing their bodies. In so doing, Scharlieb removed the veil of prudery from physiology and hygiene, while making sure that her female readers were provided with the correct terminology, via a final glossary of terms, to discuss their conditions scientifically and appropriately. For Scharlieb, contemporary social advances should mean health was at the foundation of every woman's life, and preparation for and understanding of physical changes would underpin progress. Medical women's knowledge and the passing of that information onto their own sex was an inherently feminine process.

On the contrary, Walter Rivington believed that women were adapted neither for medical, and far less for surgical, practise, by 'frame, temperament, and mental constitution'; women's 'disabilities' were too many and they were 'too heavily handicapped to compete with men'. It was precisely this fear of competition, however, which had caused the sorts of reactions detailed by Thorne and Pratt to women's efforts to study at the University of Edinburgh from 1869. As both Rivington realised, and Hosken Woodward's female characters explained, this sort of male professional hysteria rebounded particularly badly upon the supposedly superior medical man who had blown the situation out of all proportion. In Hosken Woodward's consideration of female employment, her character, Sir Henry, after claiming that there was no active opposition to women's work at the end of the nineteenth century outside working-class agitation, was rounded upon by Mrs Silverton and Madeline. Both brought up what had happened at Edinburgh as an example of *soi-disant* 'gentlemanly' opposition, Madeline countering with the belief that it could only be those of below average ability who reacted in this fearful way. Although Rivington did not consider more than a very small number of women capable of becoming doctors, he was far more critical of the demeaning behaviour of his own sex towards the experiment. Even those who did not think the attempt would succeed were forced to recognise that the strength of the opposition had the effect of making the profession look as weak-minded and facile as the women they were accusing.

If the opposition could appear unprofessional in their reactions, they were equally keen to stress women's distance from the values and attributes necessary for medical duties. 'Jennie June' and Hosken Woodward's Mrs Knagge both declared that they could never employ a woman doctor; two clear examples of female hostility to medical women's progress. Mrs Knagge's concerns stemmed from not having 'faith' in such a practitioner, while 'Jennie June's' fears were more fatal. The female professional, she reflected, would be anything but; she would be unkind, uncaring, and deadly through harsh over-prescription to patients of her own sex, while flirting happily with men. While the latter might not object to women practitioners, the former would and should. It is important to acknowledge that opposition to medical women from their own sex was apparent across this period, and not all welcomed the possibility of being treated by qualified females. Such squeamishness will be explored further in Volume IV. Supporters stressed regularly the opposite: the genuine need for women to examine and care for each other. Tales of dread, delay and death characterised such narratives. Indeed, they were frequently to be found in the writings of men who supported the cause. Thomas Markby, Samuel Gregory, and Edwin A. Pratt all pleaded for the necessity of female practitioners as far as the propriety of women patients was concerned. Simply the touch of a male doctor was too much for some delicate and modest sensibilities, Gregory and Markby argued: death had frequently resulted from terror in these instances.

By contrast, in *Seven Lamps of Medicine*, Mary Scharlieb sought the similarities between the characters of men and women, stressing the fundamental femininity of medical practice, where 'Gentleness' was a key lamp illuminating the stony path ahead. Indeed, male practitioners were inherently, she claimed, the 'most tender, unselfish, and gentle of their sex'. In an extension of such comments, and unlike 'Jennie June' and Mrs Knagge, for some male supporters, the bond of trust and understanding between women patient and female doctor was special and only too apparent. Instead of indifference, they saw deep sympathy and sensitivity; the 'usefulness' of women, both in advancing their own knowledge and correspondingly in benefiting the health and welfare of their own sex, was paramount. While this male support was welcome, it was not always what it appeared. Gregory and Markby, for example, were clear that they were in favour of a limited sphere of responsibility for women. Gregory's treatise was concerned with midwifery, and only tangentially wider possibilities, while Markby wanted to forbid women attendance upon any but women, girls, and boys – but only if they were under seven years of age. For Howard Marsh, who keenly voiced his respect for women's abilities as students and as fully qualified practitioners, and saw the Great War as an opportunity to extend their assistance, this period would be temporary. Although impressed with skills in the 'hardest' branches of the profession, such as surgery and anaesthetics, or the newest such as clinical pathology and bacteriology, so that women were more than capable of taking the place of men on war service, Marsh's article ended with a brief, but unmistakable imperative that things 'must' revert when they returned. The direction of the tide was going in one way, the article concluded succinctly, and yet Marsh had already pulled it back himself with a command to return to position once conflict was over.

In similar fashion to Marsh's ostensibly positive response, the *Observer* spoke to an anonymous respondent, an 'eminent authority of wide experience in the world of medicine', who attested to the lack of jealousy between the sexes by the early twentieth century and the fair distribution of practice to ensure that neither stole the bread from the others' mouths. Rather than gendered differences between practitioners, this statement drew them very much together. Such a positive depiction of the medical marketplace of the period, reminiscent of Scharlieb's deep connections between the sexes in *Seven Lamps*, was swiftly undermined, however, by the 'eminent authority's' reflection on women's capabilities. It was precisely the sensitivities towards their patients, which, as we have seen, were so praised by earlier supporters, he argued, that led to nerves and breakdowns. Rather than stoically accept that things go wrong and that they had tried their level best to assist, women were too introspective, and this would, consequentially, affect their whole career. Additionally, they were too apt to lean on others, too afraid to take responsibility for their actions. 'Temperament' meant that they were, ultimately, much less effective doctors. The London School of Medicine for Women's secretary, Miss Douie, was also asked for her opinion on the question of 'nerves'. Her response had a very similar ring to that produced by Arabella Kenealy in the 1890s or Beatrice Harraden in the 1910s. All stressed women's strength and adaptability in the face of circumstances and denied that their reactions were any different to men's. If anything, indeed, they were less likely to succumb to problems. This was a constant refrain amongst medical women across the period and it involved reestablishing distinctions and competition between the sexes. In this instance, the similarity between supporters and detractors was all-too evident.

REPUTATIONS

In 1915, Howard Marsh had commented that very little had been seen of 'defects and handicaps' in women's practise. Eight years earlier, the 'eminent authority', however, reminded the *Observer*'s readers of a recent case which had only served to highlight the problems women had experienced in medicine. The strenuousness of women's own responses, as characterised by Miss Douie's reactions, exacerbated the sense that not everything was fine all the time. In 1903, a former student of the LSMW and current locum house surgeon at the Royal Free Hospital, Sophia Frances Hickman, had killed herself.[1] For the 'eminent authority', this was enough evidence to prove that women could not always cope and took things too much to heart. The final section of this introduction will look at a case study of one woman doctor to show how medical women debates often ended up replacing an individual for the whole, to the benefit or detriment of the female practitioner.

One of the most internationally controversial medical women of the nineteenth century, Mary Edwards Walker, is represented in this volume by her anonymously published work *Unmasked, Or the Science of Immorality* (1878), written 'To Gentlemen By A Woman Physician and Surgeon'. This is a bizarre, messy, and rambling treatise, which has, understandably, received very little attention from historians, or, perhaps more surprisingly, Walker's medical contemporaries.[2] This could be explained by its content, which was very different to that of Mary Scharlieb's advice manual, and its provocative address to men. Concerns for women's rights were shot through with odd pronouncements about the female body, for example, such as the origins of hermaphroditism in abuse, the 'humbug hymen theory', the prevailing force of maternal impressions, and the vaginal resistance, leading to a castrating effect, of women born of marital rape. Indeed, most children were products of the latter, argued Walker. These ideas were all wrapped up in exhortations that radical dress reform, propounded by Walker's own designs for appropriate attire, was an excellent way to promote health, prevent unnatural sexual excitement, but also protect against rape. 'Unmasking' such issues, and providing a secure foundation for progress in healthy bodies and minds, claimed Walker, would abet reform of all kinds. While this argument was similar to Scharlieb's it was constructed and responded to a very different way. *Unmasked* received attention via word of mouth – Walker's predominantly – and was recommended by her and for the close reading of men, especially law-enforcers, with whom she came into contact. The *Washington Post* branded it the 'most revoltingly obscene and disgusting book we have seen for a long time'; the medical press appeared to have ignored it.[3]

From the 1860s, Mary Walker became a constant figure of fun across the globe due to her outspoken pronouncements, of which *Unmasked* was only one lengthy example, and her increasingly masculinised garb. Her status as a medical woman gave her both the confidence to write and speak about contemporarily controversial topics, but also, more interestingly, allowed her to be used as an example in the debates surrounding women's right – or otherwise – to practise. Walker's outlandishness ensured that she was regularly compared to other medical women. When she visited London in 1866, and stayed for a year pursuing various speaking engagements, the British press followed her with an awareness that she was one side of what an emancipated, professional woman could become. This soon became a fundamental way of seeing her. For the British press, it was her odd and perceived Americanisms which grated and distracted; her accent or her tone provoked annoyance for most onlookers. The *Englishwoman's Review*, a periodical engaged with investigating social and industrial questions, as they concerned women, was dismayed by Walker, because she did not focus enough on such important issues. In early 1867, the *Review* lamented the need to consider the subject of Walker, but as it was their remit, it was necessary. Rather than explore her experience as a medical woman, Walker strayed into dress reform, which brought ridicule upon her, and by extension, both her sex and her profession. In opposition to Walker's belief, detailed later in *Unmasked*, that reform could only stem from the foundations of the body, they were two separate topics for the *Englishwoman's Review*. For this periodical, Walker added nothing to the cause: she represented neither medicine nor women.[4] This eccentricity was also dangerously close to the hybridity so feared by detractors of the medical woman's abilities – the inability to connect medicine and women because of their innate differences. As William Dale noted in an irate letter to the *Lancet* in 1869, consolidating his opposition to the quackery glimpsed in the frontispiece to *The Present State of the Medical Profession*, women could never become doctors unless 'they discard all the natural and most valued characteristics of their sex'.[5] Mary Walker exacerbated this sense because she was both petite and feminine-looking, but wore trousers. Disappointingly, for the British press, she was more interested in the trousers than in her representative status of the 'race of female doctors', as the *London Review* put it.[6] It was Mary Walker's singularity that dominated coverage of her stay.

And yet it was precisely this individualism that encouraged, paradoxically, support for the rest of the 'race'. There were thousands of words expended on Walker's doings and sayings in the late nineteenth and twentieth centuries, but it was not her medical prowess with which the press were concerned. When medicine was mentioned in relation to her name, however, it was to distance her from fellow practitioners – male or female. For the *Lancet*, she started off as a 'professional sister', but upon greater acquaintance, descriptions of her battlefield endeavours became 'feminine', the focus on dress 'feminine vanity', while she appeared to remove herself from surgical action. By the end of the report, Dr Mary Walker had become a 'fair lecturess', providing sanitised depictions in which she smoothed pillows rather than involved herself in 'the stern requirements of actual service, the physical labour and mental exertion of tending wounds, and deciding when a wrong decision may mean death'. In actuality, listening to her 'prosy' lecture, she was certainly not the medical woman, or 'professional sister', anticipated theoretically.[7] The American medical press struggled too with Walker's fixations; so much so indeed that they could not think of her in any intellectual fashion, for due to her harping on 'pantaloons', 'head is never thought of'. 'This restless little spirit', argued the *Pacific Medical Journal*, 'has done more to bring derision and reproach upon female physicians than all the women-haters of the other sex collectively'; progress could only be achieved through her retirement into a convent.[8] The New Hampshire Medical Society heard a paper at their 1877 congress which lauded the deepest research and scientific acumen displayed through the publications of colleagues' Mary Putnam Jacobi and Susan Dimock's devotion to understanding the diseases of their sex. But these and other learned medical women were examples of 'true womanhood', rather than the 'unsexed monstrosities' embodied by Mary Walker. Such singular types, continued the author, A.H. Crosby, in a strong defence of women professionals,

> cannot and *will not* prevent a modest, intelligent, well educated, and cultured woman from taking her proper place in life, whether it be as the wife and mother, a crown to her husband, or whether, after due preparation

> and strict examination, she sees fit to stand shoulder to shoulder with us in the eternal conflict we are waging against the forces of pestilence and disease.[9]

For the lay press, too, Walker was very far from the 'most commendable discretion', noted the *Athenaeum*, of female aspirants to a medical career. Those 'fair English' compatriots led by the 'high priestess', Miss Elizabeth Garrett, and represented in the periodical's review by the writings of Isabel Thorne, were bolstered by arguments which were 'sensible and convincing' and ultimately 'difficult to refute'.[10] The *Athenaeum*'s comment that 'She is amongst us, but not of us' summed up the contemporary debates surrounding Dr Mary Walker. One medical woman, as the New Hampshire physician, A.H. Crosby, made clear, could not prevent others from banding together with their male contemporaries in the heroic battle against disease and suffering. Ultimately, it was Dr Mary Walker's individual alterity which had the paradoxical result of bringing other medical women, at least in theory, into the professional ranks as equals to men.

Notes

1 For more on this case, see C. Brock, 'The Disappearance of Sophia Frances Hickman', *History Workshop Journal*, 80:1 (Autumn 2015), pp. 161–182.

2 One recent exception is K. Schuller's *The Biopolitics of Feeling: Race, Sex, and Science in the Nineteenth Century* (Durham, NC: Duke University Press, 2018), which places Edwards Walker alongside Elizabeth Blackwell to consider white women's corporeal capacity for sexual agency as biopolitically normative.

3 'A New Party', *Washington Post*, 19 August 1879, p. 2; quoted in S.M. Harris, *Dr Mary Walker: An American Radical* (New Brunswick, NJ and London: Rutgers University Press, 2009), p. 167.

4 'Dr Mary Walker', *Englishwoman's Review*, II (1 January 1867), pp. 110–112.

5 W. Dale, M.D., 'Women Doctors', *Lancet*, 94:2413 (27 November 1869), p. 761.

6 Reproduced in *Englishwoman's Review*, (1 January 1867), pp. 111–112.

7 'Medical Annotation', *Lancet*, 88:2253 (3 November 1866), pp. 501–502 and 'Dr Mary Walker', *Lancet*, 88:2256 (24 November 1866), pp. 593–594.

8 'A Word About Dr Mary Walker', *Pacific Medical Journal*, excerpted in *Hospital Gazette and Archives of Clinical Surgery*, 4:12 (19 September 1878), p. 239.

9 A.H. Crosby, 'Orthodoxy and Heterodoxy in Medicine', *Transactions of the New Hampshire Medical Society (Eighty-Seventh Anniversary) Held at Concord, June 19 and 20, 1877* (Concord, NH: Republican Press Association, 1877), pp. 77–92; on p. 91; emphasis in text.

10 'Review of *Medical Students of the Period* by R. Temple Wright, M.D. and *Prize Essays on the Evils Exposed by 'Search'* by Mrs Thorne', *Athenaeum*, 2083 (28 September 1867), pp. 393–395; on p. 394.

Editorial Headnote

Samuel Gregory, *Letters to Ladies In Favor of Female Physicians For Their Own Sex*, 3rd edition (Boston: New England Female Medical College, 1856)

Yale-educated Samuel Gregory, M.D. (1813–1872) was best known as the founder and Secretary of the Boston-based New England Female Medical College, the first institution devoted to the education of women in medicine. His medical title was honorary, but he involved himself in popular topics of the day in the 1840s, such as physiology and hygiene, and came to believe that women should attend their own sex during childbirth, for example. It was his campaigning around the 'immorality' and 'indecency' of male attendance that led to the establishment of the Boston Female Medical School in November 1848, which became the Female Medical Education Society in 1850, and the New England Female Medical College in 1852. In 1873, upon merging with Boston University, it became the first co-educational medical school in the United States of America. For John Preston Sutherland, writing about the Boston Medical School in 1905, none of this would have been possible without Gregory's 'progressive, liberal spirit, broad-mindedness, faith, earnestness and unfailing activity'.[1] *Letters to Ladies In Favor of Female Physicians For Their Own Sex* (1850) was Gregory's most popular text, priced at 12 1/2 cents and running through three editions in the 1850s; the testimonials to its success were appended to each subsequent edition. From the first edition, women's 'peculiar innate modesty and delicacy' was acknowledged by reviewers, convinced that 'in many cases', she should be attended by physicians of her own sex. As there was a 'strong movement in favor of this natural privilege', claimed the *New England Farmer*, in its conclusion to a very supportive review, every lady should read it.[2] In similar fashion, as the prefatory support trumpeted, the *National Era*'s comment that it 'should be in the hands of every American woman' and 'its great importance to society', according to the *Portland Transcript*, best explained its appeal.

In addition to his administrative work, and drawing on his education at undergraduate and postgraduate level, primarily in the humanities, Gregory was also a writer and an historian of Mexico, the author of *Gregory's History of Mexico: a History of Mexico from the Earliest Times to the Present* (1847). This was in addition to works published over a period of twenty-five years on women in medicine and female health: *Facts, and important information, from distinguished physicians and other sources: showing the awful effects of masturbation on young women* (1843); *Man-midwifery Exposed and Corrected* (1847); *Female Physicians* (1864); *Doctor or Doctress?* (1868).

The publication of the latter revealed both Gregory's desire to have medical women taken seriously, but also his awareness of their special difference from men; its reception the medical press' mixed attitude of jokey uneasiness and niggled sensitivity to female interlopers. In *Doctor or Doctress?* Gregory advocated the use of Doctress for female physicians. The *Chicago Medical Examiner* noted that '[w]e approve the plan. Let the female physician have a *feminine* title, by all means'.[3] Unlike their mid-west counterparts, the *New York Medical Journal* sniggered at Gregory's suspenseful earnestness in appealing to the press about what best to call the 'dear creatures' and 'seductive beings'. Closing with a sly dig at the impure English title of the New England Female Medical College, the periodical sat on the fence about their devotion to Doctresses.[4]

Lay press contributors, however, seized Gregory's terminology, which likened medical women to empresses or princesses. *Godey's Lady's Book* determined never to refer again to women doctors, with a masculine title: 'doctress only'. This Philadelphia-based periodical acknowledged the importance of women's position in the profession, but denigrated the confounding of them with their male counterparts, likening it to dressing women in men's clothes and hindering female 'peculiar merits and duties'. Their 'full and beautiful recognition' in this career of 'usefulness and honor, of fame and fortune' could only be achieved with the nomenclature of difference.[5]

Gregory's conservatism in his support for medical women was evident in the reporting of his death from consumption in March 1872. The *Congregationalist* drew attention to his religious affiliation with Park Street Church in Boston, while the *Medical and Surgical Reporter* remarked that he 'devoted his life to the education of women in certain branches of the Medical profession'.[6] It was this qualification which would ensure that the graduates of the New England Female Medical College, such as the first Black woman to qualify as a doctor, Rebecca Lee (see Volume III) or faculty, such as the German-born and of Polish ancestry, Marie Zakrzewska (also see Volume III), have become more well known and whose reputations have increased over time than the founder of the institution, who supported their limited right to practise medicine.

Notes

1 John Preston Sutherland, 'Boston School of Medicine', in William Harvey King, (ed.), *History of Homeopathy and its Institutions in America, Volume III* (New York and Chicago: Lewis Publishing Company, 1905), pp. 159–213; on p. 159.

2 *New England Farmer: Devoted to Agriculture and All Its Kindred Arts and Sciences*, II:1 (5 January 1850), p. 24.

3 *Chicago Medical Examiner*, IX:12 (December 1868), p. 752.

4 *New York Medical Journal*, VIII:3 (December 1868), pp. 311–312.

5 *Godey's Lady's Book and Magazine*, LXXIX:470 (August 1869), p. 176.

6 *Congregationalist*, 24:13 (28 March 1872), p. 8; *Medical and Surgical Reporter*, XXVI (6 April 1872), p. 316.

1

LETTERS TO LADIES IN FAVOR OF FEMALE PHYSICIANS FOR THEIR OWN SEX

Samuel Gregory

Source: Samuel Gregory, *Letters to Ladies In Favor of Female Physicians For Their Own Sex*, 3rd edition (Boston: New England Female Medical College, 1856).

TO THE LADIES

THESE pages are addressed to you, ladies, because it is your welfare chiefly that they were designed to promote; and upon your influence and aid must depend, in a great measure, the success of the object recommended.

By a candid consideration of the testimony herein presented, you will, it is hoped, be induced to encourage the education of suitable females to share in the duties of the medical profession, especially those that pertain to their own sex.

This course will introduce among the female portion of the community, generally, a better knowledge of the means of preserving and restoring health – a knowledge which their own physical well being, and that of the race, demands that they should possess. By thus extending their intelligence and usefulness, in a sphere so peculiarly appropriate, they will not only enjoy the satisfaction of accomplishing greater good, but will strengthen their claims to honor and esteem.

Every one, who is at all acquainted with this subject, must be aware that great inconvenience and unnecessary suffering, mental and physical, result from confining this knowledge and these qualifications to male physicians, on account of the delicate relations which exist between the sexes, and the proper regard of which is indispensable to the best interests of society.

With a deep conviction of the importance of the object presented in these pages, it is earnestly commended to the favor and support of the intelligent, benevolent, and Christian women of the community, by

THE AUTHOR.

BOSTON, January 1, 1850.

DOI: 10.4324/9781003265238-1

PREFACE

TO THE SECOND EDITION.

Great progress has been made in the cause of female medical education within the four years since the date of this letter. Institutions for the purpose have sprung up, and the object has become familiar to the public mind, and a matter of interest throughout the country. The New England Female Medical College, located in this city, and commencing its operations on a limited scale, in 1848. has become known as one of our permanent and important institutions, and, through the legislature, has received the sanction and pecuniary aid of the commonwealth. Many of its graduates are already reaping the rewards of their professional success, and it has become a settled question that the exercise of the healing art is henceforth to be a sphere of employment and usefulness for women.

The author deems it but a just and proper acknowledgment to say, that his confident expectations of the approval and aid of those to whom these pages were addressed have not been disappointed, and that this enterprise has been greatly indebted for its remarkable success to the influence and cooperation of many excellent and intelligent ladies. The written commendations and opinions of female authors and eminent teachers – Mrs. Sigourney, Mrs. Hale, Mrs. Willard, Mrs. Phelps, and others – have gone abroad, and done efficient service in securing public favor for the object; many have contributed pecuniary aid, and prompted others to do so, and the grant of five thousand dollars from the legislature is to be attributed in no small degree to the influence of the thirty or forty of the principal ladies of this city, who sent in their petition in aid of the petition of the directors of the institution.

With such proofs of their interest and influence the author, with renewed confidence, commends to the women of the country the cause of female medical education.

S. G.

Boston, September 12, 1854.

LETTER TO LADIES.

It is not a recent or hastily formed opinion on the part of the writer that there ought to be a class of females, thoroughly educated and qualified to act as medical advisers and professional attendants, in those departments of practice which relate particularly to their own sex – the daughter, the wife, the mother.

To show upon what grounds his convictions rest and to what credence his opinions may be entitled, it is perhaps necessary, and therefore excusable, to allude to the means he has had for obtaining information upon the subject and the measures that have been adopted to communicate that information to the public. It is the custom, and a very good one, too, for the graduating class in Yale College, whatever may be their prospective professions or pursuits, to receive some lectures from professors in the medical department of the institution. Under these circumstances, in 1840, the author, by the lectures and by reading, made himself somewhat acquainted with the subjects of anatomy and physiology and with the history and the principles of the healing art. From the interest thus acquired in these subjects, he has given to them more or less attention from that time to the present. It struck him as rather singular that the department of the profession termed *midwifery* – a feminine occupation, as its name implies – should be exclusively in the hands of males. But on further research it appeared that it was not so, to the same extent, in any other country, and that in our own it was an innovation, dating back considerably less than a century, and was, moreover, seriously and strongly objected to by some of the most eminent medical authorities.

In 1845 the writer prepared a small work at the request of his brother, George Gregory, by whom it was published, on the unfavorable tendencies and results of some of the existing customs, among them the employment of men in the duties in question. The next year the same publisher, who is an indefatigable promoter of this enterprise, published another pamphlet exclusively upon this subject, entitled "Facts for Married Men." These two publications, being extensively circulated, served to enlighten and convince many and prepare the way for further effort. Accordingly, in July, 1847, the writer commenced preparing a work which should more fully present the question. He also in the following month, in this city, commenced advocating the subject of female medical education in public lectures to gentlemen, and separately to ladies. The work mentioned, the present title of which is "Female Midwifery Advocated," was published in the following January; since which time twenty thousand copies have been put in circulation.

This, with numerous lectures in various cities and towns, and the aid of many of the public journals, (for which the writer here expresses his heartfelt thanks,) has to some extent introduced the subject to public attention.

The demand thereby created for professional women required, of course, that something should be done towards providing a school for their instruction. A number of women were found to form a class; and, with the expenditure of much time and effort, a physician of suitable qualifications and of approved standing in the profession was engaged as lecturer; and the first term commenced November 1, 1848, and continued three months. The second commenced in April following. Twenty women have been instructed; and they have attended above three hundred cases of midwifery, and with the most satisfactory success.

A tenfold larger number of women might have been collected into the classes and instructed but for the want of the means to make the subject known to the public, to furnish the lecture room, and to carry forward the enterprise generally. In fact, to accomplish what has been done has required pretty much the entire sacrifice of the author's time and labor for the past two and a half years. But the way is in some measure prepared; a demand has been created; and, if a thousand women were this moment qualified, they would receive a cordial welcome and liberal encouragement in the cities and towns of New England alone.

Such is the increasing reluctance to call on gentlemen for these services that danger may be apprehended from trusting to ignorant and incompetent women if others are not provided. The following incident will serve as a specimen of the feeling that exists: –

> The wife of a young gentleman, a member of one of the prominent families in this city, being about to be confined some months since, was unwilling to employ a man to wait upon her, and she feared that she should give offence to some of the medical friends by employing one of the professional midwives. In these embarrassing circumstances she asked her nurse if she would not officiate, so that it might appear accidental. The nurse shook her head, and said she would not dare to; she had, to be sure, been with physicians a good many times on these occasions, and, *having been caught* in two or three instances, she had had to manage alone; "but," said she, "that was vastly different from *taking* the responsibility." "Well," replied the heroic young woman, in a position infinitely more serious to her than was General Jackson's to him when he uttered a like expression, – "well," replied she to the nurse, calling her by name, "if you will stand by me, and do as well as you can, *I will take the responsibility*." She did; and all resulted fortunately. The husband called on one of the medical friends and said to him, "Well, doctor, we have an heir at our house. The affair came off rather suddenly, and I believe is pretty much over; but the folks would like to have you call in and see them, if you please." The physician called, and, having made proper inquiries, expressed his gratification, addressed the nurse by his own title, and took leave by saying, "All right: good morning, doctor."

Now, without any implied reflection upon those who do not take such responsibilities as this lady did, it must be allowed that she exhibited a most lovely and admirable trait of character; and any physician who should not be better pleased with it than with a *fee* ought not to call himself a medical *gentleman*.

One more example, from many others that have come to the knowledge of the writer. A slight and delicate young woman, in Augusta, Maine, whose friends thought from this circumstance that she must have a medical man attend on the occasion of her confinement, resolutely refused to consent, and said "*No*" to all their entreaties and fearful prognostics; and finally, to put an end to their unreasonable urgency, she very emphatically said to them, "If you bring a man into this room, and I have strength, when he comes in at one door I shall go out at the other." They then, of course, desisted; and she was carried safely through her trials by the matron, who gave me the fact. There is a promise in the good book – "She shall be saved in childbearing if she continue in faith, and charity, and holiness, with sobriety."

The Bible only declares, "In *sorrow* shalt thou bring forth children." This torture of modest sensibilities is a wicked and superfluous infliction, for which no sanction can be found in the examples or precepts of Scripture; no, nor in the customs of any nation of heathendom. It is neither Christian, pagan, nor human.

A book has been published on the women of the Bible; but it omits to mention some of them who are worthy of great commendation. The names of two of these are Shiphrah and Puah, who Dr. Clarke, the commentator, thinks were the instructors and superintendents of the "Hebrew midwives" generally. Pharaoh, it will be remembered, commanded them to destroy the male children at birth. It could have been very easily done, when the faint spark of life is almost ready to go out of itself unless cherished into a flame. Possibly, if the attendants had been *men*, less sympathizing, courageous, and conscientious, they would have been terrified into obedience to the barbarous mandate; "but the midwives feared God, and did not as the king of Egypt commanded them, but saved the men children alive. Therefore God dealt well with the midwives, and the people multiplied and waxed very mighty."

Noble examples of true women, who rarely quail when duty and humanity call them to face danger; who have not only *fortitude* to *endure*, but *efficiency* to *act*, when occasion demands. These were women of the Bible, whose profession it would be most becoming and honorable for some of the Bible women of America to follow.

There is no other country in the world where females are so dependent upon the opposite sex for assistance on these occasions as in our own. Even the women of China, so low in the social scale, have the honor of managing these affairs. The women of ancient Greece enjoyed a like exemption from the meddlesome interference of the lords of creation. The Romans would not have been more startled to see Lucina, the patron goddess of childbearing women, haranguing the assembled gods or launching the thunderbolts of Jove than they would have been to see his majesty presiding in the puerperal chamber.

Let us now attend to the testimony of an eminent medical author, who speaks from great knowledge and experience, and who cannot be supposed to present any other than the most candid and truthful statements.

TESTIMONY OF DR. MEIGS, *of Philadelphia.* – Within two years past, two large works – "Females and their Diseases," and "Obstetrics" – have appeared from the pen of Charles D. Meigs, M. D., professor of Midwifery and the Diseases of Women and Children in the Jefferson Medical College at Philadelphia.

Though Dr. Meigs may not have intended to encourage the medical education of females for the departments that come under his professorship, he has incidentally furnished proof of the urgent necessity of such a course, and has admitted its practicability by the high commendation he has bestowed upon foreign medical ladies of acknowledged eminence as authors and practitioners. His work on Females, &c., is in the form of a series of letters to his class after they had left the institution, and is written in so intelligible and interesting a style that females themselves might get the knowledge directly from its pages instead of obtaining it through the young gentlemen to whom it is addressed.

In his second letter, comprising "General Remarks on Conduct," the professor writes as follows: –

"The relations between the sexes are of so delicate a character that the duties of a medical practitioner are necessarily more difficult when he comes to take charge of a patient laboring under any one of the great host of female complaints than when he is called upon to treat the more general disorders, such as fevers, inflammations, the exanthemata, &c. So great, indeed, is the embarrassment arising from fastidiousness on the part either of the female herself, or of the practitioner, or both, that I am persuaded that much of the ill success of treatment may be justly traced thereto.

"It is to be confessed that a very general opinion exists as to the difficulty of effectually curing many of the diseases of women; and it is mortifying as it is true, that we see the cases of these disorders going the whole round of the profession, in any village, town, or city, and falling at last into the hands of the quack; either ending in some surprising cure, or leading the victim, by gradual lapses of health and strength, down to the grave, the last refuge of the incurable, or rather the uncured. I say uncured, for it is a very clear and well-known truth, that many of these cases are, in their beginning, of light or trifling importance.

"All these evils of medical practice spring not, in the main, from any want of competency in medicines or in medical men, but from the delicacy of the relations existing between the sexes, and, in a good degree, from a want of information among the population in general as to the import, and meaning, and tendency of disorders manifested by a certain train of symptoms.

"It is perhaps best, upon the whole, that this great degree of modesty should exist even to the extent of putting a bar to researches, without which no very clear and understandable notions can be obtained of the sexual disorders. I confess I am proud to say that in this country generally, certainly in many parts of it, there are women who prefer to suffer the extremity of danger and pain rather than waive those scruples of delicacy which prevent their maladies from being fully explored. I say it is an evidence of the dominion of a fine morality in our society; but nevertheless it is true that a greater candor on the part of the patient, and a more resolute and careful inquiry on that of the practitioner, would scarcely fail to bring to light, in their earliest stages, the curable maladies which, by faults on both sides, are now misunderstood because concealed, and consequently mismanaged and incurable. In fact, what is there in the human body that can become disordered so secretly as to elude the exploratory powers of a well-educated medical man who is allowed to make the necessary inquiries?

"It is an interesting question as to what can be done to obviate the perpetuity of such evils – evils that have existed for ages. Is there any recourse by means of which the amount of suffering endured by women afflicted with peculiar complaints may be greatly lessened?

"I am of opinion that the answer ought to be in the affirmative; for I believe that, if a medical practitioner know how to obtain the entire confidence of the class of persons who habitually consult him, – if he be endowed with a clear perceptive power, a sound judgment, a real probity, and a proper degree of intelligence, and a familiarity with the doctrines of a good medical school, – he will, as far as to the extent of his particular sphere of action, be found capable of greatly lessening the evils of which complaint is here made; and if these qualities are generally attached to physicians, then it is in their power to abate the evil throughout the population in general."

Such are some of the difficulties which Professor Meigs terms "embarrassments in the practice." And he goes on to relate a case, with which he had just met, illustrating the point. A lady had suffered for twenty years with a painful disorder, and had been repeatedly subjected to mortifying examinations, which had not, however, till then, been sufficiently thorough to discover the true cause of suffering, on account of what he terms a fastidious delicacy on the part of the physician; and he adds, "I doubt not this lady might have been cured long ago had her malady been thoroughly understood."

These paragraphs contain a candid statement of the difficulties in question, and show the cause of a vast amount of unnecessary suffering on the part of females. The author asks, "What can be done to obviate the perpetuity of such evils?" And then, with manifest doubt and misgiving, and with many *ifs*, he states what he thinks may be an *abatement* of the trouble. But let all of his conditions be complied with, – let the physician be an Æsculapius in medical renown, a king David or apostle Paul in piety, morality, and gentlemanly deportment, – and that will not remove the objection, unless the race be restored to that moral position which knew no guilt nor shame nor required the drapery of fig leaves.

Indeed, it often happens that the more of a gentleman and a scholar a physician is, the more he is esteemed as a friend or an acquaintance, so much the more it increases and complicates the embarrassment. Hence many an estimable female, seeking relief from her distress, passes by the learned and respected physician, and commits herself to some unprincipled quack, *because* she neither regards him nor values his regard for her. Many young physicians dislike to locate themselves in towns where they were brought up and went to school.

I am aware that some affect to ridicule this inborn and indispensable sentiment by calling it *prudery, false delicacy*, or *fastidiousness*, as Dr. Meigs terms it; though in another paragraph he more justly and correctly speaks of it as a commendable degree of modesty, scruples of delicacy, of which he is proud, which evince a fine morality, and should exist though they prevent investigations necessary to the successful treatment of diseases.

The following paragraph, from the same author, illustrates still further the "embarrassments of the practice." It also contains an implied recommendation of midwives, and shows how very convenient it would be to have female physicians, if it was only to *assist* male practitioners in the investigation and management of female complaints. He is supposing the case of a young person entering upon womanhood, who should apply for advice on account of symptoms peculiar and painful, but not such as should at all indicate to the physician the precise cause of her trouble without an examination. "What," says he, "can you say, what do, what know? Is there any therapeutics for an unknown case? You can do nothing, know nothing, and you ought not to say any thing, except that you do not understand the nature of the malady, which it is, moreover, impossible to know without the taxis. Now, this is a terrible decision to come to as far as the poor patient is concerned; but it is not your fault that she is unfortunate in being so situated. If she will suffer the proper inquiry to be made, there can be little doubt of the ability to procure the needed information; and you cannot undertake to cure until you know what is the matter. Let them call a midwife, whom you can instruct as to the visit she is to make; or, if none such can be found, you can offer your own services for the occasion."

As the present system of medical practice has but little to do with *preventing* disease, and by such formidable obstacles deters females from availing themselves of its *restorative* blessings, we cannot wonder that they delay to apply till their complaints become incurable, or that medical authors so sadly lament the inefficacy of the healing art so far as it relates to the female portion of the community.

Among other duties that now devolve upon the male practitioner is a very simple affair, of no uncommon occurence, that could be managed by female physicians, and even by nurses and the patients themselves, as will be seen by the following advice of Dr. Meigs to his class. He remarks that the medical man should attend to it, "or, what is far better," says he, "leave a proper catheter in the hands of the patient, first instructing her to apply it for her own relief. There are many persons who could be trusted to do this little operation, which is a saving both to their own feelings and those of the medical attendant; for there is scarcely a more disagreeable operation to be performed – an operation which, I should think, every gentleman would be glad to commit to other hands than his own."

Notwithstanding this, there are not unfrequent instances, as the author *knows*, where men have been employed, and have rendered this service daily for weeks and months. Really, it is pitiful, and a reproach to the whole community, that the female portion of it, with all their education and intellectual elevation in other respects, should be so utterly ignorant and helpless in matters like these.

THE PRACTICE OF MIDWIFERY. – From the preceding remarks, I think it will appear that females should participate in the practice of medicine. It will now be shown somewhat more fully that they should be the chief actors in the department of obstetrics.

When we come to add to what Dr. Meigs calls "the great host of female complaints" the tenfold greater host of the ordinary and natural cases of births, all inconveniently attended by males, we see what an awkward and unfortunate state of things results from confining the knowledge of medicine and midwifery to men. It is embarrassing to the patient, and consequently attended with increased suffering and peril; it is embarrassing to the medical attendant, often constraining him to withhold needed services. Dr. Meigs says, "I have many times been kept out of my house all night, in order to be near a patient supposed to be in labor; and having been refused the privilege of making the examination until morning, after so tardy an admission of my request, I have been obliged to announce, not only that the patient was not in labor, but that she had not reached the full term of pregnancy by ten days or a fortnight. It is exceedingly vexatious thus to be baffled by the unreasonable backwardness of the patient to submit to an operation which she knows to be necessary and inevitable."

The thought occurs, If this eminent professor, of above thirty years' practice, and justly enjoying the esteem and unlimited confidence of his patients and the public, finds so frequent vexations of this kind, as appears throughout his writings, how much greater the difficulties to be encountered by the multitudes of young men annually sent out from the medical schools of the country to take charge of these delicate departments of practice!

The objection to the employment of males in the ordinary duties of midwifery is strengthened by the disagreeable necessity that women are frequently under of employing several on different occasions, owing to removals, decease, absence, or engagement at the moment in some of the various duties of the general practitioner which are inconveniently connected with waiting upon ladies. A gentleman in Newburyport, whose family is not very numerous, stated to me that the advent of his children into the world had been presided over by *seven* different medical men. In a family of the author's acquaintance, now in this city, the same number of physicians have been employed in the capacity of midwife, (and no two on one occasion,) though there have been but nine children.

DISTINGUISHED FEMALE PHYSICIANS. – That women may become eminent as practitioners and medical authors there is ample proof. Professor Meigs, in his Letters to his Class on Female Diseases, speaking of a topic on which it is difficult for males to obtain information, says, "I am ready to pin my faith in this matter to the sleeve of a person better qualified to judge of it than you or I. I mean the late Madame Boivin, author of the *Memorial sur l'Art des Accouchemens*, long sage-femme en chef of the Maison des Accouchemens at Paris, and author of the admirable *Treatise on the Diseases of Women*, &c. Her writings prove her to have been a most learned physician; and, as she enjoyed a very large practice, her science and her great clinical experience, as well as her own personal knowledge, are more to be relied on than that of all the male physicians together."

Surely women of intelligence and philanthropy should take courage from this noble tribute to one of their sex, and believe the truth, that they, too, may become useful in the exercise of the healing art among delicate females and tender infants, and contribute also to the advancement of medical literature.

Madame Boivin, in her work on Midwifery, reports 20,517 births that occurred in her practice in the Hospital of Maternity.

Madame Lachapelle is another celebrated medical author and practitioner, "whose vast experience," says Dr. Meigs, "gained while at the head of the Maternité Hospital at Paris, is valid claim to speak as from authority, and whose thorough knowledge of the theory of midwifery must confirm those claims as rights." She reports as having occurred under her superintendence, from 1812 to 1820, 22,243 births.

Most appropriate for these distinguished persons is the term *sage-femmes*, (wise women,) given to females who pursue this honorable profession in France. How great their usefulness! – to have superintended the nativity of forty-two thousand human beings; to have comforted, cheered, sustained so many of their sex through their hours of fear and suffering as none but women can; for they have sympathies in common, a language and sentiments which seem to be made for the purpose; their sorrows and joys are the same. It is not the peculiar regard or the strong arm of a *protector* that the suffering woman wants at such a time, but the sympathy and ready assistance of one like herself, to whom she can without reserve commit her thoughts, feelings, person. The compassionate devotion on the one hand, and the deep emotions of gratitude on the other, which are so strongly elicted in passing through these scenes of suffering and danger, are then, of course, wholly unmixed with those other sentiments with which the Creator has endowed opposite natures for different purposes – the protection, and not the invasion, of the sanctities of connubial life; to make, and not to mar, the bliss of the domestic relations.

The author is aware that this is a tender point, and that some may take it unkindly, however gently it is touched upon; but the testimony of medical authors, and many proofs that have come to his knowledge, show it to be a consideration of too much importance to be silently pased over in this connection. It is not the design of these pages to cast reflections and reproaches upon individuals of either party for that which the present custom sanctions and even commands, but to show that this custom is unnatural and wrong, and should give place to one which not only insures greater safety to life, but is in every respect unexceptionable.

The embarrassment and nervous agitation which even the sight of the medical man often occasions increase the duration and severity of suffering, and consequently the peril to the mother and infant. There is a fearful calamity which sometimes happens to the parturient woman, termed *puerperal convulsions*. Out of 16,416 labors under the care of Dr. Collins, superintendent of the Dublin Lying-in Hospital, one patient in 547 was attacked in this way. Out of 96,903 presented in statistics collected by Dr. Churchill, there was one case of convulsions in 609. In Madame Boivin's 20,000 and more cases, less than one patient in 1000 was afflicted with this alarming disorder.

Medical authors are not agreed as to the exciting causes of these attacks, which may occur in a very plethoric or a very exhausted state of the system. Dr. Collins says, "I conceive we are quite ignorant as yet of what the cause may be; nor could I ever find, on dissection, any appearance to enable me even to hazard an opinion on the subject."

May not one of the causes be so simple and natural that these deeply scientific authors have overlooked it – viz., *female delicacy*, grievously shocked by the presence and personal attentions of gentlemen? Their statistics point to this as a cause. Dr. Meigs states that, of seventeen cases of convulsions in his practice, ten were those of women in their *first* confinement – the time of all others when their mental sufferings and embarrassments are the greatest, though their safety requires that they should be the least. Dr. Collins states "that, of nineteen cases of puerperal convulsions recorded by Dr. Joseph Clarke, sixteen were of females with their first children. Of thirty-six by Dr. Merriman, twenty-eight were first children. Of thirty by himself, twenty-nine were first children." These facts, in connection with the circumstance that in the very extensive practice of Madame Boivin a much smaller proportional number of such cases occurred, should have due weight in recommending the more natural and safe administration of females in these affairs.

The question will arise in the minds of some, How are females to get along in cases of extraordinary difficulty and when surgical aid may be needed? The eminent *sage-femmes*, Madame Boivin and Madame Lachapelle, did not need the aid of men even on such occasions. All manual assistance they could, of course, render with greater convenience and dexterity than male attendants; and equally skilful were they with the appliances of art. There is very rarely needed great physical strength; too much of it has ruined thousands. It fortunately happens that Nature, when not disordered or thwarted in her operations, never needs the aid of art; and but seldom even in the present degenerate condition of the race, especially when women, Nature's handmaids, preside. Out of the twenty thousand five hundred and seventeen cases of births under the care of Madame Boivin, only three hundred and thirty-four required to be assisted – leaving twenty thousand one hundred and eighty-three children born by the unaided powers of Nature. Had she been obliged to give up to the surgeon every one of the cases of slight or serious difficulty, how grateful to this noble woman must have been the reflection that she had saved so many thousands of her sex from the mortification, ay, and humiliation, of being subjected to the *needless* interference of male operators!

Obstetric surgery will not necessarily devolve entirely upon female practitioners, though a sufficient number of energetic and resolute women could be found who would be competent for *all* cases; but there can be in every city and large town a sufficient number of this class of male surgeons who might be called on when needed; which will very rarely happen, if the professional women have the education and experience. This is said to be the course pursued in China; and it is to a great extent adopted among ourselves. The majority of physicians in Boston and other cities, having a very limited practice in midwifery, mixed with their miscellaneous duties, and feeling their incompetency to manage extraordinary cases, send for those who are more exclusively engaged in this branch of the practice.

Any thing requiring promptness of action – hemorrhage, for instance, which is considered the most alarming of the unfavorable accompaniments – can be managed as well by qualified females as by males. In cases requiring surgical aid, there is abundance of time to send for it. Medical authors advise the practitioner not to take his mechanical agents with him, as there will always be time to procure them, even in the most urgent cases, as one writer remarks. Physicians, in such circumstances, take time to call in counsel: midwives can do the same.

It may be replied, that this plan will answer for the city, but never for the country. But in country towns women are now accustomed to rely much more upon each other, as it would be unsafe to depend wholly upon the uncertain arrival of the physician, who might be in some distant part of his extensive professional jurisdiction, administering to the halt and the lame, the bruised and the broken, the sick and the dying. As midwives could live on a smaller income, there could be a larger number of them and more conveniently located. These would be the familiar advisers and instructors of those who might consult them; and thus this knowledge would become diffused among the female portion of the community generally.

There is no reason why *all* women should not possess the little knowledge and ability which would enable them to render their sex needed assistance when a professional person is not at hand. There is now such a lamentable ignorance upon this subject, and women are such a profound mystery to themselves, that the most foreboding anxiety takes possession of the minds of many for months previous to their time, lest the doctor should fail to be there or should arrive too late. And well it may be so; for, in his absence, numberless mothers and infants have miserably perished, surrounded by a room full of terrified and useless women, any one of whom ought to have been able to save them.

Many physicians, from having often been witnesses of the helplessness and groundless alarms of the women present on these occasions, have doubtless come to the honest conclusion that the sex is so deficient in ability as to be incapable of managing such responsible affairs; whereas they should rather blame themselves for having taken from women their occupation, the knowledge, and the practice, and thus reduced them to such a pitiable condition. The change, then, in country towns and villages, so far from diminishing, will greatly increase the safety of those concerned.

But says one, "Female attendants cannot get about in wind and storm, night and day." Women will go where duty and humanity call, – to the frozen shores of Greenland or the burning climes of Africa, to the loathsome dungeon or the battle field, – not only as angels of mercy, but sometimes, as the noble Hungarian ladies, as ministers of destruction to their country's foes. So far as relates to this profession, they do go now, in city and country, as nurses or *second* assistants. Let them be qualified as *superintendents*, and they will be waited upon with more distinguished consideration.

Rev. Mr. F., in a town which the writer visited in Maine, remarked, that it was a source of sad regret and great affliction to his wife, in prospect of maternity, that it was necessary to have a gentleman attendant. He said if there had been any way to avoid it, any competent woman in his village, or had he known any in Boston for whom he could have sent, he should not have hesitated a moment in obtaining her. Such would be the feeling of every humane husband, possessed of a correct and delicate regard for his wife; and there will be ways and means for these doctresses *to get about.*

The following illustration of the point and the spirit of the last two paragraphs occurred since the publication of the first edition of this Letter. In the summer of 1851 the author was applied to by a gentleman of intelligence and influence, at the present time (1854) a member of the legislature of Vermont, from a town in that state bordering on Canada, who came to Boston expressly, as he stated, to engage a female physician to attend his wife in confinement. Several months after, in midwinter, the person engaged went on her distant professional visit, and performed her responsible duties with the highest degree of satisfaction to her employer, having carried the patient safely through her critical period; although two sisters of this lady had lost their lives in similar circumstances under the care of male physicians, and she was apprehensive of a like result in her own case. In December, 1853, the same professional woman a second time performed this journey of some 300 miles to attend the same lady, and with results alike satisfactory. This female physician has twice been called to attend cases in Newport, Rhode Island – thus having patients near 400 miles apart.

Perhaps the argument most relied upon against female practitioners is, that they have not the coolness of judgment and firmness of nerve requisite for cases of great difficulty. Let us look at this point. Suppose physicians were as ignorant upon this subject as females now are, they would then be easily alarmed and incapable of rendering efficient aid in a case of emergency, as young doctors often are, and non-professional gentlemen almost always are; so that the fact of being one of the stronger sex does not render one competent. On the other hand, if females had, in addition to their natural qualifications, the acquired knowledge of the physician, they would act with coolness of judgment and with efficiency.

In every accident or difficulty which can happen in the practice, the rules of action are plain and definite, and only need to be followed to insure the greatest possible safety. Two things will enable a weak man or a nervous woman to act with firmness and effect in trying circumstances; viz., 1st. To know just what to do; and, 2d. To know just how to do it. And to acquire this knowledge is not at all above or beyond the capacities of the female mind; but, on the contrary, it is in a measure intuitive with them, and something in which they can greatly excel.

But, says the objector, the midwife must be inferior to the physician, because she is not acquainted with all departments of the profession of medicine. Well, then, if it is necessary, let the *sage-femme* study medicine and midwifery three years or more. There is a surplus of twenty thousand females over the number of males in New England; and hundreds of them would be willing to devote any necessary length of time to qualify themselves for a useful, honorable, and remunerating occupation. It is the duty of the public and of wealthy individuals to *give* them the education, if they have not the means to obtain it, and let them use it for the good of their sex and the race.

But there are decided advantages in having a class of women devoted exclusively to this department of practice, whatever may be the extent of their collateral knowledge.

Excellence in various departments is obtained by a division of labor. In the medical profession this is carried to a much greater extent in other countries than in our own. It is related, as an illustration, that a gentleman passing through the streets of Paris slipped down and broke his right shoulder. He was taken up and carried into the office of the nearest surgeon, who looked at him, and excused himself from operating by saying that he only attended to the setting of *left* shoulders.

This may be an extreme of division and subdivision of professional duties; but it is not more absurd than the opposite extreme that prevails among us, where the term *physician* is so very comprehensive. The following *sign* enumerates a very few of the duties that pertain to an American "doctor." This particular specimen may be a quack; but, if he is, he does not differ from the honored profession in respect to the *variety* of his accomplishments and his disposition to render himself *generally* useful. This medico-literary curiosity is taken from the Boston Post.

"*Queer Signs.* – The following is a *verbatim et literatim* copy of a sign which may be seen any day in the eastern quarter of this city: –

Consult
Doctor
Waller
(Accoucher)
On All Diseases
Particularly
Midwifery And Diseases of
Women And Children
Fevers And Agues
Diseases of the Skin
Bone Setting. Sore Legs
Tooth Drawing
Squinting Cured."

Add to this specification, clubfoot, consumption, corns, and cholera, – in short, "all diseases" which afflict mortals, male *and* female, – and you have an idea of a modern *accoucher*, as this son of Æsculapius styles himself.

Rather an incongruous and inconvenient vocation, which calls one in so many directions often at the same moment – requiring in every thing great hurry and despatch, tempting the impatient man of multifarious duties to terminate lingering labors by the stimulus of ergot or by instruments.

It is gratifying to learn from the following that there is an improvement in respect to the abuse of this timesaving drug, spurred rye, in one city at least. "The use of ergot," says Dr. Meigs, "has very much diminished in Philadelphia in the course of the last ten or fifteen years. Few practitioners, when I was first engaged in business in this metropolis, were unprovided with a portion of ergot, which was given in almost every case of slow labor. The number of stillborn children, I doubt not, was greatly increased by this pernicious practice."

The attendance of females, being more natural, would remove a common source of difficulty and delay. Dr. Dewees, of Philadelphia, states, in his work on Midwifery, that he was once called to attend a lady whose midwife was absent; and the moment he entered the room her labor pains ceased, and did not recommence till a fortnight afterwards. "Every accoucheur," says he, "has witnessed a temporary suspension of pain on his first appearance in the sick chamber." A physician in Woburn attended a lady; and, perceiving that his presence had a retarding influence, he very candidly told the friends that the best thing he could do for the patient was to go away and leave her. He did so, and the favorable result proved his absence the best of prescriptions. Mental emotions, operating through the nervous system, have a powerful influence, as Dr. Dewees justly remarks, in exciting or suspending uterine contraction. A physician in Weymouth, having expended much time with a patient, pronounced the birth impossible without the aid of art, and started home for his forceps; but, before he returned, Nature, relieved from her embarrassment, had anticipated his services, and dispensed with his skill.

It has been urged in favor of retaining this practice exclusively in the hands of physicians, that they need the ordinary cases to qualify them to manage the difficult ones. Medical students will of course continue to study this branch, as they now do surgery, though some may never have occasion to set a broken bone; and if a physician should be called to render surgical assistance in obstetric cases, and was not so familiar with the minutiæ of the art, the *sage-femme* would be present with her knowledge and practical skill, and both together would manage difficult cases better than they are now conducted. If the question is, whether this practice should be confined *exclusively* to males or females, the arguments greatly preponderate in favor of the latter.

The greater facility with which women can obtain this sort of knowledge, especially the practical part of it, must be obvious to every one. It is so difficult for medical students to *get cases*, that they often graduate with mere book knowledge, having little or no practical skill, unless they have access to a large hospital. And it seems rather cruel and revolting to take advantage of the poverty of women to make them obstetric *subjects*, in a hospital or out, for the education of young men in affairs which humanity and morality demand that women should manage among themselves. Females, during their course of education for this profession, could very conveniently and usefully attend with ladies thoroughly versed in the science and practice, and officiate under their direction. They would thus graduate much better qualified than are young physicians.

Some may ask, If there are such advantages attending the exercise of this art by females, why has the practice almost entirely passed into the hands of males, especially in our enlightened New England? Is it not the result of the progress of the age? All change is not improvement. While society has made progress in most things, it has lost ground in many. The answer to the first question is this: While the various sections of the public have been absorbed, each in their own affairs and interests, the medical profession have very naturally been mindful of theirs; and of course they had no objection, so long as nobody else raised any, to letting women remain ignorant, and allowing this whole business, with the honors, and emoluments, and influence it confers, to slide into their hands.

The kings and autocrats of Europe, in the exercise of their paternal care, have made provision for the more dependent portion of their subjects; but in this country, the public, on whom devolves the duty of taking care of themselves, having omitted to provide the female portion of the community with any instruction upon this subject, and allowed all the practice to be taken from them, they have been growing more and more ignorant and helpless, as to their own affairs, from the landing of the Pilgrims to the present time. The following record will show how this subject was viewed by our ancestors, and what trouble one Dr. Rayus fell into by getting out of his "appropriate sphere."

We are informed, in the first volume of the "Collections of the Maine Historical Society," that the General Court, held at Wells on the 6th of July, 1646, "presented Francis Rayus, *for presuming to act the part of a midwife*. The delinquent, examined by the court, is fined fifty shillings for his offence; and paying the fees, five shillings, is discharged."

In the town records of Rehoboth, in this state, it is recorded that, on the 3d of July, 1663, the town voted to invite Dr. Samuel Fuller, of Plymouth, to come and reside and practise among them. "It was also voted and agreed that his mother be sent to, to see if she be willing to come and dwell amongst us, to attend on the office of midwife, to answer the town's necessity, which at present is great."

It appears that the good people of Rehoboth did not think it would at all "answer the town's necessity," in this latter respect, to have a male physician only among them.

Mrs. L. H. Sigourney, in her work entitled "Examples of Life and Death," thus speaks of Mrs. Ann Eliot, of Roxbury, wife of the "apostle to the Indians:" –

"Among the multitude of employments which a systematic division of time enabled her to discharge, without omission or confusion, was a practical knowledge of medicine, which made her the guardian of her young family. Her success in the rearing and treatment of her own children caused her experience to be coveted by others. In her cheerful gift of advice and aid she perceived a field of usefulness opening around her, especially among the poor, to whom with a large charity she dispensed salutary medicines. But her philanthropy was not to be thus limited to the children of penury. Friends and strangers sought her in their sicknesses; and she earnestly availed herself of the best medical works that she could obtain, to increase her knowledge and her confidence in its application." On the occasion of her death, which occurred in 1687, the town voted to erect a ministerial tomb, and passed a unanimous resolution, that "Mrs. Eliot, for the great service she hath done this town, shall be honored with a burial there."

In Blake's Annals of the Town of Dorchester is this record among others for the year specified: "1705. This year Died Feb. 6th Old Mrs. Wiat, Widow, being 94 years of age, having as a Midwife assisted ye Births of one Thousand One Hundred & odd Children."

This was quite an extensive practice, considering the country location and the more sparse population at that time; but the following example, furnished from the author's native state, is somewhat more remarkable.

The account, which is contained in Thompson's History of Vermont, relates to Mrs. Thomas Whitmore, who, with her husband, went to the town of Marlboro', in that state, in 1765. It reads thus: "Mrs. Whitmore was very useful to the settlers both as a nurse and a midwife. She possessed a vigorous constitution, and frequently travelled through the woods, on snowshoes, from one part of the town to another, by night and by day, to relieve the distressed. She lived to the advanced age of 87 years, officiated at more than two thousand births, and never lost a patient."

It is true that the less healthy females of our cities and populous towns, at the present day, may need more scientific assistance than did those "women of the revolution." And they will have such; for the female practitioners are to be thoroughly educated for their profession – what has never yet been done in this country. The artificial state of society, so far from being an argument in favor of male attendants, is the opposite. The patient is delicate in health, sensitive, nervous, especially at such times. So much the more need of avoiding all unnecessary annoyances. The terror and alarm thrown over the scene by the formidable parade, haunting the imagination for months beforehand; the shuddering ideas associated with the scientific and dignified surgeon, and the implements of his art, together with his ergot, inhalers, and bottles of oblivious ether or chloroform, and all the "meddlesome midwifery" of the present day, – surely this is enough to appall the most heroic woman and jeopard the life of one of ordinary "nerve."

The Princess Charlotte, of England, young and accomplished, lost her life in confinement with her first child, in 1817. She was attended by the usual parade of royal physicians and distinguished friends, with ministers of state and others assembled in adjoining apartments. "All this brought on," as a medical author writes, "anxiety of mind and excessive fatigue, followed by hemorrhage and convulsions, terminating in a fatal syncope, which all their united skill could neither prevent nor cure."

This event cast a cloud of sorrow over the nation. It was the theme of every tongue and the burden of every heart. An English gentleman, who was in London at the time, informed me that Mr. Hume, member from Scotland, declared, in his place in Parliament, that it was his candid conviction, that, if she had been spared the useless parade, and attended by a good Scotch midwife, she would have then been a living woman.

But to come nearer home. A clergyman who lived in this city at the time of the occurrence, three or four years ago, informed me that his wife, young and acutely sensitive, was attended on the occasion of her first confinement by a skilful and excellent physician; but, when she came to be subjected to the preliminary measures to ascertain whether it was likely to be a natural labor, it was more than her philosophy could bear. She burst into tears and sobbed like a child. Of course she was wholly disconcerted; the nerve force, which was all needed for accomplishing its appropriate office, was dissipated, exhausted. After some delay and a consultation of physicians, mechanical means effected what Nature's efforts might have done had they not been paralyzed – a healthy, well-formed woman as the patient was. In consequence of the extreme nervous excitement and the mental and corporeal suffering, inflammation and fever set in, and in two days she went with her infant to the grave.

O, ye mothers, who have delicate and carefully trained daughters, will you not do something to save them from such a trial, and, it may be, such a fate as this!

Thomas Moore, the poet, in his journal, as edited by Lord John Russell, under date of May 24, 1823, makes a memorandum of his wife's accouchement, speaks of the successful attendance of the midwife, and says, "The physician did not arrive till an hour after all was over, to Bessy's great delight, who has a horror of his being even in the house on these occasions."

A lady of great intelligence and moral worth, having perused the first edition of this Letter, communicated to the author the following case, with permission to use it, if he should wish, in a future edition: –

"*A Case.* – A lady of good constitution, nurtured in simple, industrious habits, and of nervous system under good control, approached her first accouchement. She was remarkably destitute of apprehension with regard to the event, and on terms of friendship with the gentleman physician who was to officiate. When the time arrived, quite an array of friends surrounded her; and, having had no information or idea of the style of examination that was pronounced necessary, she felt a revolting and horror that it was impossible to subdue, and the vigorous action by which Nature was about to pursue her operation was suspended. Pains occasionally returned, but produced no effect, seeming to be spasmodic, and wasting themselves upon the system at large. Ergot was repeatedly and copiously administered. Eighteen hours passed, and the patient seemed to be sinking. Though in a bath of perspiration, coldness seized the extremities and sight forsook the eye. Then the physician hurriedly, and with great exertion of manual strength, used the forceps; and a very fine infant, weighing nearly eleven pounds, was brought into the world, but never breathed, its head having been fearfully compressed by mechanical force. There was here neither malformation, nor malpresentation, want of vigor, nor previous disease. The only cause that seemed assignable was the sudden overthrow and terrible revulsion of a long-cherished, deep-seated delicacy. Afterwards, when the same person had similar anticipations, it was her earnest prayer that she might be saved from the revolting intervention of men; and her only two living children were both happily born before the arrival of the physician."

A clergyman of this city remarked, in conversation, that a family in his society employed a distinguished physician as accoucheur. After some delay, he decided, in consequence of the pressure of other engagements, to use the forceps. He did so, and in a few days the mother and child were no more. The gentleman said the family had ever felt that it was an entirely unnecessary sacrifice of life.

But, to remove all doubt as to the existence and extent of the dangers which attend the present officious system of midwifery, some eminent medical authority from the Universities of Edinburgh and of New York will here be presented.

In a work entitled "A Comparative View of the State and Faculties of Man with those of the Animal World, by John Gregory, M. D., F. R. S., Professor of Medicine in the University of Edinburgh, and First Physician to his Majesty in Scotland," is the following passage: –

> "Every other animal brings forth its young without assistance; but we judge Nature insufficient for that work, and think an accoucheur understands it better. What numbers of infants, as well as mothers, are destroyed by the preposterous management of these artists, is well known to all who have inquired into this matter. The most intelligent and successful practitioners, if they are candid, will own, that, in common and natural cases, Nature is entirely sufficient, and that their business is only to assist her efforts in case of weakness of the mother or an unnatural position of the child."

Dr. James Gregory, son of the author just quoted, and also professor of the Practice of Medicine in the University of Edinburgh as late as 1821, thought women abundantly competent to assist in childbirth, and strongly protested against the employment of physicians.

The following is an extract from a lecture by Gunning S. Bedford, A. M., M. D., professor of Midwifery and the Diseases of Women and Children in the University of New York, to his class of medical students, November 1, 1845: –

> "Allow me, in the most solemn and emphatic manner, to caution you against an error which, unfortunately for suffering humanity and the honor of our profession, has too generally prevailed. I allude to the indiscriminate and unpardonable use of instruments in the practice of midwifery. If the grave could speak, how fearful would be its revelations on this topic! how monstrous the guilt of those who revel in innocent blood! No more than six weeks since, I was visited by a medical gentleman who had been in practice but a short period, and in the course of conversation the subject of operative midwifery was introduced; and he observed to me that he had enjoyed the best opportunities of becoming familiar with the use of instruments, for his preceptor had performed the operation of embryotomy on an average sixteen times a year! To you, gentlemen, an announcement of this character may appear a romance; but I have myself witnessed in this city scenes of blood sufficient to satisfy my mind that this is not an exaggerated picture; and I will take the liberty of citing one case, among several others now fresh in my memory, to show you that I

do not speak without cause when I protest against the unholy acts of men who were intended neither by Heaven nor Nature to assume the sacred duties of the lying-in chamber."

The professor then proceeds to relate a case of thrilling horror – a piece of "atrocious butchery," to quote his own words. When he arrived in the room of the patient, "the perspiration of death was on her." "In her death agony," says he, "she supplicated me to save her, and said, with a feeling that none but a mother can cherish, that she was willing to undergo any additional suffering if she could only be spared to her children." After narrating the case, the doctor proceeds: "The question may now be asked, Why was embryotomy had recourse to in this case? I never could ascertain. There must have been some secret reason for it – the burning love, perhaps, which some men have for bloody deeds. There was no deformity of the pelvis; the head of the fœtus was of the usual size; and, as far as I could learn, it was an ordinary labor."

The professors of midwifery manifest a commendable degree of humanity in exhorting their pupils to beware of rash and hasty resorts to mechanical aid; but, so long as the absurd and unnatural practice of posting a man at the bedside in parturition prevails, so long instruments *must* be used. When Nature, shocked and paralyzed, cannot perform her office, her work must be accomplished by the poor substitutes of art.

But the sacrifice of life is not all. The shock to modest sensibilities, and consequent suspension of labor, frequently render necessary the countervailing force of ergot or the employment of instrumental or ill-adapted manual aid; and from these result numberless injuries, which sometimes render the life of the sufferer miserable, and go to make up that "great host of female complaints," the vain attempt to investigate and cure which constitutes quite a share of the present medical practice.

Many ill-fated infants are by the same cause put in peril of life and limb. Conversing with a gentleman in East Thomaston, Maine, he called his little son, about six years of age, and wished me to place my hand upon his wrist, the cords and joint of which were rigid and almost useless; upon his arm, which had been broken, and healed with a projecting callus at the fracture; upon his shoulder blade, which was warped out of shape; upon his side, where was an indentation of several ribs, – all of which disasters he experienced at the dreadful hour of his birth. The gentleman said, that since that occasion he had employed a plain sort of a matron to wait upon his wife, and no trouble whatever had occurred. He was, as we might well suppose, most decidedly in favor of female assistants.

An army might be collected of poor, crippled, deformed creatures, to whom life is a burden instead of a boon, in consequence of their never having been born, but calamitously introduced into the world by the resources of science. Well may it be said of such, "Better is the day of death than of one's birth."

Multitudes of infants are now lost, who by more suitable assistance, or by none at all, might have been saved to become the joy of their parents and ornaments to society. A wealthy gentleman present at one of the author's lectures, in Boston, said that he employed one of the most celebrated physicians that could be obtained to attend his wife in three instances, and every child was lost. On the fourth occasion a female practitioner officiated, and there was much less inconvenience and suffering, and a living child, now a fine lad, in whom centre the hopes of his parents.

A person of great worth and influence in this city gave me an account of a case of disappointed expectations and blighted hopes in this respect, instances of which are not uncommon, though, from the delicate nature of the subject and other reasons, they are wholly unknown to the public. The case was as follows: –

A young lady was taken in labor; and, though every possible assistance was rendered by the young medical gentleman who attended, yet after a long period of suffering the infant was born lifeless. This was a cause of extreme sorrow to the parents and friends – so much so, that in prospect of her second confinement the greatest anxiety was expressed that a similar misfortune might not occur. On account of the faithfulness and skill manifested by the young physician, his attendance was considered indispensable. His anxiety was increased by that of the friends, with whom he deeply sympathized; and of course he felt a heavy responsibility. The time arrived; and, to make assurance doubly sure, at the desire of both parties, the presence of an eminent professor was obtained. After a tedious and distressing labor, and considerable aid from art and operative skill, the child was delivered – alive! Pain and anguish were forgotten, and the most rapturous joy was expressed by the young mother, in which physicians and friends participated with the most lively sympathy and satisfaction. But alas! alas! the little one showed signs of distress and of ebbing life; and in consequence of an injury to the spine, discovered on a more careful examination, its brief existence was soon over, and unutterable grief as soon succeeded to transports of joy.

MIDWIFERY PRACTICE IN BOSTON. – The number of stillborn children in Boston has been for the past few years something over three hundred annually. There are, of course, various causes of this absence or loss of vitality, some of them wholly independent of good or bad midwifery practice. But it is well known that many children are born lifeless in consequence of protracted, distressing, exhausting labors, occasioned by the circumstances before mentioned, and that many are destroyed by the various means used as substitutes for the natural powers.

In the author's work, "Female Midwifery Advocated," published two years ago, it was given as an opinion that three hundred stillborn children was a very large number for this city, and indicated an unsuccessful system of obstetric practice. It could be given only as an opinion, the whole number of births not then being known or registered; but we now have data by which to ascertain *comparative* results. The city registrar informed me, early in December, that efficient measures had been taken to ascertain and record the number of births in Boston in 1849; and it would amount to 4000, and might be something over. If we suppose it to be 4200, and call the deadborn 300, (to say nothing of the large number that perish in early infancy,) it gives one in fourteen. In 21,502 births in the Hospital of Maternity, in Paris, under a female superintendent, the number of stillborn was 783 – a fraction over one in twenty-eight, or about half the ratio in Boston, where the proportion would have swelled this number of 783 to more than 1500.

The fatality to mothers, – the "childbed" cases, – it is probable, is proportionally as great as that of infants.

Some allowance should, perhaps, be made for the greater skill and more prompt assistance in a well-conducted hospital; but, on the other hand, it would seem that in this "new world," in the salubrious city of Boston, whose population is, to a great extent, made up from the healthy stock of the country, there ought not to be a greater mortality in the incipient stage of existence than there is in an old, luxurious, and effeminate city of Europe.

For some reason, the number of "stillborn," though recorded as usual in the bill of mortality at the office of burials, has for a year or more been omitted in the weekly reports through the newspapers, and in the Medical and Surgical Journal, where it has appeared for twenty years or more. On inquiring of the registrar the occasion of the omission, he replied, that he only knew that such were the directions. It would seem that it was a matter of as much interest and importance to the public to know how many human beings perish at birth, as to know how many leave the world after a stay of a few hours, days, or weeks, and are reported under the head "infantile diseases." At any rate, there are as good reasons for it now as there have been in time past.

From the data furnished by the new registry of births, some other important considerations can be presented. There are three hundred physicians in this city: 4200 cases of midwifery would give them on an average fourteen each – not enough to make them adepts in the art; but, on account of the repugnance to employing young physicians in these duties, they have less than their share of cases, next to none at all, while the older and more celebrated are overwhelmed with applications; so that some cannot do justice to their patients for the want of skill, and others for the want of time. As the *age* would not be a matter of so much consequence to female practitioners, the business would be more equally distributed among them.

I am very well aware that the medical profession, in consequence of an over supply of members, has but a poor remuneration from all the duties that now pertain to it, and I regret as much as any one the inconvenience that may result to some physicians from restoring the practice of midwifery to females; but a measure recommended by so many and weighty considerations should receive the support even of those who may be temporarily discommoded.

Suppose, now, that these forty-two hundred cases of childbirth, instead of being attended by three hundred gentlemen, were intrusted to forty-two good women every way qualified for the office, – and surely Boston could furnish that number of females, of just the right description, to be educated and employed as sage-femmes, – one hundred cases in a year, or about two a week, would be a moderate practice without attending to other departments. They could, of course, devote ample time to their patients, and would never be interrupted by the miscellaneous duties of the medical practitioner.

The number of females being considerably larger than that of males, in consequence of the recruiting of armies and navies, the loss of men at sea, and, in this section, the constant emigration, women need all the occupations for which they are adapted. So their performance of these duties, instead of being a loss of labor to the community, would relieve the widow and her children from want, and the relatives or the public from the necessity of sustaining hundreds and thousands of females who have both the ability and the disposition to support themselves if they could only have the opportunity.

But man, the lord of creation, has the world before him, and can choose his profession or pursuit – war, politics, agriculture, commerce, mechanic arts, mercantile affairs, (not excepting ribbon and tape,) and a thousand vocations and diversions; and, not content with these, he must wrest from the long-suffering and ever-yielding sex the more responsible and dignified of their duties, deprive them of the honor of presiding over the nativity of mankind – a calling which Heaven and Nature designed them, and them alone, to pursue.

There are said to be forty thousand physicians in the United States. Twenty thousand of these ought to give place to this number of women, and turn their attention to pursuits better adapted to their strong muscles and strong minds than is this waiting with ladies from two to twenty hours, and this simple, mechanical routinism of midwifery. Indeed, physicians of good intellectual and scientific attainments do consider it beneath their qualifications; and when circumstances permit they are glad to be rid of it, and devote themselves to departments better calculated to exercise their mental capacities.

In addition to providing for the self-support of twenty thousand or more women, this change would release that number of men, and secure to the country the benefits of their mental and manual industry – quite an item in our political economy and national wealth. Of course this very desirable change cannot be brought about so suddenly as to create any great disturbance in the established order of things, even if the enterprise is carried forward with all possible vigor; so that physicians now in the field need not be greatly alarmed in prospect of female competitors.

There are probably three thousand young men annually assembled in the medical schools of the country. Let half of the prospective pupils turn their attention to other pursuits, and the same number of females be put in a course of training, and the proper division of professional duties will gradually be established between the sexes. If at first but a quarter of the male should give place to female pupils, (and there ought to be that number at least,) the change would be still more gradual. But, in fact, every one ought to wish that the whole business of midwifery could be immediately transferred to women; for every instance of the real or supposed necessity of employing a man in such a case is an unfortunate occurrence and one to be lamented.

There is not all the necessity which some people imagine for these severe trials of female sensibility. In the Southern States, the colored women perform these services to a great extent, and that without knowing the first letter of the alphabet. An editor of this city, during a temporary residence at the south, employed one of those natural Ethiopian doctresses to attend his lady in confinement, and with the most satisfactory results. A gentleman who had resided in Arkansas remarked to the writer that one of his neighbors there owned a famous practitioner of this description, who spent her whole time in riding from the residence of one planter to another, and was a source of quite an income to her master.

Thomas Ewell, M. D., of Virginia, a distinguished physician, honorary member of the Philadelphia Medical Society, and an eminent author, appeals to the ladies upon this subject in the following graphic and earnest manner: –

"In some parts of our country the negro women, feeling their ignorance, and fearful of harming their mistresses, hesitate in acting until they accidentally discover the powers of Nature: they then obtain great reputation in the practice of midwifery, rivalling the most renowned doctors of the trade. They soon discover the secret that Nature does all the business, and that they have only to keep themselves quiet and pocket the credit of the operation.

"Indeed, considering the extraordinary facilities which Nature has provided for the birth of the humankind, considering the numbers who bring forth daily without suffering, it seems wonderful how so many ladies on these occasions can make such an ado about the affair, can so idly injure themselves with unhappy conceits, can apprehend any thing but the most fortunate termination of their case.

"But the cause of all such groundless fears may be traced to the arts and ignorance of designing persons. A thousand times more notice is taken of one little irregularity of the attendants than of the many cases Nature conducts without aid. This operates on the fears of the women; each considers that the worst may be her case; assistants at extravagant rates are sent for; and they pocket commonly very handsomely for the folly of the patient. I beseech you, for the sake of decency, of justice to your attendants, of charity to poor women, abandon such improper infatuation. Believe the truth, that, in ten thousand instances to one of the contrary, women can render you all proper assistance without the meddling of men operators. Their hurry, their spirit for acting, have certainly done more harm than all the improper conduct of women, of which they are so fond of talking."

When physicians, whose own interests and that of their profession would lead them to sustain the present system, speak in this strong manner against it, women ought certainly to believe their testimony.

A SUCCESSFUL MIDWIFE. – The following inscription, taken from a gravestone in the Old Burying Ground, in our neighboring city of Charlestown, will show in what high esteem these professional women were held in this vicinity less than a century ago: –

> "Here lyes Interred the Body of Mrs. Elizabeth Phillips, wife to Mr. John Phillips, who was Born in *Westminster*, in Great Britian, & Commissioned by John, Lord Bishop of *London*, in the year 1718, to the office of a Midwife, and came to this country in the year 1719, & by the blessing

> of God, has Brought into this world above 3000 children. Died May 6th, 1761, aged 76 Years."

From this it appears that midwifery, in the true signification of the word, is no new idea in this section, no untried experiment, and that this movement aims at no innovation or revolution, but simply to *restore* this office to its natural and rightful possessors, in whose hands it was and ever should be.

A great change has taken place in the customs and manners of New England society since Mrs. Phillips's day. In reference to these matters, the order of ideas is directly inverted. There was then much less affectation of modesty. A whole town could exhibit so great a want of *refinement* as to put such a record as the above in a public place! Accompanied with true delicacy and purity of mind was an honest frankness, that called things by their right names. Neither prospective maternity nor midwifery, when alluded to, was considered an occasion for a smile or a blush; nor did the women deem it necessary to avoid observation by secluding themselves from the green earth, the sunlight, and the pure air of heaven for weeks and months previous to their confinement, to the detriment of their own and infant's health and future well being; but, when the important occasion arrived, they showed their *real* refinement by allowing no male intruders within the sacred precincts of the lying-in room.

Now all these things are changed; and a practice which our ancestors punished as an offence against propriety is glossed over with circumlocutions and French phraseology, and compliance with it enforced by the code of fashion.

Mary Wolstonecraft, in her vindication of the claims of females to some of the more responsible and remunerating duties of life, thus speaks upon this subject: –

> "Women might certainly study the art of healing, and be physicians as well as nurses. And midwifery decency seems to allot them; though I am afraid the word *midwife* in our dictionaries will soon give place to *accoucheur*, and one proof of the former delicacy of the sex be effaced from the language."

MORAL CONSIDERATIONS. – This view of the subject has hardly been alluded to; but I should feel that one of the most serious and weighty reasons in favor of female physicians was omitted if this were passed over in silence.

It is not necessary to say that physicians, as a body, are an intelligent, honorable, and most useful class of men. Nothing is farther from the author's desires or intentions than to depreciate their worth in the estimation of the public, or to discourage sound and thorough medical education. Among the profession he has many valued friends and agreeable acquaintances, classmates and others. It is not that he regards their interest less, but the general good more, that he thus strongly urges this matter.

Far be it, too, from the writer to affirm or imply that there is not now a high-toned female delicacy in New England and the country; indeed, the assumed existence of such delicacy is the main ground of his argument. The good opinion he has of the abilities of his countrywomen leads him to believe that the object aimed at is not an impracticable one; and his faith in their good sense and elevated principles makes him believe that they will not be offended at, but will rather approve, the plain and faithful manner in which he has felt it his duty to present this subject.

The unfavorable tendency of the present system of medical practice, in a social and moral point of view, does not necessarily presuppose a want of virtuous, or even of religious, principle; for there is no one who cannot properly utter the petition, "Lead us not into temptation." When it is considered that a profession of forty thousand or more men in the country – not all of whose hearts can be reasonably supposed to be the shrine of probity – are obliged, from the necessity of the circumstances, to have the most intimate and confidential relation to the female portion of the population, especially those in married life, it is impossible to doubt, even were proofs wanting, that it must be a source of not a little domestic unhappiness, wounded feelings, alienation, and sometimes the dispersion of an otherwise happy fireside circle.

The following, from the "Code of Medical Ethics adopted by the National Medical Convention in Philadelphia, June, 1847," will show how directly at variance is the medical with the moral code and the conventional forms of society. After speaking of the necessity of perfect frankness, both as to mental ailments and bodily diseases, lest concealment should prevent a cure, it says, –

> "A patient should never be afraid of thus making his physician his friend and adviser. Even the female sex should never allow feelings of shame or delicacy to prevent their disclosing the seat, symptoms, and causes of complaints peculiar to them. However commendable a modest reserve may be in the common occurrences of life, its strict observance in medicine is often attended with the most serious consequences," &c.

A system of practice which renders it necessary to treat thus lightly that natural reserve which the Creator has implanted to be *observed* between the sexes cannot but tend to lower the general tone of delicacy and weaken the safeguards of public virtue. And who can say how much the employment of men, in services which women only should perform, may have assisted in causing the great deterioration from the Puritan morals of past generations?

Many clergymen – those who possess a reasonable share of general intelligence – understand the bearing of these things, and have felt it their duty to encourage and assist this movement to restore, or establish, a code of medical ethics more in harmony with the code of the Bible and Nature. They perceive that they have been laboring with indifferent effect as conservators of public morals, in consequence of having (according to the present system of medicine) expended their efforts on chronic and incurable complaints instead of attending to causes and prevention.

Rev. Wm. Hosmer, editor of the Northern Christian Advocate, Auburn, New York, in speaking of the subject in his widely-circulated journal, in the following paragraph expresses his views of the evils and the remedy: –

> "Medical Education of Females. – An institution has lately been started in Boston under the patronage of the American Medical Education Society. From the circular of this society, forwarded to us by the secretary, Samuel Gregory, – a well-known lecturer and author of many valuable works, – we learn that 'the object of the association is to educate midwives, nurses, and female physicians.' This is a most laudable enterprise, worthy alike of the philanthropist and the Christian. There are hundreds of females in the country, who could in no other way be so useful to the world as by qualifying themselves for medical practice among their own sex. All who know any thing of the matter know full well that the modern practice of medicine too nearly overlooks the distinction of sex, and that there is no remedy for this evil but the medical education of females. Nature suggests it, reason approves it, and religion demands it."

The French, who, as it is well known, are not noted for being over-particular in relation to the ceremonies between the sexes, are altogether in advance of us upon the subject of providing their women with female attendants, as will be seen by the following paragraph from the Boston Medical and Surgical Journal of 1845: –

> "Instruction of Midwives in Paris. – According to the new regulations regarding the instruction of midwives in Paris, it is required that they shall present testimonials of good character, be at least eighteen years of age, and able to read and write correctly the French language before they can be admitted to the clinical lying-in hospital. It is only after having diligently attended this institution for twelve months, and taken two full courses of lectures on the Theory and Practice of Midwifery, that they can present themselves as candidates for the degree."

Rev. Dr. Jenks, in speaking (in the *Comprehensive Commentary*) of the Hebrew midwives and of institutions for educating these professional women among the ancient nations, says, "The French government wisely support such schools at the present day."

According to L'Union Médicale of August 26, 1847, there were 480 licensed midwives in Paris. The French are certainly good judges in this matter, taking the lead, as they do, of all the world in medical affairs.

The editor of the Boston Daily Bee, who has resided sometime in Paris, speaks as follows: –

> "We would call attention to a paragraph headed 'American Medical Education Society,' among the local matters, in another column. One

> cannot walk through a street in Paris without seeing the portrayed sign of a *sage-femme* with a young infant in her arms; and we have heard French surgeons of eminence say that, except in cases of great difficulty, females, properly educated, (as they are there,) were far preferable to male practitioners. No one who has the good of the community at heart should refuse his aid to this commendable undertaking. Liberal donations will doubtless be made."

But, not to rely upon French example alone, let us look at other European countries. The following is a translation of a diploma, the original broad parchment of which I have in my possession, having received it from the lady herself, now a resident in this city. She remarked that the king was accustomed to bestow some of his royal charities in sustaining annually half a dozen midwives in the institution. The certificates must have amounted to a great number by this time. The document indicates the custom in that noble and virtuous nation, Sweden.

"I, Peter Gustavus Cederschjold, physician and surgeon, professor of midwifery in the Medical and Surgical Institute and director of the General Lying-in Hospital in Stockholm, hereby give notice that Fredrica Wilhelmina Mellgren has this day been examined before the medical faculty, and has given evidence of a very good knowledge and understanding of all the branches pertaining to Midwifery, and by this letter she is accepted as a practitioner, and has all the rights and privileges which the law gives for the exercise of this profession.

I therefore affix the stamp of the common Lying-in Hospital seal and sign. Stockholm, June 29, 1826. By authority of the Faculty. P. G. Cederschjold.

No. 1233 Midwives' Certificate, for F. W. Mellgren.

A. F. Idstrom, Doctor of Medicine, and Adjunct."

It is the custom throughout Europe to educate women for this practice. John S. Crawford, M. D., of Galena, Illinois, in a letter to the author, dated June 20, 1849, and enclosing a remittance in aid of the object, expresses his cordial approval of the effort making in this city for the education of professional women, and adds, "This course has been pursued by many, if not all, of the Medical Schools of Europe for some years; and during the time of my attendance in the Dublin Lying-in Hospital, there was a class of females attending for instruction, to whom, as well as to the students from the 'Schools,' a Certificate or Diploma, of having attended three full sessions, was given, and an examination made of their competency to practise midwifery.

In Russia, as I am informed by a gentleman who has resided there, principally in St. Petersburg, ten years, the government provides institutions for educating females for this profession; and they are employed by all, from the Empress to the wife of the serf. The gentleman said he had occasion to employ one of them for his lady; he was much pleased that measures were in progress to provide female practitioners among us, and gave something for the object.

Rev. Dr. Baird remarked to the writer, that the employment of females in this office was the general custom of Europe; said he had stepped into an institution where a lady was lecturing upon the subject at the time. He expressed himself in the strongest terms against our system of midwifery, and said if his influence would aid this enterprise any he would most cheerfully give it. He accordingly made himself a member of the society, and gave a strongly written recommendation of the object.

If the women of Russia and other European countries can manage these affairs, most certainly American, New England women can; for they are altogether better informed in other respects, and our system of female education is every year growing more solid and thorough.

ETHER AND CHLOROFORM. – In the author's work, published two years ago, the opinion was given, and sustained by the best authorities, that the use of these agents in childbirth was unnecessary and unsafe. Since that time proofs of this point have been multiplied. Professor Meigs, in his recent work, Obstetrics, says, "Having carefully studied the reports upon etherization and chloroformization, whether those in this country or those produced in Europe, I remain as yet unconvinced, either of the necessity for the method or of its propriety. I am a witness that it is attended with alarming accidents, however rarely. As to its employment in midwifery here, notwithstanding a few cases have been mentioned and reported, I think it has not begun to find favor with accoucheurs." In dentistry and surgery people had better do without these noxious influences on slight occasions; but in severe cases of surgery their judicious use is a different matter, as the injurious effects of employing them might be less than would arise from the shock to the system by the pain of amputations, the excision of tumors, and other formidable operations. A strong reaction has already commenced against the use of ether, chloroform, and all their modifications.

With regard to the "American Medical Education Society," it is proposed to have it incorporated by the legislature at an early day.* And it may not be thought unworthy of pecuniary aid from the state, and perhaps such assistance will be rendered, unless the public and individuals of wealth should anticipate legislative action on this point, and prevent the necessity of it. Certainly, no literary, scientific, or agricultural institutions can be of greater importance to the public weal than an establishment for qualifying midwives, and female physicians, to administer to the wants of women and children, and nurses for the responsible office of attending the sick generally. The Maternity Hospital, to be connected with the College, will not only serve for educational purposes, by affording the pupils practical knowledge, but will be a most important charitable institution for the accommodation of large numbers of *virtuous* poor women, who now have to pass their critical periods amid poverty and distress, in damp and unwholesome residences of the city.

The following very handsome and – so far as relates to the *object* – very judicious paragraph, is clipped from the Boston Post, of March 8, 1848. The editor having been present on the occasion of one of the author's lectures, remarks, "his lecture last evening, in the lower hall of the Tremont Temple, was fully attended by gentlemen, and his observations upon the impropriety and injurious effects of the present custom of employing males in the offices of midwifery were marked with sense, shrewdness, and discretion, and attended with general approval. His positions upon this subject, and upon others immediately connected with it, were logically enforced, and need only notoriety to be followed by a propitious legislative action. *Progress* is the watchword of the times, and when manifested in causes akin to this in substantial and practical good, none but the conventionally dull will regret it."

Female Practitioner in Boston. – Thirty years ago Mrs. Janet Alexander, from Edinburgh, where she was educated for the profession of midwifery, was introduced into practice in this city, under the auspices of Drs. John C. Warren and James Jackson. She had an extensive and very successful practice for twenty-five years, among the most intelligent portion of the community. It has been the pleasure of the writer to meet with many, and to learn of a still larger number of heads of families, among the wealthy citizens, who had employed this lady, and were therefore most decidedly and understandingly in favor of educating females for the office generally.

For some time after Mrs. Alexander arrived, as I was informed by her daughter, her prospects of success in this city were rather discouraging, and she decided to remove to New York; but a number of the influential ladies of the city immediately interested themselves, and made up a purse of $1200 for her, and encouraged her to remain.

A clergyman remarked to me, that he had always employed Mrs. Alexander in his family, as had most of his society. He said that when she died, (in 1845,) it was a time of heartfelt mourning with all the women who had known her great worth and eminent usefulness. A lady, now acting as agent in this city for the Medical Education Society, reports that she meets with very many of the friends of this gratefully remembered woman; and finds not only them, but other ladies, with hardly any exceptions, most cordially in favor of the objects advocated in these pages. Many of the more favored in point of wealth, on giving their names and something *to help along*, kindly and encouragingly remarked, that when the plans were fully matured, their more substantial aid should not be wanting. No, the influence and aid of the ladies *cannot* be wanting; for it is woman's nature to be ever humane and benevolent, and "ready to every good work."

Source Endnote

* The association was incorporated by the Massachusetts legislature the same year, 1850, by the name of Female Medical Education Society, and in 1856 its name and organisation were changed to that of New England Female Medical College, the institution being previously conducted by the society.

Editorial Headnote

William Dale, *The Present State of the Medical Profession in Great Britain and Ireland, With Remarks on the Preliminary and Moral Education of Medical and Surgical Students* (London: A.W. Bennett, 1860), frontispiece image of 'The "Upas" of the Medical Profession'

Little biographical detail can be gleaned about William Dale, M.D. (London), M.R.C.S. (England) (1821–post 1895; fl.1860s–1870s), who was employed in Plymouth, Devon, later became Honorary Physician to the West Norfolk and Lynn Hospital, and finally as the 1895 *Medical Register* recorded, ended up at a Health Resort, in Bishopsteignton, South Devon. Dale's writings on the contemporary state of the medical profession peppered the marketplace from 1860 to 1875. From a Licence of the Society of Apothecaries in 1853 and a midwifery licence two years later, he appeared to have made slow progress ascending the medical ladder, from registration in 1859 to a M.D. in 1865 and membership of the Royal College of Surgeons.[1] Unlike double winner Walter Rivington, extracts from whose reflections are to be found elsewhere in this volume, Dale was not a successful, but was a repeated, entrant for the Carmichael Prize. His first attempt in 1860, from which the current image is excerpted, failed because prizes were not awarded that year. As the Preface to this version explains the work for the volume was 'snatched' from sleep and the fruit of early rising, considerable labour and much thought. Unwilling to allow 'the labour of his hands' to disappear, he believed that his production would be 'highly useful' to those interested in the topic discussed. Interestingly, Dale wanted readers to engage with the text both immediately and in the future, and offered a fascinating material feature to ensure that developments were recorded. By offering deliberately blank leaves at the end of the book, Dale hoped that changes and alterations in practise by educational and examining bodies could be added to ensure that his work was a 'trustworthy guide to the medical profession for many years to come'.[2] The 1860 version was noted as 'just published' in early February 1860 at an affordable 2s 6d, indicating the intended audience of potential or actual medical students.[3] It did not receive much critical attention, but the *Medical Critic and Psychological Journal* noted in rather a terse and oddly back-handed compliment in July 1861 that it was a 'sober, thoughtful pamphlet, the object of which is best expressed by its title-page'.[4] An advertisement for Dale's work in the *Lancet* reproduced two equally unpropitious comments. The first was from the *Dublin Medical Press* about it being a 'serviceable guide', while the second, extracted from the *Western Morning News*, remarked only on the 'good deal of humour' in the frontispiece.[5] Rather than using the end pages for their own notes, reviewers did not progress that far through Dale's reflections.

Dale took his own advice for additions to his project to heart, however, and added to comments on the state of the medical profession throughout the next decade and a half. He tried again for the Carmichael Prize in 1868, but once more was unsuccessful. When Dale published this version in 1869, the Preface now accused the winner of the 1868 Prize, Edward Dillon Mapother's attempt, as null and void. As a member of the Council of the Royal College of Surgeons in Ireland, as well as someone who forwarded a printed and irrelevant essay, rather than a manuscript, claimed Dale, Mapother should have been disqualified. Dale's response was a far more 'faithful delineation of the present state of the Medical Profession in Great Britain and Ireland', as the Prize stipulated.[6] Again he drew the reader into this debate, appending the rules and regulations of the Prize, and asking them to decide. In a non-review, the *Athenaeum* dismissed Dale's writing, by suggesting that it did not contain 'much that will be new to the members of the medical profession in the United Kingdom', before launching an attack on the whole edifice as not fit to grace a 'free and enlightened country'.[7] Debate, at least, had been stimulated by Dale's work. Two other reviews were more impressed, citing, in particular the low cost of the volume, and Dale's Christian thoughtfulness surrounding the moral training needed for medical students.[8]

Dale achieved second place in the Carmichael Prize in 1873, and published the result two years later.[9] Despite the developments that had occurred since 1860, one bugbear lingered from his original attempt at outlining the present state of the profession: women who wanted to study medicine. This was one area he evidently wished his readers could not update on the blank leaves of his volume.

Notes

1 UK Medical Register 1867; 1887; 1895.
2 'Preface', William Dale, *The Present State of the Medical Profession in Great Britain and Ireland, With Remarks on the Preliminary and Moral Education of Medical and Surgical Students* (London: A.W. Bennett, 1860), pp. iii–iv; p. iv.
3 *Athenaeum*, 1684 (4 February 1860), p. 185; *Lancet*, 77:1962 (6 April 1861), unpaginated.
4 *Medical Critic and Psychological Journal*, 1:3 (July 1861), p. 504.
5 *Lancet* (6 April 1861).
6 'Preface', *The State of the Medical Profession in Great Britain and Ireland* (Dublin: Fannin and Co., and London: Longmans, 1869), p. iii.
7 *Athenaeum*, 2187 (25 September 1869), p. 406.
8 *Wesleyan-Methodist Magazine*, 15 (June 1869), pp. 548–549; *London Quarterly Review*, 33:65 (October 1869), p. 257.
9 William Dale, *The State of the Medical Profession in Great Britain and Ireland* (Dublin: J. Atkinson, 1875).

2

FRONTISPIECE IMAGE OF 'THE "UPAS" OF THE MEDICAL PROFESSION', *THE PRESENT STATE OF THE MEDICAL PROFESSION IN GREAT BRITAIN AND IRELAND, WITH REMARKS ON THE PRELIMINARY AND MORAL EDUCATION OF MEDICAL AND SURGICAL STUDENTS*

William Dale

Source: William Dale, *The Present State of the Medical Profession in Great Britain and Ireland, With Remarks on the Preliminary and Moral Education of Medical and Surgical Students* (London: A.W. Bennett, 1860), frontispiece image of 'The "Upas" of the Medical Profession'

DOI: 10.4324/9781003265238-2

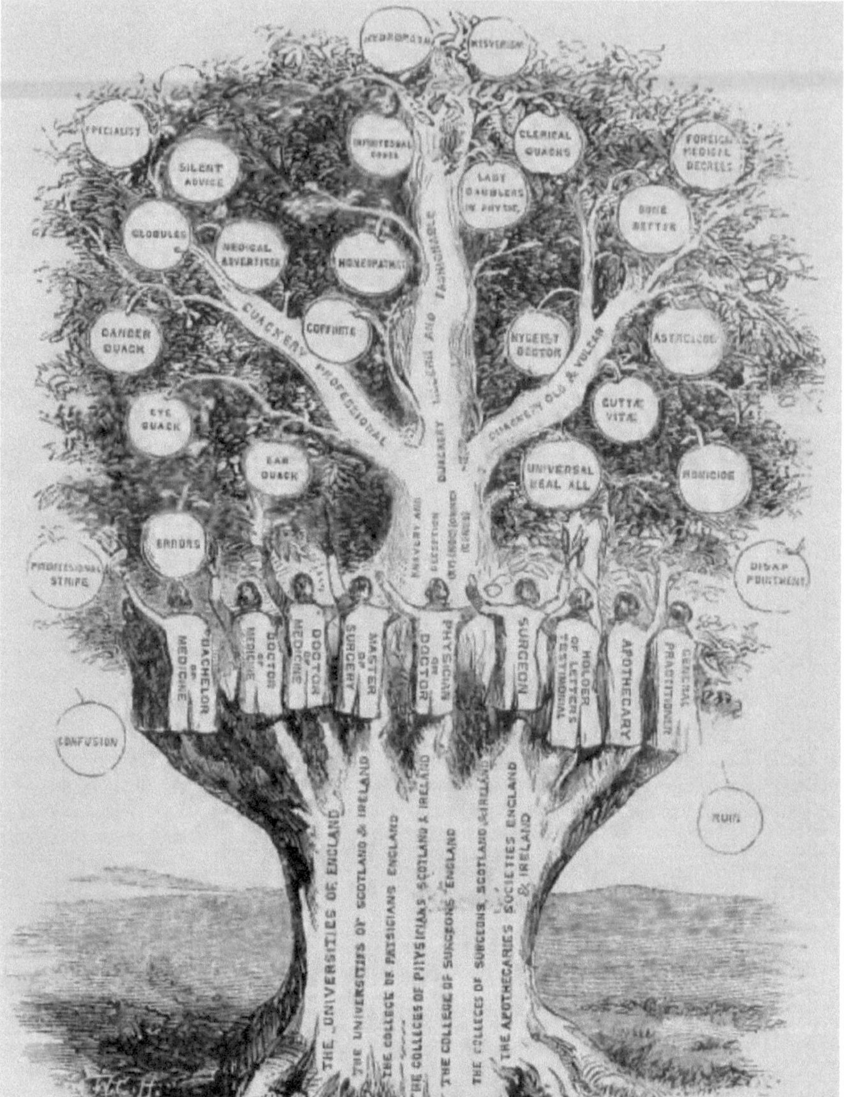

THE "UPAS" OF THE MEDICAL PROFESSION.

"The appellations, 'Doctor,' 'Surgeon,' &c., are not distinctive of qualification, and hence the land is filled with Charlatans and Impostors. In England, we have in practice men holding Foreign Diplomas, which may be purchased for a few pounds, and a certain amount of false swearing. We have men practising without diplomas as Homœopathists, Hydropathists, Prescribing Druggists, &c. We have Specialists, as Aurists, Oculists, Cancer-curers, &c.,—all known to, and employed by, the public as 'Doctors.'"—*Vide pp.* 20, 21.

Editorial Headnote

'Lady Doctors', in Jennie June, *Jennie Juneiana: Talks on Women's Topics* (Boston: Lee and Shepard, 1864), pp. 115–117

'Jennie June' was the pseudonym of prolific journalist and writer, Jane Cunningham Croly (1829–1901), who was born in Market Harborough, Leicestershire, but lived in New York and Massachusetts after her family emigrated to the United States of America in 1841, when she was twelve. Fifteen years later, she married David G. Croly, who was a reporter on the *New York Herald.* Cunningham Croly was soon supplementing her husband's fourteen dollars a week with her own contributions to papers such as the *New York Tribune*, *World*, *Times*, *Noah's Sunday Times*, and the *Messenger*, honing journalistic skills that had been apparent since youthful productions had entranced the audience of her brother's Massachusetts parish. Editorial work followed in the 1860s for the *Sunday Times*, *Demorest's Magazine*, *Godey's Magazine*, the *Home-Maker*, and the *Cycle*, which she balanced alongside a busy domestic and social life. In a posthumous collection of articles and tributes, Cunningham Croly's brother, John Cunningham, D.D., remarked upon 'Jennie June's' leadership of the global 'new woman' movement, which he defined as not the 'monstrosity' so beloved of satirists, but the 'rise and development of a better, nobler type of womanhood'. 'Gifted women' in their thousands, claimed Cunningham, were now able to voice their opinions in poetry, dissertation writing, fiction, and journalism because 'Jennie June opened the path for them. Womanhood was her watchword, and God, duty, faith and hope the springs of her life'.[1]

'Jennie June's' support for her sex was consolidated when she set up 'Sorosis', a woman's club based in New York City. One of the key catalysts in the flourishing of this movement in postbellum America, Cunningham Croly, incensed at being excluded from a press dinner to celebrate Charles Dickens in March 1868, established Sorosis as a space for women to develop literary and artistic tastes, express these outwardly in lives and work, and to discuss 'new facts and principles, the results of which promise to exert an important influence on the future of women and the welfare of society'.[2] Though conservative in aim initially, such clubs soon began to involve themselves in wider civic concerns and philanthropy.[3]

Before Sorosis, however, Jennie June was already debating women's topics in her various columns and in collections such as *Jennie Juneiana.* Due to the author's visibility in the press and numerous areas covered, *Jennie Juneiana* was mentioned and reviewed across an array of publications from the serious, well-respected *Atlantic Monthly* to 'The Very Best Children's Paper in America!', the *Little Pilgrim: A Monthly Journal for Girls and Boys* via professional periodicals such as the *California Teacher*. Jennie June's conception of 'women's topics' range from seasonal amusements, with sections organised for each part of the year, alongside meditations on 'Patch-Work Quilts', 'How to Lean on a Gentleman's Arm', and 'How to get Married'. The topical mêlée is interspersed with more serious reflections on contemporary concerns, such as occupational difficulties and, as excerpted here, 'Lady Doctors'. The *Round Table* labelled the sketches 'disconnected', but praised the 'plain speaking' tone, which addressed 'the plainer sort of people' but would be advantageous to those from higher echelons.[4] Similarly, the avoidance of 'big, coarse, and masculine subjects' and the 'sense and pleasantness' of an author who talked 'like a woman upon woman's topics' unlike other female writers of the day attracted the bi-monthly *American Literary Gazette*.[5] The *Atlantic Monthly* despaired, alternatively, at the attempts not to appear 'strong-minded', disparaging the 'prevalent American newspaper-style' and 'very silly things' contained within.[6] Jennie June's attitude to 'Lady Doctors' was identified by the *Atlantic* as particularly nonsensical. What the other reviews missed in not mentioning this article, and the *Atlantic* drew attention to, was the ease with which women's place in medicine could be mentioned as both a topic suitable for women to discuss amongst a variety of others, as well as its everyday position in debates of the 1860s.

Notes

1 John Cunningham, D.D., 'A Brother's Memories' in; *Memories of Jane Cunningham Croly 'Jenny June'* (New York: G.P. Putnam's Sons and London: The Knickerbocker Press, 1904), pp. 3-12; on p. 11.
2 Mrs Croly, *Sorosis: Its Origin and History* (New York: J.J. Little & Co., 1886), pp. 8–9.
3 Allan Nevins, *The Emergence of Modern America, 1865–1878, Volume VIII of A History of American Life in Twelve Volumes* (New York: Macmillan, 1927), pp. 342–343.
4 *Round Table*, II:3116 (July 1864), p. 69.
5 *American Literary Gazette and Publishers' Circular*, III:7 (1 August 1864), p. 208.
6 *Atlantic Monthly*, XIV:LXXXIII (September 1864), pp. 387–388.

3

'LADY DOCTORS'

Jennie June

Source: Jennie June, 'Lady Doctors', in *Jennie Juneiana: Talks on Women's Topics* (Boston: Lee and Shepard, 1864), pp. 115–117.

WE saw, in a country paper, a paragraph to the effect that, in Chili, the Spaniards found as many eminent physicians of the *female* sex as of the *male*. And "so should it be, it seems to us," said the sapient editor. Possibly he might like it, but so should not we. Lady doctors! from such the Lord deliver us! The increase of deaths among women would be frightful. There is a natural viciousness among women towards each other which is totally incompatible with strict justice, and especially mercy. They would purge, and blister, and drug, without feeling the first softening influence from the milk of human kindness within their breasts. Hard and stony, they would have no sympathy with nervous headaches, general debility, incapacity for exertion, or complete prostration. Who would want to detail one's pet weaknesses to the rigid figure, with harsh and uncompromising aspect, who, dark and grim, takes a little hand between her bony fingers, and feels the pulse as if she was trying to discover the juice in an ancient lemon? Or, to a fancy professional, in janty hat and feather, and balmoral boots, who would sit twirling her dainty cane, and, while making a pretence of listening to your aches and pains, privately reflect on the tender squeeze of the hand received from the last male patient, and wonder if it was prompted by gratitude for her services or in admiration for herself. No, no; lady doctors might answer for the masculine half of the community, and, no doubt, they would consider them vastly agreeable, but if it did not keep six men on the sick list where there is at present one, we confess to being much mistaken; and any woman who owned an individual in such a case, would possess an unusual degree of confidence who neglected to be present at all professional interviews, or who acceded personally to any request to procure unheard-of medicines from distant points, even although urged to "prevent mistakes."

Women are nearly all treacherous and cruel to each other. In a boarding-house, it is for the men they save dainty little dishes, or keep hot the tender steak or cutlet; and in stores it is the man who receives polite attention from saleswomen, while women, who comprise at least two thirds of the patrons of such establishments,

DOI: 10.4324/9781003265238-3

are frequently compelled to submit to impertinence and neglect. Lady doctors might do in other countries, where women are under greater restrictions, and compelled by necessity to undergo a business training; but here, where they rely for their bread and butter upon any body to whom they can attach a claim, and are accustomed to indulge in whims and caprices to any extent, the whole and sole limit being their inclination and prejudices, – a graduating class of intelligent young kittens or old cats would be just as serviceable to the community in the shape of doctors.

Editorial Headnote

Thomas Markby, *Medical Women* (London: Harrison, 1869)

The Reverend Thomas Markby (1824–1870) was a writer, educator, editor of Francis Bacon's *Essays* and *Advancement of Learning*, and headmaster. Most importantly, for nineteenth-century developments in the education of women and the proto-university extension movement, he was Secretary of and examiner for the University of Cambridge Syndicate for Local Examinations (established in 1858) from 1866 until his untimely death at the age of 46 four years later.[1] Such a position gave him an insight into the benefits of women's capacity and enthusiasm for learning. He was a regular contributor on educational issues to the *Contemporary Review* in the 1860s, debating burning topics such as joint education; something he believed useful in rudimentary years, injurious to both sexes in teenage years, and beneficial at tertiary level. This was later posthumously excerpted in James Orton's edited transatlantic volume, *The Liberal Education of Women: The Demand and the Method; Current Thoughts in England and America* (1873). In other *Contemporary Review* articles, Markby extolled the advantages of the local examination system, which enabled students to select their own subjects, as well as since 1865 the granting of girls under eighteen access to the examinations; a process in which he had been heavily involved. Towards the end of his life, the cause of women's education dominated his publications, and he supported the extension of the local examination system to a more advanced stage, signing both petitions sent to the Vice Chancellor of Cambridge in the spring of 1868 recommending the opening of assessment to the over eighteens and to women teachers. Also, in 1868 he published *Practical Essays on Education*, a book-length compilation of articles from the *Contemporary Review*. The *Pall Mall Gazette* found Markby an intensely 'Cambridge' man, knowledgeable, but caught up in the precise and practical workings of his own university's systems.[2] Although approving of female education from his own experiences in Cambridge, Markby took a decidedly suspicious view of women's rights' advocates, part of his disdain for those who were not experts in their chosen political or educational field. While Markby supported women's right to an education, ultimately, for him, their vocation was and should be wifedom and motherhood. As with many other supporters of women's rights in this period, Markby's ideas were founded upon a desire to help women become sufficiently educated to fulfil their natural roles.

Unsurprisingly, medical periodicals were not impressed with Markby's ideas, and the *Lancet* attacked his hostile attitude to the profession's support of the Contagious Diseases Acts, but ignored his views on women doctors.[3] The *Medical Times and Gazette* reviewed *Medical Women* in an editorial of August 1869, fearing its 'womanish tone', adopted by 'a Cambridge clergyman, an active promoter of better education for women, who once was considered a man of sense'. With this new publication, claimed the *Gazette*, Markby talked and argued after the fashion of those who mixed far too closely with women's affairs: an example of the 'ambition of the androgynous'. The reviewer despaired at 'see-saw arguments' and hysterical, incoherent contradictoriness about co-education, rightful patients, and the inherent badness of unfeeling medical men. Ultimately, claimed the *Gazette*, and turning his own bugbears back against him, Markby was as guilty of 'writing on a subject about which he knows nothing about', as those who wrote without experience about education.[4]

Markby's *Medical Women* received surprisingly little critical attention otherwise. This can be explained perhaps by his death so soon after publication, but also its timing. In 1872, two years after the death of Markby, a more famous work with the same title by Sophia Jex-Blake was published. The second *Medical Women* has overshadowed the original thanks to Jex-Blake's contemporary notoriety and later key role as medical woman and co-founder of the London School of Medicine for Women. Jex-Blake did, however, cite Markby's original, albeit in a footnote, to illustrate the 'profound purity of science'. The art of healing, the acquisition of medical knowledge, was acceptable to audiences of both sexes, she insisted, using Markby's words, and would indeed forcefully confirm rather than belie innate goodness.[5]

Notes

1 S. Raban (ed.), *Examining the World: A History of the University of Cambridge Local Examinations Syndicate* (Cambridge: Cambridge University Press, 2008), p. 17.
2 'Practical Essays on Education', *Pall Mall Gazette*, 1095 (14 August 1868), pp. 9–10.
3 *Lancet*, 95:2422 (29 January 1870), pp. 163–167.
4 *Medical Times and Gazette*, II (14 August 1869), pp. 191–192.
5 S. Jex-Blake, *Medical Women: Two Essays* (Edinburgh: William Oliphant & Co., and London: Hamilton, Adams, & Co., 1872), n. 1, p. 131.

4

MEDICAL WOMEN

Thomas Markby

Source: Thomas Markby, *Medical Women* (London: Harrison, 1869).

MEDICAL WOMEN.

More than one attempt has been made of late by earnest women to obtain admission into the medical profession. I believe that in the United States of America several ladies are already practising as physicians, with what success I am not able to say. In England, one lady, Miss Garrett, has found a door open to her, and is exercising her art with distinguished usefulness to her sex, and with no less honour and, as I trust, profit to herself. To many minds this may appear – I confess it does to my own – to settle the question of the admission of women into the ranks of medical practitioners. If one woman can usefully exercise the healing art, there can be no conceivable reason why thousands should not follow her example. More than that, there are so many cases requiring medical help which seem specially to call for the attendance and advice of women, that one is fain to wonder, not that they demand permission to learn and practise medicine, but that they should not have been long ago invited to do so. In the sufferings of women and children there is much which seems to a layman's eyes fitter for feminine than masculine minds to deal with. In childbirth, above all, I can understand the presence of any man, except her husband, being at once odious and mischievous to the labouring woman: odious because it is one of those bodily functions which her nature teaches her to keep as far as she may out of the sight of men, and hence mischievous, because her muscles answer to her instincts, and, revolting from the presence and touch of man, refuse that easy play and ready action which is best calculated to shorten her pangs and save the life both of herself and her infant.* At the same time I fully admit that it is possible, I may even go so far as to say commendable, for a woman to avail herself of the advice and skill of a man under any suffering her nature may impose upon her. She may argue with equal truth and modesty that in times of sorrow and pain sex is forgotten; that she meets the leech who helps and heals her on the ground of common humanity; that she sees in him nothing but a kind and health-giving hand, busy in a work which stands

DOI: 10.4324/9781003265238-4

next to the ministry of the Gospel in Christian dignity. And it would be a wicked injustice to omit full acknowledgment of the merits of the medical profession in this department of their duty. Nothing is rarer than for a woman to find in the conduct or deportment of her attendant anything which can give pain to her mind. I believe that, as a matter of fact, any fault in that direction is almost without example. I think I can assert – and my means of knowing the state of the case have not been inconsiderable – that women would with one voice bear testimony to the desire shown by the great body of medical men to be regarded by them in the light of God's ministers, sent to their bedsides on errands of humanity and mercy. Nor do I in this speak merely of the heads of the profession, or of married men of mature age. I have seen a little of one or two hospitals, and to the best of my belief there exists among the bulk of medical students a right and becoming sense of the gravity of their ministry. It is, therefore, far from my purpose to find fault with medical men in this matter. If by degrees practice has fallen almost exclusively into their hands in ailments wherein it would often be better for women to be attended by women, it is due to a silent and scarcely perceptible course of events over which they could by no possibility exercise control. For the existing state of things was brought about by no sudden change, made in obedience to the theories or discoveries of some leading teacher; it has come to pass simply and solely through the slow and irresistible influence of fashion. The only effectual means of stemming the tide available to the individual practitioner was to refuse to visit a woman asking his aid in her extremity. I should hope, and I honestly believe, that no medical man of respectability was ever known to do so. But what I do say is, that many women cannot bring their minds to receive the services of men with equanimity; that if they cannot do so, to force on them the choice between such services and unaided suffering is a cruelty; further, that it is a cruelty of that kind which it is a peculiar shame to men not to seek to relieve them from without an hour's delay. Every one understands how much in affairs of this kind depends on a woman's will. Many things, right and laudable with her free and intelligent consent, become in the absence of that consent cruel and wrong. I say that this is one of such things, and I desire to call the attention of my countrymen to it. If I am asked why I come forward, I reply that circumstances have, by a kind of accident, made me better acquainted than many of my contemporaries with the feelings and sorrows of women. Indeed, I say, frankly and unreservedly, that on this subject I am but a voice; but I say too, that I am in it the voice of much anguish; of how much let the following extract serve for a specimen: –

> "I hope you will, when opportunity offers, give to other men the impression I convey to you, for I wish men should know what women think; but it is a subject so hard to speak of, that women are mostly silent on it. This, however, I *must* say, that I think the compulsory attendance of men on women in special ailments is one of the bitterest and shamefullest cruelties which the stronger sex has ever practised on the weaker. We women dare not speak, but, O God, what we have suffered! God has endowed

> women with a peculiar sensitiveness, or sense of modesty, so acute that I think a man can scarcely understand it. That this sensitiveness, – these pure, fine, delicate feelings, which were part of our Creator's dower to us for wise purposes, – should be lacerated, torn, put to exquisite torture, and then, in many cases, at last deadened and killed – tell me, can this be agreeable to the will of God? I have known sweet young girls who pined away and died from the shock of such treatment. One, who had been put into a doctor's hands for special treatment, was cured physically, but her parents were so terrified for her mind, and she wept so constantly over the shame, that they had to take her about to travel abroad, and divert her in every way to try to obliterate the memory. Again, I knew a dear dignified lady who, in middle life, chose death rather than male attendance. She calmly said: – 'It is as well to die one way as another. The treatment I should have to undergo from a man would kill me through my mind.' There are (the writer continues) people who pretend that women do not feel as they do about it. Of course, every woman will try not to shew that she is wretched under it – *she will try to make herself into a stone*."

These are the strong words of a woman writing out of her agony. Few men, I trust, can read them unmoved. I do not see how any man can refuse to acknowledge that the burden rests with those who deny medical education to women, to shew cause for that denial. Nature, in accents that cannot be mistaken, emphatically demands a woman's care for a woman's suffering. Are men so bold as to contradict nature, and say she lies, or is a fool? Surely not. Assuming, therefore, as I am confident I may do without hesitation, that there is a great and growing cry for medical women from their own sex, I will at once proceed to address myself to the only two questions which appear to arise upon this assumption. These are, first, whether there are women willing and able to adopt medicine as a profession; second, whether opportunities of learning the art can be opened to them. I hope to be able to give an affirmative reply to both.

To the first, at any rate, women have themselves replied by acclamation. I suppose there is scarcely a medical school in England, France, Germany, or the United States, to which women have not in the course of the past ten or twelve years either directly applied for admission, or inquired through friends whether, if asked for, it was likely to be granted. The difficulties Miss Garrett encountered, and the self-denying perseverance by which she overcame them, are well known to the world. Miss Sophia Jex Blake is earnestly striving to overcome similar obstacles, with what alternations of success and disappointment – a disappointment fraught with dark omen of the hard measure the rising generation of young men are likely to mete out to women – is equally notorious. Nor do I think any one is likely to deny that these ladies may fairly be regarded in the light of representatives of a large number of their sisters. Miss Jex Blake says: – "Several of the American Medical Schools for men have at different times granted degrees to women, and there are now established special colleges for that purpose. I have already stated that the President of the Washington University in St. Louis maintained the views that I have just advocated, he having professed to me his readiness to examine and grant a degree to any woman, who by private study had duly qualified herself to receive it. The University of Göttingen some years ago conferred the degree of Doctor of Philosophy on a female student, afterwards Frau Doctor Rodda, and two ladies have recently studied Medicine at the University of Zurich. I believe, indeed, that many more instances might be adduced, had any one the inclination and the leisure to collect them; but these will probably suffice at least to show the direction in which the tide is already setting." (*Visit to some American Schools and Colleges*, p. 249.)

Nor, if what Miss Blake further says be well founded, can the opposition to the admission of ladies into the ranks of medical practitioners be very formidable. She writes: – "If women care enough for learning to conquer all difficulties in its pursuit, and simply ask that, when successful, their success shall be acknowledged, do national universities fulfil their trust in refusing the petition? That the time is coming when they will openly acknowledge such a position to be untenable, is made hopefully apparent by the fact, that the University of London recently refused, *by the Chairman's casting vote only*, a woman's petition for a medical degree." – *Ibid*, p. 248.

If this be really the case, and I suppose, although Miss Blake does not give the date or other particulars of the meeting referred to, she must have taken care to assure herself of the correctness of her statement, the opening of the medical profession to women cannot be far off. For the Senate of the University of London contains a very large number of physicians and surgeons; indeed, if I am not mistaken (I have not a copy of the London University Calendar at hand), a large majority of its members are one or the other. Many of the voters, therefore, on this occasion must have been medical men. I suppose they can scarcely have been all arranged on the one side and an equal number of laymen on the other. Some, therefore, must have voted for, some against, the admission of women to their school. One would be glad to know the reasons which weighed with the latter. Let me say frankly that I do not believe they were mercenary. I do not say that there are no greedy doctors – so long as human nature is corrupt, that will be impossible. But if the books of the profession in general could be laid open to the world, I believe nothing would surprise people more than the large proportion of their work which is done for little or even nothing. Every one knows that the most eminent physicians and surgeons in London – men, every moment of whose time is money – constantly reduce their fees, or even remit them altogether, in favour of needy patients. So among their less fortunate brethren; many a country doctor rides hundreds, aye thousands of miles, visiting poor patients, for attendance on whom he gets hardly enough to pay for the keep of his horse, much less himself. Indeed, so exemplary is the charity of the profession in this particular, that if it did enter into a voter's mind that midwifery constituted a lucrative part of his practice, he could scarcely be blamed. The right answer to the argument of loss to practitioners, already ill paid, seems to be, that in the long run the profession would not suffer. That it is not rapidly increasing in numbers is easily shewn. It is enough to print the following returns: –

1851.– Males of all Ages.	
Physicians	1,771
Surgeons.	13,470
Other *Medical Men* ..	3,949
	19,190

1861.– Males of all Ages.	
Physicians	2,385
Surgeons, Apothecaries.	12,030
Medical Students, Assistants	3,566
Dentists	1,567
	19,548†

That is to say, that while the population has multiplied at the rate, I suppose, of something like 1 in 5, the medical profession has scarcely advanced at all. Medicine herein is only partaking of the lot that has fallen to other professions. Men will not encounter the certainty of hard work and the possibility of starvation, when trade and emigration with open arms invite them to come in and find a certainty of abundance. Will any man try to stop this process? He might as well set to work to sew the Eildon Hills together again. In the ministry of the Gospel, bishops are learning to meet a great and growing diminution in the numbers of the clergy by ordaining lay-agents and deaconesses: doubtless, a mere return to the will of their Master. So it will be with the heads of the medical profession. They must before long become alive to the fact that, while the work increases with the population, the number of hands to do it is nearly stationary. Now, in trade it might be said, increase your charges. But this the doctor in a poor district cannot do. As the population in his neighbourhood multiplies, so do the calls on his time multiply, while his purse is but slightly swelled by a number of small fees, which scarcely pay the actual cost of drugs and the means of conveyance from place to place. Even in wealthy districts he is not able to defend himself so strongly as might be supposed. For competition naturally flows towards rich neighbourhoods, and young men, eager for practice, are not always over scrupulous about popularity hunting. On the other hand, a man can seldom reckon on being supported by his patients against a pushing rival. For little as it is to their credit, the plain truth is, that the last person the richest people will pay is the doctor. No charges are more haggled over and grumbled at than his. On the whole, I honestly believe that the profession in general might turn over a large part of their present duties into other hands without ultimate loss, and that their average incomes would be better than at present, because the diminution in receipts would be more than counterbalanced by the diminution in numbers and in labour of recipients. No one, I apprehend, will deny that women can be fairly remunerated at less cost than men. Now, I do not pretend to anything like a scientific knowledge of political economy, but surely unaided common sense cannot be wrong in coming to the conclusion, that to employ the more costly labour, where less costly would answer the purpose, is bad for all parties. Take nursing: I suppose no one would maintain that to employ men instead of women as nurses would be good economy. Carry the rule then a little farther, and if there be other departments of the healing art which may safely be entrusted to women, hand them over accordingly. As far as money is concerned, I cannot but think the result would simply be, that there would be fewer men in the profession, each doing less work and each getting better paid for it. The only class who would really suffer would be that of *ladies' doctors*, as they are called. These the changes proposed would probably exterminate, and, I cannot help adding, a good thing too. I confess I have not a grain of faith in these specialties. A man devoting himself to a single and limited branch of any profession – medicine perhaps more than any other – is apt to become narrow and morbid in his views. In particular, he is almost sure to get a sort of trick of referring every affection to those causes which have chiefly occupied his attention. I think I am not wrong in stating that young men of the highest ability and promise, when beginning to rise into large practice as physicians or surgeons, strive hard to avoid being consulted on one class of maladies alone, and that they do so on this very ground.‡ I confess that if I had any sufferer akin to me, whose case required further aid than that a lady like Miss Garrett could give, I should be far more willing to take her to a physician or surgeon in general practice, than to a ladies' doctor, if only on the ground of probably superior skill and better success in treatment. But to return. I put out of view mercenary motives, which I repeat I do not lay to the door of the profession, and inquire what are likely to have been the grounds of opposition. One, and that a main one, probably was a fear lest if women were admitted they would trespass on the proper domain of men. I fear if I were to say that men have trespassed on the domain of women in medicine, and that they ought therefore not to complain if the sex retaliate upon them, I should fail to disarm the adversaries. Nor, indeed, did so shameful an argument possess the smallest weight with any mind, would I condescend to use it. I own at once, and without reserve, that for women to attend men might possibly introduce evils as great as those with which I am at present concerned. I do not see, however, the smallest reason to fear that, in this country at least, any woman would venture upon an unseemliness of this kind. What in the all but universal *bouleversement* of decency and nature which appears to prevail in Paris (not, I trust and believe, in France generally) just now, may come to pass there, I cannot tell, any more than I can tell what the defiant boldness of a section of American women may adventure; but assuredly, whatever we do or do not do in this matter will not affect either one or the other one iota, and not one word has been said by any English lady indicating the slightest tendency to a hankering in that direction. All the communications I have received agree in one point – in speaking only of being permitted to treat women and children. More than that does not appear so much as to pass before the minds of applicants. Besides, nothing can be easier than to prevent any possibility of further license. Let a clause be inserted in every diploma granted to a woman, forbidding her to attend any patients but women and girls, with boys under seven years of age. With this precaution I cannot help thinking it would be on the lowest grounds prudent for the medical profession to open their doors to women. For now that one or two have found their way in, that abundance more will climb over the wall after them, unless the door be opened pretty soon, I take to be as certain as that the sun shines in the sky.

A subordinate reason for objection, we may suppose to have been a doubt whether women would have the nerve to endure the sight of and contact with suffering, or the intellect to grasp a competent knowledge of medicine and surgery. The former inquiry I confess would never have occurred to my own mind, and I only mention it because I have heard it seriously adduced as an argument against medical women. I should have thought a larger proportion of women than of men able to train themselves to this kind of endurance. I take it that laymen, as a rule, are not only more unnerved by pain in their own persons – a fact I fancy no one will question – but by the sight of it in others, than women. I remember a young married lady standing by the side of a very eminent surgeon while he performed a troublesome and delicate operation on the foot of a youth staying in the same house with herself. She rendered him such assistance as was in her power, received his compliments on her courage, saw him to the door, and fainted. Now, what she did at the end I take it most men would have done at the beginning of the business, and that this is just the difference between the two sexes. A woman screws herself up to do what is wanted, and defers her feelings till afterwards; her brother is useless for the first few times, and by degrees gathers courage to see and deal with suffering with, not indifference but, unflinching nerve. However, such may not be the case, I have not experience sufficient to enable me to give an opinion on the question; but that women can be trained to all that can possibly be required of them, I cannot for a moment doubt. If in time of war a woman can spend days and nights in a military hospital – shrieks and groans of wounded men ever and anon ringing in her ear, pain and anguish such as eye never sees elsewhere, relieved only by death in the most awful forms, ever in her sight, and walk in the midst of all with a bearing so calm, so peaceful, so godlike, that her very shadow brings comfort to the sufferer: will any one persuade me that no woman will have nerve to help a sister through her travail, prolonged and painful as it may be – will have the strength of mind to console both the patient and herself

> "With thought, it must be, 'tis love's fruit, the end for which she lives,
> The mean to make herself new-born: what comforts will redound"?

I cast such doubts to the winds.

Of the peculiar fitness of women, provided they can acquire the requisite skill and knowledge of medicine, for dealing with the infirmities of their own sex and of children, I feel I need say nothing. That will probably be admitted on all hands. A reserved patient does what he can to defeat the doctor. Unless he has full faith in him, and tells him with perfect truth and frankness all he knows about himself, his chances of amendment are, to say the least, considerably lessened. Now it is tolerably certain that none but a woman can find her way to the recesses of a girl's heart. Take a maiden of seventeen or eighteen to consult a man, and rely upon it she will tell him no more than she can help. To shew again the wide extent of the reluctance, nay, the absolute refusal in many cases, of women to submit to the inquiry of men into the details of infirmities incidental to their sex, I will give an extract from a letter that has been put into my hands. It was written by one lady to another. She says: –

"I assure you, there is hardly a word in your letter which I could not most heartily re-echo. There are many things which, if I spoke the whole truth, I should have to put in darker colours than you do. Only scattered instances have come before you. I have seen them almost by hundreds, and know many things to be true which you can only think likely; as for instance, the amount of suffering that goes untreated when men-doctors are only available.

"But it seems to me that the peculiar hardship of our case is, that we cannot put before the public in plain words the facts which would make it quite unanswerable. We cannot say straight out, 'It is simply indecent that men should come into the absolute physical contact with women that is required in treating cases of uterine disease. It is monstrous to ask pure-minded girls to submit to what cannot but be to them a personal indignity of the most horrible kind.' That is the simple truth."

The writer in the same letter goes on to speak of a case that had come under her notice, of a girl "who, after undergoing one examination, felt the fancied shame too acutely to remain at home." I cite this expression to show that the lady from whose letter I quote is no bigot. She perfectly understands that the poor girl committed no sin, and need have felt no shame. She only feels, what I think every one will admit, that it is a matter in which a woman's will ought not to be forced. Within fair limits, old Sir Hildebrand was not far wrong in morals when he exclaimed, "It shall ne'er be said there was but one woman in Osbaldistone Hall, and she died for lack o' her will," If in such a matter as that with which we are dealing, by forcing a girl's will you make her miserable, I say you commit a cruelty; if you make her brazen, you do her a wrong. And unless she submits with the full and free consent of her will, one or the other result must follow. Admit women to treat women, and all these troubles and difficulties melt away. Concede that the feminine intellect is strong enough to acquire, and give it the opportunity of gaining, the requisite knowledge of medicine, and the whole grievance is removed. Even supposing that in some respects a woman's services would be inferior to a man's, she can claim some compensating advantages. Her delicacy of touch and quickness of perception would enable her often to detect symptoms which might escape a man. In dealing with infants, unable to make known their feelings by articulate speech, this seems to the unprofessional mind to open a way to singular usefulness. Let it be remembered, too, that all women ask is freedom of choice. They do not say, "Forbid men to attend us." What they say is, "Do not force us in our affliction to have recourse to men on pain of death if we refuse."

I do not anticipate that any one will seriously maintain that women are incapable of the mental effort required to learn the art of medicine. They have of late years "given their proofs," so to speak, in great abundance. Do not let me be misunderstood. I do not for a moment believe that women can rival men in powers of mind any more than in powers of body. Nor will any sensible woman be reluctant to confess, or disposed to complain, that it has pleased God to bestow on her endowments different from, or less than, those of her brother. She will doubtless feel that unless the difference between the minds of men and women were as great both in degree and kind as between their bodies, the intellectual intercourse of the sexes would lose all its zest. Either sex has its proper excellence, and neither reason to complain of God. But because you cannot accomplish the ascent of Mont Blanc, it does not follow that you cannot climb up the slopes of Snowdon. No more does it follow because women are not likely to be great poets, or to make grand discoveries in science, that no woman can be a poet at all, or enter into many of the secrets of nature. Granting that women are not likely to rival Hippocrates or Sydenham, I own I do believe that many, if they only had the chance of learning, would prove at least as sound practitioners as a good many men who have reaped both fame and profit in their time. The question arises, then, no doubt the most important and difficult one we encounter in the whole inquiry – How are they to be taught?

The establishment of separate Medical Colleges for the instruction of young women seems to me out of the question. Supposing even that, once set going, a number of female students could be got together sufficient to maintain them, where are competent lecturers to be found? A man may be a tolerably trustworthy practitioner without being in the least fit to become a teacher, and indeed ability to teach is by comparison so rare, that it is notorious that the existing Medical Schools find it no easy matter to keep up their staff of lecturers. Nor is it likely that a man, having lectured one class in his subject, will come and do his work over again for a fresh set of students who might just as well have been present before. No man could find either leisure or spirits for such a task. The only resource left seems to be that the two sexes should learn together. As this proposal may startle some minds, I will venture to state at length some of the arguments which may be adduced in favour of it, without confining myself altogether to the case of medicine.

When I first heard mixed schools, as they are called, proposed for this country, I felt as much opposed to them as any man could have done. But I own that in the course of the last two or three years my opinions have undergone a change. I am free to acknowledge both that such schools appear to open the way to solving some difficulties in providing for the education of both sexes, which seem otherwise almost insoluble, and that, with some limitations, the objections which presented themselves at first sight do on more ripe consideration crumble away. To begin with, one has to encounter the invincible logic of facts. I have on another occasion cited the example of Rivington School, Lancashire.[§] To this I may now add the case of a school at the opposite extremity of the kingdom. At Callington, in Cornwall, the exertions of the rector of the parish have succeeded in establishing a mixed school of the most useful character. It was examined this summer by one of the Fellows of Trinity College, Cambridge. This gentleman tells me that in his opinion the system works admirably. There was a famous race between a boy and a girl for the place of Captain of the School. The boy beat by a little. "The boys," he said, "seemed to him to have gained in delicacy by the admixture of sexes, and he could not discover that the girls were in any way coarsened by it." Indeed, he even thought that there was a higher standard of propriety among the girls than, if report speaks true, exists in most girls' schools. No one seemed to think it at all strange that boys and girls should sit at their lessons together. In short, the experiment was, in his judgment, entirely successful. Again, there is the example of National Schools. In great town parishes, it is often possible to separate boys and girls entirely. Their means, as well as the number of their scholars of either sex, enable them to have separate buildings and separate staffs of teachers. But this is far from being the case in many country places, where, although there is nominally a master for the boys and a mistress for the girls, they are obliged, in order to cope with the task before them, to mix their work a good deal. The folding-doors are often flung back in order that one may take the general superintendence of the school, while the other gives the eldest or the youngest scholars of both sexes some special lesson. Now it does not appear to be the opinion of the clergy, or of the general public, that the growth of National Schools has injured either the manners or morals of country parishes. There is one excellent point – one indeed that should never be lost sight of in this matter – in the management of National Schools: the boys are distinctly placed under the master; the girls under the mistress. Both, therefore, receive their chief training, whether in learning or discipline, from teachers of their own sex. I do not see, therefore, on the whole, why it should be said, as it is commonly said by the opponents of mixed schools, that they are too alien from our national habits and views to succeed. And after all, are they not simply a return to the order of nature? Nature has not ordained that one marriage shall produce none but boys, another none but girls, but makes most fruitful of both. Why should we not say that as boys and girls are brought up together in the family, so they may be brought up together in the school? It requires some much stronger argument than the accident of our present habits to prove that this will not do. Under the pressure of great difficulty, it is scarcely ever wrong to go to nature for guidance. We are, as a nation, unquestionably at this moment under a great difficulty in regard to the education of our youth. Use the means well and we have plenty for boys, but for girls above the rank of servants scarcely any. What is to be done? To my mind, it is not easy to show that it is unwise or immoral to have recourse to the order of nature and teach both under one roof. At the same time, I am very far from saying that there should be no limitations to the rule. Every one, I think, will grant that it is not desirable, if it can be avoided, to let women teach schools consisting exclusively of boys, or men of girls. Again, to say nothing of the different studies likely to be pursued by persons able to prolong their education beyond fifteen or sixteen years of age, the close quarters of school life are better avoided in the case of young men and women together, at all events while profligacy in the former is condoned as it at present is by society. But I cannot see what objection can be raised to the professorial teaching of Universities being addressed to audiences consisting of both men and women. At Cambridge, the lectures of many of the Professors have been, for many years past, indeed for anything I know from time immemorial, regularly attended by ladies. I have been accustomed from childhood to hear much of University affairs, and I never heard so much as a whisper of objection to the presence of women in the lecture rooms. Yet there must have been numberless occasions on which the professor was compelled to enter upon topics requiring quite as careful and delicate treatment as any that could occur in lectures on medicine. The truth is, there is no branch of moral or natural science that may not be kept pure, or made prurient, at the will of the expounder. If any one doubts this, let him see how some French writers have contrived to deal with botany. In treating of the purest and loveliest of all the natural sciences, they have contrived to suggest such filthy thoughts that their books are simply disgusting to every right-minded reader, man or woman. But surely this is not necessary. Secure purity of thought and propriety of expression, and there is nothing which may not in fit time and place be spoken of between men and women. Are wives ashamed of being seen to be with child? Does any mother shrink from speaking of the birth of the infant in her arms? Or was the plainspokenness of the Virgin Mary unmaidenly, when she said to the Angel, "*How shall this be, seeing I know not a man?*" I am bold enough to say that there is nothing in the art of healing which may not fitly be spoken of before an audience of both sexes, provided there be a generally good tone prevailing among them, and the lecturer be of a pure and manly spirit. Indeed, I will go farther and say that his example in treating subjects of the kind incidental to his work with equal purity and courage, will be far from the least valuable part of his teaching. It will bring home to the hearts of his hearers, with more force than any other argument, the truth that every creature, every ordinance of God, is good and pure. Probably the chief objections to the admission of women into the craft will lie in the dissecting-room. Without question the work that must there be done is at once most necessary and most revolting to the tiro. Equally without question, would it be unseemly to permit students of both sexes to frequent this room together. But there could be no difficulty in setting apart hours for the attendance of female students, or, should the school be a large one, a separate room. If a woman could not be found competent to undertake the office of demonstrator, it must be entrusted to a man of approved character and discretion. Soon, no doubt, there would be plenty of women competent to the task. But take it at the worst, let it be supposed that women can never be employed as demonstrators in anatomy to their own sex, is the teaching of anatomy by men to women comparable in unseemliness to what under the present system may happen, and probably does happen, daily? There is nothing to prevent a young practitioner of five-and-twenty conducting the most delicate examination upon the person of a living girl of eighteen. Yet this is thought decent, and a thing which the profession is not called upon to take steps to render unnecessary, or forbid altogether, while it is held intolerable that a woman should be in the same room with a man in the presence of a piece of earth – for after all a corpse is no more than a piece of earth. If this be not Pharisaism, I don't know the meaning of the word. Or is any one prepared to go so far as to say that anatomy is under all circumstances a study unfit for women? If so, I would reply by the inquiry, Can it be God's will that the secrets of the human frame should be made known to men and hidden from women? In point of fact, acquaintance with them is evidently of far more general importance to the latter than to the former. For men may, and very often do, go from birth to the grave without ever experiencing more than the most trifling disorders of any vital function. It is no exaggeration to say that, as a rule, the less a layman knows about his own body the better. Whereas every woman that lives – wife, mother, or maiden – is always exposed to infirmities that go to sap her very life.

I feel, however, I have said enough. I have gathered up as well as I can the reasons for the admission of women to the medical profession. If stronger ones can be produced against them, I am ready to be convinced. If, on the contrary, a door can be opened to women I shall rejoice, partly because it will be a relief to many who pine in secret and untold suffering, partly because it will open to the sex a new resource for earning bread. Upon this part of the subject I do not propose to dilate at any length. Every one knows that the order of nature is at present upset in this country, that women largely outnumber men; that this disproportion is greatest in what we may call the professional classes; and that consequently it is there that want of daily bread is most pressing among women. People say, "Why don't they become governesses?" The answer is, that it is impossible to find situations for so many as one hundred thousand governesses, while there are nearly three millions of women in the United Kingdom who have to support themselves by their own exertions. Of these it may be estimated that fully one-sixth are born in a rank of life which makes menial labour a trial almost worse than starvation. Even if it be argued that a woman always does right in earning honest bread, it may be replied, while we concede it, that it is hard she should be forced to sink in the social scale and live in the kitchen with footmen and housemaids, while her brother is under no such necessity. For while nothing is harder than for a single woman, well born and bred, but without means of her own, to maintain herself in the rank due to her birth, nothing is easier than for a single man to do so. Poor indeed he may be, but with fair industry and tolerably good health, a decent coat and sufficient food are always within reach. How far different the case is with women, let any man use his own opportunities of inquiring. If he does not feel that what he finds is a sin, and a shame to men, I can only say I am very sorry for him. Unhappily, the apathy with which men have too long regarded this state of things is already bringing a bitter curse on the country. That debauchery can ever be rooted out of the land I am not rash enough to hope, any more than to say that there are not women as well as men wilfully and determinedly dissolute. But I do say, that when there are thousands upon thousands of women who have to make the dreadful choice between want and the streets, it is time for men to look about them. It will not do to fold our hands and say that this is the natural fruit of civilization, or with worse than ostrich-like folly to seek to drive the plague out of sight with a policeman's truncheon. The first thing to be done is to treat women in a different spirit. Hitherto we have used them as children, kept them in pupillage and imposed upon them so many restrictions that if we bid them earn their own bread they may well retort upon us and say that, with Egyptian tyranny, we bid them eat while we take the meat from their mouths. Has not God given them talents to improve against the Great Day? Has He, at the same time, denied them discretion how to use them? I believe that if we opened to women every calling not distinctly unfeminine, we should be in the end, from every point of view, gainers. Take divinity. Of how much drawing-room theology we should get rid if women had the opportunities of study so freely open to men, and if their presence were regularly recognized in divinity lecture-rooms. Or, how are deaconesses to be fitted for their office if every means of learning how to discharge it remain closed to them? Christ, at all events, was not deterred from admitting women to His teaching by any fear lest they should intrude themselves upon duties unfitted for their sex. That they are not less eager now-a-days to know His doctrine than they were when He was on earth is clear to any one who does not shut his eyes. It is women who crowd the churches of popular preachers, women who are caught by ritualistic gewgaws and rush to the secret orgies of the confessional. They do it in innocence; the guilty are those who mislead them. To sum up all in a word, – Women throughout Europe are earnestly beseeching men to open to them the door of knowledge. Shall we reply by locking it in their faces and taking away the key? God in His mercy on the world forbid!

HARRISON AND SONS, PRINTERS IN ORDINARY TO HER MAJESTY, ST. MARTIN'S LANE.

Source Endnotes

* I cannot say how long it has been customary for childing women to call in the help of the doctor. I have been told, I know not with what truth, that the fashion was set by one of Louis XV's mistresses. The word *midwife* of course shows that it must have been unknown to our ancestors; yet there is no reason to think that childbirth was more destructive of life in their day than in our own. Indeed, as midwives now-a-days practise almost exclusively among the poor, and it is notorious that poor women get through their hour of trial more easily than their wealthier sisters, the balance of safety seems to incline to them. Medical men always say that in difficult cases women are useless. But it is probable that the number of such cases is more than met by the number of those which are rendered dangerous by the presence of a man.

† *Census,* 1851 – *Table* xxv. iii. 3. 1861 – xix. iii. 3. *Summary of Population Tables, Ages, Civil Conditions and Occupations of the People in England and Wales.*

‡ It will be observed, that to decline to meddle with cases with which a man feels his ordinary course of practice has unfitted him to deal, is another thing. Thus, for example, I have known able surgeons refuse to touch the eye, on the ground that operations requiring much physical strength and involving comparatively rough work, destroy the subtlety of finger necessary for operating on so delicate an organ.

§ *Practical Essays on Education,* p. 293.

Editorial Headnote

A Woman Physician and Surgeon [Mary Edwards Walker], *Unmasked, or The Science of Immorality. To Gentlemen* (Philadelphia: Wm. H. Boyd, 1878)

Mary Edwards Walker (1832–1919), known more familiarly to contemporaries as Dr Mary Walker, was born in Oswego, New York, into a family that encouraged progressive ideas, and formed Walker's lifelong beliefs in women's rights and abolitionism. She was educated at Syracuse Medical College, graduated in 1855, and practised in Columbus, Ohio; later moving to Rome, New York. Here she began to wear male attire, which contrasted with a 'distinctly feminine, petite' appearance and a 'gentle' demeanour.[1] In 1862, Walker graduated in hydrotherapy from Hygeio-Therapeutic College, New York.

Walker's subsequent role as a surgeon in the Civil War has been debated for over a century and a half. After assisting with the wounded in Washington and with increasingly strengthening attempts to secure a proper commission, Walker was contracted as an assistant surgeon to the Union Army in 1864. She was taken prisoner in April that year, and sent from Georgia to Richmond, Virginia. Walker remained prisoner until August, when she was exchanged with a Confederate surgeon. Stints in Louisville, Kentucky at the Women's Prison and finally in Clarksville, Tennessee at the Refugee House concluded her army career, at her own request, in June 1865. Due to eye damage sustained while imprisoned, Walker was unable to practise surgery to the same extent as before. In November of that year she was awarded the Medal of Honor by the President, Andrew Johnson. She was the only woman ever to receive this recognition.[2]

Abashed by her achievements, the press was keen to disparage her medical skills. The *New York Medical Journal* published a letter from Roberts Bartholow, formerly assistant surgeon (Captain), who wrote about his experiences of this, as he put it, 'medical monstrosity' when she came to demand employment as a medical officer. She was deemed to have 'no more medical knowledge than any ordinary housewife'. Despite these considerable doubts, she was ordered to be sent to the front. Bartholow concluded that the War Office had hoodwinked the army medical staff to place Walker as a spy to be captured.[3] Contemporary reassessments of Walker's credentials have been kinder, with one recent journal focusing on her lifesaving, *avant garde* techniques of wound care through hygiene rather than amputation.[4]

The British struggled, bemusedly, with Walker when she visited the Social Science Congress in October 1866, and spoke on topics ranging from infanticide to women's rights, and her appearances were commented on in newspapers and periodicals from America to Australia. Reams of newspaper print covered her stay, fascinated by her opinions, but most intrigued by her attire. As *Punch* summed up, it 'would be incorrect to call Dr Mary Walker a physician in petticoats'.[5] By the last decade of the century, and the advent of the bicycle, the *Girl's Own Paper* could remark that the 'semi-masculine garb' of Dr Mary Walker would barely be noticed in current times, where women had innocently adapted their costumes to the machines they rode.[6] Although her experiments no longer shocked, it was fascinating how much they had entered social and cultural terminology in the last third of the nineteenth century. As the *Women's Penny Paper* put it succinctly in 1897, 'Dr Mary Walker's name was a bye-word when most of us were children'.[7] What was most interesting, however, was that Walker's behaviour encouraged the British press to consider her alongside their own new and would-be-medical women, as the introduction to this volume discussed.

Despite, and perhaps because of the extent of her lecturing from the mid-1860s onwards, *Unmasked* was only Walker's second full-length work after the volume of essays, *Hit*, appeared in 1871, discussing issues dear to Walker's heart such as dress reform, tobacco, temperance, and the franchise. *Unmasked* was published on the first day of 1878, and was frank in its graphic depictions of sexual intercourse and its potential consequences for women. Produced anonymously, but with the sex and occupation of the writer evident, Walker confirmed that she was the author whenever she appeared in public. Despite threats to take the work out of circulation, mainly by the police, it remained in print and even reached a second edition.[8]

As a consequence of her sartorial choices and her Civil War experience, Walker was one of the more contemporarily notorious medical women who caught the eye of the popular press in the nineteenth and early twentieth centuries, and continues to do so today. She was recently chosen as one of Hillary Rodham Clinton and Chelsea Clinton's studies of inspirational 'Healers', alongside Elizabeth Blackwell (see this volume) and Rebecca Lee Crumpler (see Volume III), for example, in *The Book of Gutsy Women: Favorite Stories of Courage and Resilience* (2019).

Notes

1 K.C. Hurd-Mead, M.D., *Medical Women of America: A Short History of the Pioneer Medical Women of America and a Few of Their Colleagues in England* (New York: Froben Press, 1933), p. 66.

2 J. Bellafaire and M. Herrera Graf, *Women Doctors in War* (College Station, TX: Texas A&M University Press, 2009), pp. 7–21.

3 Bartholow letter reproduced in 'Article IX: Dr Mary Walker', *American Journal of Dental Science*, 1:4 (August 1867), pp. 201–203; on p. 202.

4 K.M. Klifto, A. Quan, and L. Dellon, 'Mary Edwards Walker (1832–1919): Approach to limb salvage therapy', *Wound Repair and Regeneration*, 27 (2019), pp. 285–287.

5 'A Plea for Pantaloons', *Punch*, LI (22 December 1866), p. 9.

6 Dora de Blaquière, 'The Dress for Bicycling', *Girl's Own Paper*, XVII:823 (5 October 1895), pp. 12–14; on p. 13.

7 'Current News', *Women's Penny Paper*, VII:165 (25 February 1897), p. 12.

8 S.M. Harris, *Dr Mary Walker: An American Radical, 1832–1919* (New Brunswick, NJ: Rutgers University Press, 2009), pp. 161–162; p. 182.

5

UNMASKED, OR THE SCIENCE OF IMMORALITY, TO GENTLEMEN BY A WOMAN PHYSICIAN AND SURGEON

[Mary Edwards Walker]

Source: A Woman Physician and Surgeon [Mary Edwards Walker], *Unmasked, or The Science of Immorality. To Gentlemen* (Philadelphia: Wm. H. Boyd, 1878).

CHAPTER I.

Introduction.

A number of "private treatises" have been written "to women exclusively," by men physicians. This was before women were regular M.D's., or before any woman had many years' practice in the profession.

If women generally can be benefited by such books, it is but fair to suppose that men generally may be benefited by women physicians writing "private treatises" to men, embodying advice, facts, observations, discoveries, etc., that are all important for men to learn in a pure way as matters of science, instead of acquiring with the most degraded ideas of life, and only such parts as are demoralizing and filled with the grossest errors.

It is very evident that the great need of light among men has not been properly met by men; no man has elaborated on important points in the direction that is most vital, and hence it becomes the duty of whomsoever can peer into the darkness with a light, to do so with all speed, even if such light be no larger than a glow-worm, it may be the humble means of guiding many a weary one into a lost path, and of preventing myriads from losing the path of rectitude who are now approaching manhood, to say nothing about those in the great future, whose need for light shall be as great as those now traveling in the bewildering paths of existence.

Knowledge must ever be the basic principle upon which the purest morals are founded. It is upon this corner stone of life's monumental building that grand towers of soul reach the zenith of human excellence in middle age, and are crowned with the beautiful verdure of ripe years' real worth.

With all the strides that have been made in art and science for the past one hundred years, the philanthropist must view with the deepest sorrow that but little progress has been made in morals, so little, that the men who even make *pretensions* to purity of manhood are conspicuously few. The majority of men have no high moral standard, but without shame assert that they are as good as any other men, and carry the idea, that, as they have become self-complacent, women ought to be satisfied with whatever standard of morals men choose to be reconciled to for themselves.

Men would be amazed if women should assert that such a standard was a low one and did not correspond with a true woman's ideas of noble manhood, and that it was just as good a standard for woman's *morale* as it is for men's, (a position that is just as fair for women to take as for men, as any one with logic must admit.)

Women feel this inequality most poignantly, and deplore the low position taken by men, as few men can ever understand. Woman's silence upon the subject mislead men into the idea that they are indifferent to man's morals. Men never hear the eloquent speeches of women of all ages when this subject is discussed in the homes of all grades of women, and the despair that settles over their faces as the want of pure manhood is felt by them with no hope of ever having the general ideas of men any better, and women being compelled to marry *such* men if they ever marry at all. While men are so ignorant of the real aspirations of women they will continue to wrong them.

Men assume a right to have all relationships with women outside of marriage because they are *men*, and then assume the right to desert such women as beneath their contempt, and illogically reasoning both ways, assert that such women were not equals with them, because they yielded when unable either mentally or physically or financially to resist them.

Every art, often not at all understood by woman, is used to entrap her into such relationship when she does not fully understand the strength of her own passions and certainly not of men's, and she is placed in a position where she cannot possibly be forewarned; if not forewarned in a manner to make her disrespect all manhood, in a word, to be constantly on the alert believing every man a seducer. If he is not such, it is not for want of encouragement from the great masses of men in the following way: The arts and traps of seduction are talked over by men before boys, and so the youths grow up in the belief that there is something smart in taking advantage of women, and that it is the most telling evidence of manhood possible. Brought up in such a school it is more a misfortune than a fault that men as a mass have so little moral conscience, for there is little or no direct influence to counteract such schooling, and the lessons in defective conscience and low ebb of soul are so often given, that the most poisonous and deleterious stuff becomes a part of the man.

It is true that pernicious teachings are graded to some extent among men and boys in the different classes of society, but the same ideas of their immoral rights that men believe to be their prerogatives as *men*, that all other men are called upon to respect *as* rights and women to tolerate, are the bases of jokes, good-natured slanders and pleasantry.

Men tacitly acknowledge each other's right to their own code of morals, and an exclusive right to their own victims is asserted with threats, fists and bullets. Such decisions of the rights of weak-moraled men to weak-minded women are heralded almost every day.

The thieves of woman's self respect have wide ranges of "codes of honor." Such men call those who live better lives than themselves, fools, and those who live worse ones, brutes, which is an insult to the brute creation, since no animal can be found that is as bad as some men.

The masses of men do not believe that one man ever lived, except Christ, who did not exercise what he deemed "manhood rights in degrading some woman," and there are men who even doubt Christ's pure life in this regard.

There are many restraining influences with men, but the greatest is fear, without which the exercise of the basest passions (or rather the violation of the natural laws) would be so great that the race would soon become extinct. But the "fear" is not concerning the results on the soul or body of their victims, but that their own bodies may suffer from some law that shall be enforced in the shape of disease, or of some human law that is administered by individuals in the shape of cold lead globes, or sharp pointed steel if not in prison cells, or in hemp circles.

Where no common law prevails, men treat women as though they had not a single right of existence, and but for their living, adding to men's sexual gratification, they would not be allowed to live at all.

Where common law does prevail, women are constantly writhing under the inequality of law as regards sex, and men are so annoyed that to have peace, more and more just laws are enacted by them. Laws are made by men who have not a remote idea of living up to them, believing themselves clever enough to infringe them without publicity, and thus pass for much better men than they really are, while the selfish making of protection laws is for the double purpose of protecting their victims for their own use, whether such women be wives or mistresses.

And yet men have failed to enact laws of this character that are sufficiently potential to do away with the necessity for individual administration of bullet or knife law. A certain class of men are restrained by nothing less potent than this kind of law, and but for such law being occasionally administered by the relatives of women or by the victimized women themselves, there would be much more of iniquity than there is at present, although one is almost led to exclaim, how can the world be *much* worse than it is?

There is a fearful moral confusion that certainly appalls one who looks upon every grade of society as it really is.

While every man has his code of honor in relation to women, nearly all of these codes can be summed up in the following list.

1. The code of a pure life, where no sexual wrongs to himself or to a woman have ever existed, but where every woman is treated with the same deference as though she was his honored mother or sister, where his wife is treated with all the acknowledged rights as though she were physically stronger than himself, and perfectly independent of him in all regards.

That there are so few with this code, is why there is so much of contention, strife, rapes, seductions and murders. There can be none of these evils where men live up to the noble standard of true manhood.

2. The code of "sowing wild oats" and then marrying a pure girl and settling down, and priding himself on being one of the very best of men, never once dreaming that there can be any better specimens of manhood, or thinking that he has any obligations to that pure girl, in keeping himself pure for her, as she has been keeping herself for him.

3. The code of living life No. 2, being equally careful not to have any slanders in the shape of illegitimate children, and like No. 2, boasting that they "never visited a public woman, or seduced a girl." – But all through life having relationship sexual with so-called respectable women, married and single. Sometimes men with this code marry and sometimes do not, but always living the same life, making their marriage a convenience, if they ever do conclude to marry, and with their associates talk jocosely over the convenience of having a wife, when there are reasons why it is not policy or pleasure to go elsewhere. They use every art to keep their wives in the belief of their faithfulness to them, and laugh at the idea of a jealous thought in them, or frown and become angry at such a suspicion.

4. The code of this class is to visit reputable houses, talk up marriage, court several different girls, (taking precaution to have them in different places, or in different circles of society,) seduce under promise of marriage through force or fear, help them out of *enceinte* condition, carry on the game until he wearies of his victim, or she finding he will not marry discards him. Those of this class boast that they are "as good as any men" among their chums. They boast of their conquests and get rid of some of their victims by getting some other fellow to play the same game and then twit the girl with unfaithfulness to them as a cause for desertion.

5. The code of this class is to visit disreputable houses, make bargains and sales, and would despise seducing girls, or invading other men's families – pure sexual gratification is the one idea, and the quality is little to be considered. More married men than single ones patronize such houses. We shall give the reasons therefor hereafter

This class treat respectful women with much more deference than the seducers who boast of never going to a bad house.

6. The code of this class is to be constantly on the alert for victims, and their thirst for variety leads them into the most dishonorable means to accomplish ends. Rapes are committed by them and even small girls are victims.

CHAPTER II.

Equality.

If men would only reason, they would very soon understand that the true position of women is always one of equality with themselves in all the relations of life. This is true, taken not only from the most just, humane and noble standpoints, but from the most interested and selfish ones, for not only are the children stronger, healthier, more intellectual and less irritable, having a stronger hold on life, but from the merest *sensual* motives, this is true: where the wife is simply a grown up governed child, always more or less under the dominant will of the husband, she can never give the strength and satisfaction to the husband in the sexual relation that she would if an individualized woman, with all the distinct magnetic power that only such women can impart.

The more of selfhood a woman possesses, the greater the ability to concentrate all of nerve power in the relation which she willingly engages in for reproduction in a pure monogamic love that is not robbed of the fineness of the relation by the degredation of partial or complete compulsion. While such a relation is not *love*, there must be love with it, or it is an injury to both parties in the transaction; with love and respect there comes a peaceful satisfied condition of both body and mind. Excess, however, brings irritability and unrest. This would be avoided by sleeping separately. Much of the disgust that at times is so unbearable would be avoided if the matters of making and un-making toilets were done in separate rooms. Few people are so bound together in soul that there is not an ill-concealed disgust for private toilet matters, and even the ordinary arrangement of the clothes.

However pleased with the person when clothed, the dressing and undressing transition, after a little time, becomes an endured unpleasantness.

Several cases have come to our knowledge where women could not void fluids when their husbands were in the room, no matter how dark the night or how long they had been married. Women have suffered much, and made an effort to do so for an hour at a time, and although in severe pain because of the necessity, it was impossible to be relieved until they were entirely alone.

Men have had to partially dress and stand outside of their own rooms in hotels, before their wives were not able to get relief.

Children are often severely punished for not attending to the calls of nature before retiring, and invariably doing so as soon as put to bed and left alone. If they were tied in their toilet chairs and left alone for a few minutes the result would be accomplished.

This is a peculiar condition of the system that few grown people understand. They can understand their failure to respond to the calls of nature, when they enter a closet that is so disgusting that the inclination of nature immediately leaves them.

Fistulas often result where a person so disgusted is placed where there is no alternative but to visit such a closet. Every house however small in towns and cities ought to have closet plumbing where water flows abundantly, so that the calls of nature would not be so dreaded and postponed.

It is found that constipated bowels caused by postponement of the calls of nature so irritates the organs of sex, that much of immorality is the result. There must be an equality of rights of the organs of the human system. If one is free to eat and drink, there must also be freedom to evacuate the solids and fluids in order to have peace in the system.

All should know the evils of exciting influences on the organs of reproduction, and both boys and girls should be equal in such knowledge.

Men as well as women suffer from inequality of knowledge as well as of rights and privileges in the various relations of life. Men who deny any rights to women on account of their superior physical strength, sooner or later have their own rights as men interfered with, because the sentiment of tyranny is ever encroaching more and more; it is not safe to deny any one rights that belong to all.

In the middle ages men were mutilated (castrated) so that they could sing like women in their choirs. They would not admit the women in the choirs at all, and the great injustice to women was visited upon the sons of men, because they must have the voices of women and could not get them without mutilating men when they would not acknowledge woman's right to sing.

Mutilated men are devoid of fine sensibilities, and are harsh and unfeeling and even cruel.

These cruel men were, and are to this day, the guardians of the women of the Harems. They accompany them whenever they are allowed to go out, and hold them under constant surveillance. Women herded in this way bear children that are tyrants from birth, being marked by those who tyrannized over them. Their failure to make advances in civilization, is owing to the manner in which the women are treated. But a few years will elapse before the men of this country will be able to see themselves reflected in the glass of as gross inconsistency as the men to whom we refer. Men may laugh at the idea of women singing in public, or even uncovering their faces being "out of woman's sphere, and out of the delicate proprieties of life, and making women unfit to be wives or even good enough to be called *women*," but let men remember, that it is only a piece of the same barbarism that allows men to be the dictators of women in *anything* that relates to existence.

Nothing less than perfect equality of rights will ever result in the greatest happiness, and the grandest possibilities.

Enlightened women look upon any interference with human rights of women, whether as regards a failure to pass a law to protect woman in her clearly expressed right of suffrage in the Constitution, or any human rights, as being as great a barbaric wrong, as men can possibly deem the mutilation wrongs of men. They differ only in *degree* but not in kind, for both stab in the same direction. Both seek to be the masters of the special functions of sex.

A marked instance of oppression to women, resulting in cruelty to boys is apparent in the Turkish Harem, where boys from 10 to 15 years of age are kept in large numbers for licentious acts in the rectum, which results in agonized death from inflammation.

Enlightened countries are becoming more just to women, but still we are shocked with facts like the following that will soon be obsolete in England, as they are already in America, owing to the advance of public sentiment beyond the codes:

Not many years since an English court decided that a man might beat his wife with a stick not larger than his little finger, continuing to legalize this relic of barbarism.

If a woman was untrue to her husband in Athens, he could take away all her property, beat her, and sell her at auction, but he could do what *he* pleased.

Mohammed ordained that untrue wives should be buried alive, but afterwards decided that they should be stoned to death.

In Egypt an untrue wife's nose was cut off, while in Germany her hair was cut short.

In the Polynesian Islands the wives are not allowed to eat the same food as the husbands, or cook it at the same fire.

In China, the women have so many disadvantages that they are constantly praying that in the next world they may be men. Husband and wife may mutually agree to separate, but if the wife leaves without his consent, he may strangle her. Talkativeness, or a disregard of parents in law, are causes for a man's divorce.

All of these inequalities of sex have their penalties. But we have neither time or space to elaborate truths that need but a mention. It is because of the inequality of rights of sex, that so much of outrage is perpetrated by men of all ages. Rapes on little girls of but two or three years of age, are attempted by young men often giving them venereal disease. Boys from a dozen to eighteen years of age, are often found attempting to outrage little girls, and as boys commence so young to pursue the vices so well understood by the constant talk before them of men hardened in crime, no boy is too young to read this book, and his special attention should be called to the chapters on Pure Manhood, and the Language of the Nerves. Small boys should learn that vice so degrades the *boy* that the man is capable of outrages far worse than murders, and that by "slow degrees the tempter wins; then step by step they give up all," and become perfect demons; and as an illustration the following is related:

In the war with the Larmates, Emperor Proclus, in fifteen days, violated one hundred virgins who were his captives.

American men will violate their wives while menstruating, which even an American *Indian* is never guilty of doing. Perfect equality of men and women in all the relations of life would produce the best results to *men* as well as *women.*

CHAPTER III.

Pure Manhood.

We have searched books in vain for any description of a pure man. We expected that in works devoted exclusively to men, where the virginity of woman is so freely discussed, that the virgin man would have a descriptive mention, but in such books as in all others, we have failed to find any mention of the physical signs of manhood virginity. Such a neglect in works advocating either pure marriage or continence, is, to say the least, most remarkable. But a scientific and metaphysical writer cannot let the subject rest until investigation proves whether or not woman alone has signs of a virgin condition, whether such signs are not equally marked in man. It would not need much thought to conclude that any portion of the body put to new use would be likely to be changed in some measure, and particularly a portion of such importance as the procreating organs.

The signs of virginity in woman is a topic that all writers on private treatises, whether to men or women, always speak of and make a theme of the greatest importance in proving the chastity of women, as though man had any more right to expect to find a perfectly chaste wife, than woman had to find a chaste husband, and not until within a few years has the world been very well enlightened upon the subject, and learned that even in some marriages there has been only external copulation yet conception has taken place and a hymen as perfect as is ever found, seen by the attending obstetrician.

On the other hand, after marriage when perfect copulation has occurred many times, the entrance of the vagina has contracted so rigidly when the act was repeated, that more effort was required to complete copulation than at the first act after marriage. These facts learned from the most reliable persons, prove that the copulation signs of chastity in woman are not to be relied upon, and by so much stress having been placed upon such signs, much of wretchedness has resulted to men for want of confidence in their wives' chastity, that has been cruelly thurst into the wives' faces, who were powerless to explain the difference between a delicate little membrane at the entrance of the vagina called the hymen, that has been forced to yield so soon after marriage, that the relaxing moisture of the parts has not prepared it to yield without great effort and pain. In after conditions where the system of woman has received all of that kind of excitement that it can bear, the muscles of the vagina contract and refuse to receive more, although the woman may still desire to gratify her husband even if not at the time congenial to her. Most married men have had the hymen theory very much muddled by this after condition, at all periods in the lives of married women.

But very few men ever stop to consider their own inconsistency in demanding such purity from their wives, since, if they were themselves pure, they could not so readily doubt the chastity of women. It is strange that men can be so thoughtless as not to know that their own want of confidence in the maidenly purity of their wives, and their ability to judge of the same, would lead their wives to distrust them in their own youthful purity, for how can a young man judge of a *wife's* condition if he is not able to draw comparisons with a mistress.

Had not women studied the medical profession, and studied into this one-sided virtue business, the world might still have gone on without women ever knowing that the signs of man's virtue are *unmistakable*, although there are but few comparatively who are virtuous long enough to know themselves what are the sure signs of a virtuous man. We doubt not that by far the greater part of men in middle life and old age, believe that there are no signs of virtue in men, but that what *is* a sign, is *undeveloped* manhood, since they have not thought upon the subject enough to consider the time and cause of the physical change in the penis. Men make their wives believe "the power to make an erection and leave the franum praeputii of the penis all next to the scrotum, is simply an omen of perfect manhood that is developed with time, and gradually grows away from its attachments.

This is all false, but is a story generally told wives who are always contrasting the difference in the attachments of the cuticle on infants and the freedom from attachment of the same on their husbands, and hence the very natural question as to the *time* when the change takes place.

So firm and unyielding is the attachment, and so painful any attempt to free the same from near the head of the penis, that only under the greatest excitement, a number of times, will it tear away, and every time there will be some, more or less slight, blood discharged from the torn membranes.

Masturbation will not tear this away; sexual relations alone will do so, and when this unmistakable sign of man's virginity is generally understood, boys will, with proper training, make men that will honor manhood.

Young women who were not chaste have not dared to marry doctors, and the time has arrived when young men who are not chaste do not dare to marry doctors, for the same reasons that young women have had, and continue to have, and the time is not distant when young men will not dare to marry pure women anywhere, however young, for *all* women will be informed upon this subject.

A number of men living to be 30 years old and over, have married with unmistakable signs of having lived a perfectly pure life, and the harshness upon wedding nights that unchaste men have been guilty of, was impossible with them, because of the effects on their virginity not only, but that selfish reckless disregard of a wife, that unchaste men evince in the sexual relation is not known, but a tender regard is ever observable.

Where husband and wife are both virgins, the sexual relations on both sides will be moderate and mutual, and satisfactory, and soothing, for husband will not seek to gratify unreasonable desire, because he will not have such a desire. It will be weeks and perhaps months before the fullness of the relation is experienced by either, just as it is always some time before the fullness is reached by pure woman without regard to *whom* she has married.

Chaste women who marry unchaste men, are often three months in reaching and sometimes *never* reach a perfection of orgasm in sexual relation, owing to the fact of the husband having lost magnetic power by his unchastity, and thus unfitting himself to become a father for her children, by being unable to father the highest type of humanity that shall be superior to both parents which *should* result.

The loss of virginity in men, and the failure to live chaste lives is more a misfortune than a fault, as is often the case with women.

Men are, when mere boys, allowed to go into all sorts of chance company with little or no regard as to the moral character of the same, with no warnings as to results on soul, and seldom a word about the results on the body. Parents, mothers as well as fathers, think because the public places so low an estimate upon the morals of men, that they have few if any responsibilities regarding the morals of their sons. They cannot bear babies and bring disgrace upon them, and they have little or no organized thought about sons bringing disgrace into other people's families. Few people look away beyond disgrace, that is but the opinion of other people; they do not get a sight of the wrongs to their bodies that are not immediately perceptible. The masses of men reason but little on the most important subjects relating to social life. They are contented to know the arts relating to the attainment of passional aims, and the ordinary preventives of deleterious results; but they do not even learn the plain lessons taught constantly: what will spoil the horse will spoil the man. The variety and excess of the horse causes him to be excited beyond control at the sight of a mare, no matter of how inferior breed and how poor condition she may be in at the time. And so men lose by variety the nice sense of selection, and the power of control, and take any women they can that chances to be near, for like the horse, licentious thoughts are ever uppermost in their minds, and they conclude that there is not a woman in the world but that would pursue the same course as himself with her price paid. There are large numbers of men who cannot be made to believe that there is a single man or woman who live pure lives, because their own lives and their observations of others have led them to such a conclusion. One of the most common expressions from men when the subject of pure manhood is alluded to, is this: "Men are all about alike, some are more shrewd than others."

No man can ever tell how chilling such expressions and those of similar import are to pure women, who would love with a worshipful devotion the embodiment of pure manhood. But men cannot understand such chilling of the soul, until the best women make similar assertions about all other women – imagine such a condition ye good men, and see if, no matter what troubles you have braved like philosphers, see if, we repeat, you do not require all your brains to resist suicidal inclinations. Nothing else in life comes home to the soul with such crushing weight as the loss of confidence in sexual purity. Life seems to be robbed of the charm of all charms when the permanent friendship of uncompromising confidence has been destroyed. Only the skeleton of the individual is left. What was thought to be genuine substance proves to be but a fleeting shadow in sunshine, that is lost all together in twilight and darkness. For with a disregard of pure selfhood, saved and retained for the partner of life, there is loss of so much of fineness of soul and body, power of soul and body grandness, that it would take volumes to write out all the same in a complete manner. The horse cannot have sexual relations with a cross balky mare, a big-legged mare, one of inferior size, inferior breed, or of any description and *ever* recover from the magnetic effect. The parts having contact may be immediately washed after the relation, but there is no power to take from him the mare's impress left upon him that will be transmitted sooner or later to his posterity. So marked is this that some of the colts from the best breed of mares, sired by the best breed of horses, have partaken of the dispositions and looks of mares that held sexual relations with the horse months and even years before. The male takes upon himself these magnetisms to a wonderful extent, indeed they become as much a part of him as are his feet or any other part. So is it with men, and they take up these magnetisms and retain them in their systems, and transmit them to posterity. Men may discard the women with whom they have had sexual relations but they will find, no matter how low or degraded they may have been that their children will inherit the traits and often the looks of their mistresses.

This is a law that cannot be avoided but does not stop here. Like all other great laws, there are many deleterious effects that loom up in importance as we follow the various winding paths outside of the clearly defined one of rectitude.

The worst effects as regards such transmission comes upon *men*, because the life and power of the spermatozoa is magnetic in its unconscious life and power, and receives from the man the wonderful but as yet but partially understood impress upon the nerve centers, that time can never eradicate, and when this subject is fully understood by boys, they will cut off their right hands before they will thus wrong their own soul's tabernacle, and destroy the power to give to their posterity the sublime traits of their pure wives.

Prostitution will never be stopped until men are educated on these points, and it is because we so fully realize this that we have done what no other woman has dared to do, lectured and written to men exclusively on these important subjects.

But we have not yet reached the depths of the injury that promiscuous relationship brings. As soon as conception takes place, the blood of the spermatozoa begins to circulate in the veins of the wife, and the magnetic power of the spermatozoa also diffuses itself into the magnetism of the wife. The circulation of both increases in strength and quantity the whole nine months and so the very elements of the unchaste, that the husband has gathered up in his former relationship with those unfortunate women, is circulating in the bones and muscles and nerves of his wife, through the arteries, veins and nerves, and she can never eradicate it from her system. Not only will the children inherit more or less of all these traits, but in thousands of instances have the once pure wives had so much of the prostitute elements, or thieving elements or drunken elements pervading their system from the husband inheritance, that they have eventually been overpowered by them, and the good originally in such wives has lost the controlling power in their whole organization.

That these effects on different people are varied according to the laws of the modification of laws, as yet but very imperfectly understood must be acceded to by all reasoners. Close observation tells us that these mysterious laws can be delved into still deeper than human eye has yet peered, and that from a knowledge of what is now already clear, we may yet solve unthought of problems called "unknowables."

There are those who can never be convinced of intricate facts unless the most striking evidences are witnessed, like a blonde woman whose blonde husband has had sexual relations with a squaw or an African, becoming the mother of a genuine papoose, or a pure African child.

The law of modification often steps in and gives a specimen of a child where only the negro texture shows itself in the rigid curls of the flaxen hair, or of a complexion and hair that is midway in color.

The peculiar traits of character, disposition and predisposition are often more marked than the looks of the face, and not unfrequently the want of tenure of life is a telltale of no small moment, and the only easily discovered evidence of outraged law.

There is another depth regarding the influence of the magnetism of *presence*, that is still more difficult of explanation than even the mysterious contagious elements of disease, as seen in fevers, small pox, or epizootic, that could not have originated from any process of fear in the minds of horses, unless they have reasoning powers that they are supposed to be deficient in, or unless there is a power of mind in the human that so infused the animal hundreds of miles away, that the effects were the same as though there had actually been exposure to the disease.

We often feel most miserable in the presence of some people without any seeming reason, and feel happy in the presence of others, experiencing an indescribable something in regard to such presence, that we know not how to commence to investigate.

We feel it beyond our mental depth to reason it out, and like the mystery of mysteries that we every day behold in nature, we yield the point and plod along with a reluctant dismissal of the whole subject from our minds for the time, as the too barren results of such thoughts weary us, without convincing us that their solving is an utter impossibility. The deeper one delves into metaphysics the wider the field seems to expand.

Dr. Franklin touched the keynote of electricity for the business world; but who shall be able to so trace humanities' magnetic power, and so touch *its* key, that the masses shall heed its moral warnings?

The world must be made better by understanding the intricate laws of human development in body and in mind. For the masses to comprehend the physical effects of unchastity, outside of the production of illegitimate children or of venereal diseases, but little reading is necessary if plain language is used. But the wonderful effect upon the *mind* requires such deep methodical thought, that but few minds are accustomed to habits of clear arrangement of their thoughts so that they could express themselves intelligently on subjects that must reach the deepest convolutions of the brain.

As the sexual relation calls for the most intense nerve excitement, and the strongest and most powerful and concentrated emotions, so does it as surely call forth and receive the brain impressions, that in spite of all other considerations, are lasting and transmissable. And those who associate in the sexual relation with the low, the ignorant, the vile, the fickle, the unmethodical in thought, the undeveloped in mind, cannot avert the law of effects upon themselves that they are powerless to throw off.

Many a man of brilliant talents and fine culture has become a mere cypher in the world from this cause. Many that have attained intellectual eminence have failed to become the bright stars they might have been, but for this cause.

It is lamentable that the incentives to pure manhood are so few. Those who are the honorable exceptions in society with all kinds of codes of honor, are not the favored men of the time, because they are so rare that women do not know how to treat them. And so they look about them and see the worst rakes present the favorite beau of the evening with the purest women of all ages.

Such is the demeanor of a pure man that the women are not aware of his purity, only in exceptional instances. The purest of women with their general association with men not morally sound, do not appear the same women used to, when there was less corruption among men. Men themselves do not appear the same, if we can credit those who lived a half a century since as young men and maidens. But let us hope that we shall see no deeper degradation of sex, but that with knowledge shall come rapid strides towards a pure manhood, with those who have ignorantly degraded themselves, and that knowledge shall be so diffused that the young men shall all grow up as pure as they could wish the young women to be that they shall sometime marry.

CHAPTER IV.

Hermaphrodites.

Perfect hermaphrodites are very rare, although all cases of partial defective organs of sex are generally spoken of as hermaphrodites. Cases are related where persons after having been married as men for several years, were afterwards married as women, and in both relations there was mutual satisfaction, with the exception of there being no posterity. What were the antenatal conditions of these cases, no one is able to relate, as far as we are informed.

They are always licentious, owing to an inheritance of the same irritability of the organs of sex, and to defective moral sentiments that were antenatal conditions. They never menstruate unless they have a penis, and then the menstrual fluid is never passed except when they urinate.

The parents of children born with defective organs of sex have always felt that they were disgraced, and in some way at fault for such an occurrance although they generally have no definite idea of the direct cause.

It has been our fortune to have complete histories of such cases from our own observations, and it needs but little evolution of thought to establish principles that are axioms with such keys.

Hermaphrodites are but legitimate results of abuse of either or both soul and body. No woman's body *can* be abused without a suffering of soul, and *vice versa.*

We relate cases to prove our position in instances so marked, that the least logical cannot fail to be convinced of the correctness of our position.

Mr. – –, married a fine, healthy and beautiful girl of eighteen years of age, when he was about twenty-two. He had been living in a promiscuous manner since he was fifteen years of age, with no restraints upon his animal nature, daily cultivating the same until he lost the power of self-restraint. He had no respect for womanhood and no regard, only so far as he could be sexually gratified, and the remonstrance of his wife when menstruating, the disgust at the time, and the terrible debility and irritability after, had no effect upon him but to complain of her want of disposition to please him. (*She of course had no business to have any thought about herself.*) Herself and orphan sister of sixteen years were sole occupants of his house.

Every night he had sexual relations with his wife three or four times, except when she was menstruating, and then he, a little time after marriage, made his wife's menstrual period an excuse to force the sister into such relationship. He was so brutal and tyrannical, and such were his threats of vengeance if they either left the house or exposed him, that the matter was kept quiet. His wife bore him one child, a daughter, and both wife and sister died soon after with consumption, caused by venereal disease that he had given them.

The child is now about eight years of age, feeble and timid but utterly devoid of any vagina.

No doubt but that mother's mind was so firmly fixed on her child, (if a girl,) being protected from man's abuse, that her mental influence caused the physical defect in her daughter.

A young woman of twenty-five in this same condition, married a man in Washington, D. C., and when the discovery was made by her husband, a divorce was the finale, although she begged and pleaded for the *friendship of marriage* and consented to allow him any immoral liberties he might desire with others.

Two families of young couples in New York, were living near neighbors. Each had one child. Their intimacy resulted in one of the men taking the other man's wife and eloping with her.

After a few months they returned and the affairs were so settled that one couple again lived in their married relations. The deserted wife became *enceinte* soon after and as soon as she was sure of her situation she applied to her physician for medicine to destroy the fœtus. When we told her that we could not give her anything, she remarked with a great deal of anger, that as her husband had once deserted her, she hoped that if her child was a girl that "it would never be able to have a husband's relation, and if a boy that it would never be able to be a husband." When the time of her *accouchment* arrived we attended her and found the child entirely wanting in a vagina and anus.

The external labia were present and an enlarged clitoris that was really a defective penis, from which both the urine and the feces were voided, but there was no other developments of sex, and without any seeming cause except the painful passing of the feces the child died in about a week.

Among those who saw this strange freak of nature, was Mrs. Safrona Falley Nye, whose husband was an eminent Methodist clergyman stationed at Rome, New York.

The Author became acquainted with Miss Falley while a student years previously at an institution largely endowed and named after her parents in Fulton, Oswego county, New York. This ladies' sympathies led her to call upon the poor mother of a child whose defective organs would preclude all grand intellectual possibilities, not only, but cleverness in any direction.

1. Internal labia and clitoris forming a defective penis.
2. External labia.
3. Lower part of the malformation.
4. Leg.
5. Where vagina should be.
6. Where the anus should be.

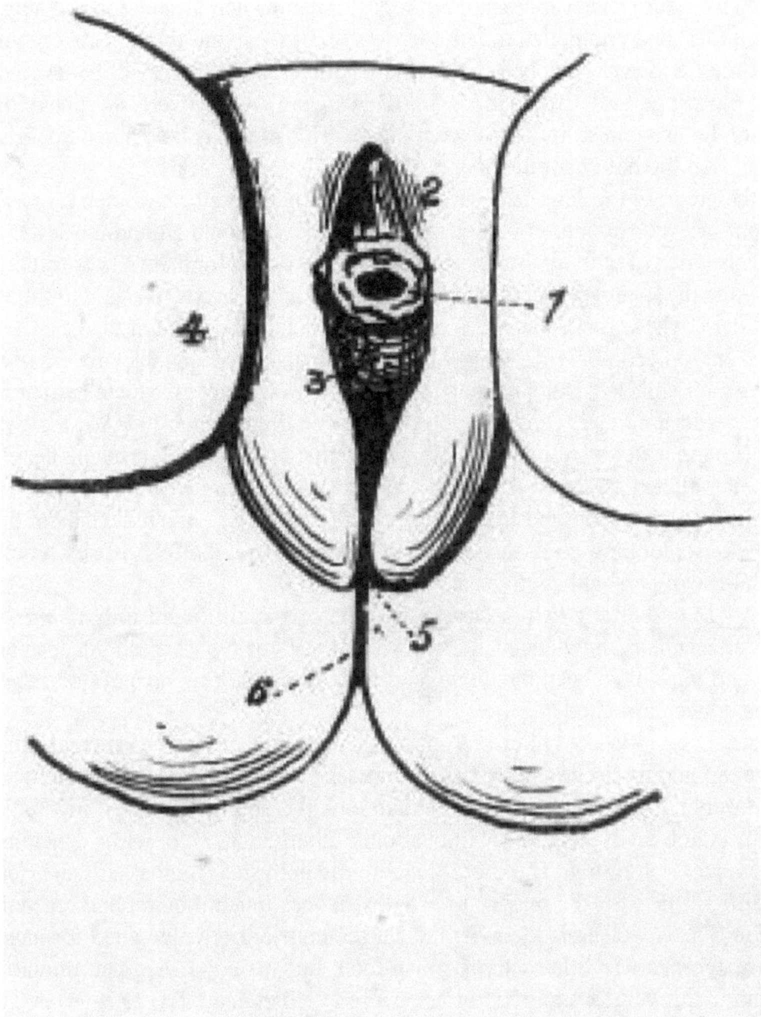

Hermaphrodite

A man about thirty, in a good position with a quiet immoral reputation, was married to a girl of twenty; one child was born before a year had passed, and a second one in a year after. This last was six or seven months old when we were called to see it. The anus was perfect as was the testes, but the penis was defective and resembled the enlarged, closed clitoris just described and illustrated.

There was no cuticle close to the pubes nor over the bladder for a space half as large as an ordinary saucer and much the shape. The muscles were and had been from birth as perfectly exposed as though the cuticle had been removed with a knife. Serum was constantly exuding so agonizing the child that no one but the mother could be induced to endure its never ceasing irritability, moaning and frequent screechings.

The father had compelled the mother to submit to sexual relations every night three times, and every day before he took his dinner, up to the day of her accouchment; pleadings and explanations of disgust and agony were all unavailing, although he used no stimulants except cigars. This man has held a position given him through the ballots of the people, (*men.*)

To the credit of the Jews be it said, that their religion protects women for twelve days out of every month. Is it surprising that so few women among the Jews will ever marry men of other faiths when there is no protection for them? These outrages are beyond the sphere of men's legislation; and when wives are goaded into suicides or murders, where can a man be found that peers into the facts of the case! Such women are too poor to fight with law for divorces, and have too much maternal love to leave their children, well knowing that men's laws will not give them to their *real* owner, because mothers cannot support them according to their judgment, of what a proper support for a child must be, forgetting that a mother will bring up her children better alone in poverty, than with a bad husband having wealth.

While we write, thousands of women are praying for death to relieve them from sexual abuse, looking no farther into labyrinths of the evil effects of sex tyranny, than their own personal agony.

Men will be better when the true principles of social life are fully *unmasked.* They reflect their knowledge of social life from their own standpoint, but how *dense* and *dark* have been the clouds through which the few rays of grandeur of soul have been reflected.

The effects upon the mind are not so clear to the masses, as mental efforts require thought to discern them, and the masses obtain more ideas from sight than from thought. Thinking wearies more than looking, and the power of methodical thought is not easily acquired without some inheritance, although it is acquired by a course of training. There are but few metaphysical minds and such learn how difficult it is for the masses to progress where much thought and reasoning are required. The clearest the most lucid arguments are often counted for naught because the average mind cannot grasp their full meaning. A great amount of systematic thinking is required to trace cause to effect and effect to cause and the masses not being methodical thinkers fail to grasp the full scope of deep reasoning, and to delve deeply into metaphysical subjects. But the facts related regarding well known cases of hermaphrodites, and the every day to be seen marks of mothers on children ought to arouse thought among men of but ordinary intelligence.

In every community there are many cases of people with clearly defined antenatal marks upon them, and some who are deformed from the same cause.

A gentleman brought a very large orange to his wife who was *enceinte* a few weeks. She thought it would seem far from generous not to divide, although she very much desired the whole of the orange. When her child was born there was an orange attached to its back with a little stem.

A young woman who was a few weeks *enceinte*, had her sympathies so aroused regarding a child about seven years old that could not talk, and, believing its mother derelict in trying to teach her, took the case in hand but failed to better her condition. When her child was born it was deaf, and at the present time, cannot say but a few words, although much older than children who talk well.

There are many cases of blood marks on the face, caused by the *enceinte* mother having a favorite animal slaughtered, or being shown an injury of some sort.

It is needless to multiply cases. Facts suggest remedies in many cases; if anything in diet is longed for, it by all means should be procured if possible, as there is some want in the system that ought to be supplied.

When unusual sights are forced upon the attention, woman ought to be instructed to place her mind upon the subject, and resolve that it *shall* not affect the child in utero, and particularly, should woman resolve to have perfect children as regards sex, that there shall be no more occasions for letters similar to the following being written:

Dr.: – At your request I furnish you the following statement:

About the year 1848, a patient in man's apparel, aged about twenty-eight years, applied at the Cleveland (Ohio) Medical College for treatment as a clinic subject. The external genital organs were those of a male, of usual development except that the scrotum contained no testicles. The subject complained at regular intervals of about a lunar month, of pains in the pelvic regions, similar to those of menstural colic, followed by a free menstrual discharge from the urethra (penis.) This monthly discharge had been regular from the days of puberty, continuing about five days, and gradually subsiding and entirely ceasing until the succeeding period.

The subject was suspected by the faculty of being a hermaphrodite, and after the lapse of a year or two an opportunity was afforded for verifying the facts, by the death of the patient.

A post mortem examination revealed the most interesting fact that there was in this individual, a complete double sex. The uterus was of normal size and form, the fallopean tubes of usual diameter and length, admitting the introduction of a small probe to the ovaries which were of natural size and structure; the fimbria was natural, the os-uteri well developed, projecting naturally into the vagina; the vagina of the average size and structure opening into the urethra about an inch, perhaps less, from the neck of the bladder; there being no external signs of a vaginal opening or vulva; the testicles were located about midway upon each side between the uterus and ovaries in a fold of the broad ligaments, and were about two-thirds the size of those of average male adults. A section showed a normal internal structure, but the microscope did not reveal the presence of spermatozoa. The pubes were more prominent than in the average male, and well clothed with the usual hirsute covering. The writer of this sketch made two plaster cast models of the external and internal organs, including the bladder and rectum and other parts in *situ*. Dr. Garlick, now living at Bedford, Ohio, assisted in the autopsy, and the specimen with one cast is now or should be in the museum of the Allopathic College, and the other cast was deposited in the museum of the Homeopathic College both of Cleveland, Ohio. Prof. H. P. Gatchell, now living at Highwood, Illinois, and Prof. Pulte, now living at Cincinnati, Ohio, were present with the undersigned when the examination was made, upon which the above sketch is based.

J. BRAINERD, M. D.

WASHINGTON, D. C., *January* 4, 1878.

[The above was furnished the author with permission to publish, by Prof. Brainerd. A number of other eminent gentlemen in the profession, besides the professor, and those mentioned by him, were witnesses of the autopsy. – THE AUTHOR.]

In closing this chapter, we are not blind to the fact, that whoever makes an attempt to elucidate principles not conceded to be such by those ignorant of the same, and others related to them, may not receive all the benefit that the author hopes for, in the immediate future, but the "leaven" of scientific truth cannot fail to be a *power* when there shall have been time for the important leavening process in the minds of the millions who err from ignorance of great principles that sham modesty has prevented them from having facilities to acquire.

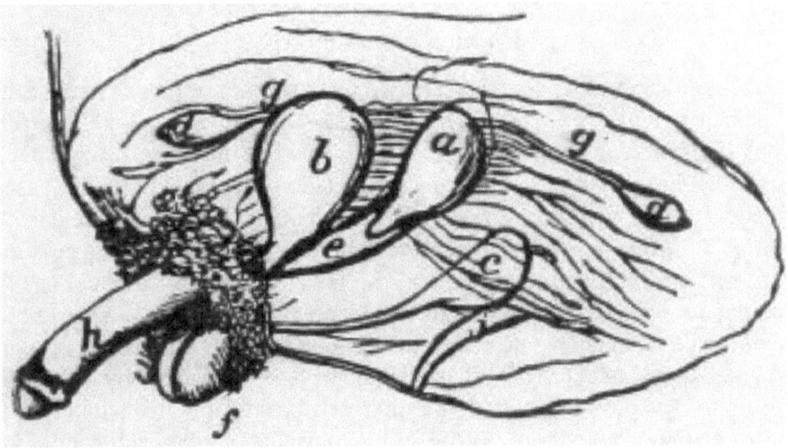

a. Uterus.
b. Bladder.
c. Testicles.
d. Ovaries.
e. Vagina.
f. Scrotum.
g. Fallopian tubes.
h. Penis.
i. Anus.

CHAPTER V.

Morning Sickness in Men.

It is well known that but few *enceinte* women escape morning sickness in the first part of pregnancy, and some suffer all through the nine months. But that the husbands of such women should suffer instead of them, has always been a mystery that has called forth no further explanation than that "it was because of sympathy." There have been instances where the first symptom of the *enceinte* condition of a man's wife was his own sickness of the stomach in less than twenty-four hours after her conception. So unvarying and so marked has this been, that a rude joke has come from other men that they could always tell to a day when a certain man would need a doctor for his wife. This has been a source of so great annoyance that men thus effected have kept as much out of the way of jokers as was possible, even to the injury of business matters. Jokes in any form in relation to the giving of life and immortality, are beneath people with any pretensions to a knowledge of the grandeur and responsibility of human antenatal development.

The sickness of the stomach is owing to the sympathy that exists between the nerves of the uterus and the nerves of the stomach. And as man has no uterus or womb, that he should suffer all the terrible nausea, and his wife be perfectly free, is owing not to an ordinary sympathy, for he could not sympathize before his wife knew her own condition, neither could he sympathize because of witnessing a deathly sickness of the stomach in her, since she does not experience any; therefore we must delve for a deeper reason, and in so doing we find that it is the wonderful fine magnetic intelligence that is communicated through her nerves to his nerves. In a word these nerves of the organs of sex, are wonderful knowing and have a wonderful power of *telling* before the brain does, and have power superior to the organs of speech in communicating such knowledge.

All married people learn of acts and motives of each other in this wonderful manner, and the freer they are from any sexual wrong the clearer and truer will be the knowledge thus gained. Unthinking, unreasoning people even, often get distinct ideas of moral wrongs through this nerve power, when they have no other means of knowing, and it matters not how much such an untrue person may protest that the true one has no cause for jealousy, the knowledge thus gained cannot be blown away by a breath of denial.

Many wives get distinct ideas of the existence of a wrong of some kind, although they do not always get distinct ideas of just the character of such wrong.

Men sometimes take the pains of their wives, and thus relieve them from suffering without any intention to do so.

It is not always a sympathy that exists between married people that causes them to take each other's pains, but a power that is not yet fully understood. As an evidence of this, a man whose wife was taken with severe labor pains in the middle of a bitter cold night, refused to go to a neighbor's for a long time, telling her she could wait until morning if she tried. He at last went in an angry mood and left the outside door wide open. His wife said she wished with all earnestness and prayed that he might have just as severe pains as she had, that he might understand her sufferings; and soon after all her pains left, and a neighbor woman came to her alone, saying that her husband had such pains that he had to lie down in the street until he got over them. These pains continued at intervals after his return home all through the night and until her child was born, while her own pains were scarcely felt. We are acquainted with parties who were themselves cognizant of the facts in the case just related.

Men who have morning sickness when their wives are *enceinte*, would find that it would soon cease if they would obey the great law of justice to antenatal posterity, by allowing all the strength of the prospective mother to be given to the child in utero, instead of making sexual demands upon her.

This is not *always* true however, for young men who run away to another part of the country, or even to foreign shores, to cure dyspepsia when they have seduced girls and left them in *enceinte* conditions, find that the world is not large enough to get away from the great law of the language of the nerves that cannot be controverted.

Every man ought to understand that much of the suffering of wives from sickness of the stomach, both while pregnant and at other times, is a result of copulation.

CHAPTER VI.

Kissing.

The above heading may at a glance surprise the reader, since the most of people treat the same as of but little moment in any aspect from which it may be viewed. It, however assumes an importance when the fact of venereal disease being contracted by kissing, is verified by observation and research. Dr. Naphey, and others eminent in our profession are firm in this belief. One would be far from an ordinary reasoner who did not concede the probability, since venereal diseases affect mucus tissues, not only in the organs of generation, but those of the nose and mouth. It matters little how a venereally diseased tissue comes in contact with sound tissue of the same texture, or quality, if the most healthy is not affected, it is because of an unusual power to resist disease, that very few people possess.

Those eminent in the profession estimate that twenty-five per cent. of the people are tainted in some degree with venereal disease. One of the best authorities in

Cincinnati, Ohio, states that thirty per cent. of the children born alive, die before one year of age, and that fully one-fourth are from some syphilitic taint.

This is but a sample of most of our cities, although some of the larger ones have a still greater proportion. The habit of kissing children is a pernicious one – for if they are tainted with the loathsome disease it may not make a positive appearance until about the time of puberty, or still later in years; still it is better to avoid danger by such familiarity On the other hand the tender and susceptible lips of the young ought not to be kissed by those of mature years who may be severely affected, although no symptoms are visible in the face, and no marked ones in the mucus membrane of the mouth, although some parts out of sight may be badly ulcerated

But aside from diseases contracted, the habit of general kissing is a reprehensible one, since it leads to greater familiarity – there are "holy kisses" from women that are far from being holy in the estimation of men who are so sensual that the least kissing or petting of any kind arouses the animal passions. Married women have said that they never dared to make the least demonstration of affection, as it aroused their husband's passions so that no matter how much they loathed sexual relations at the time, there was no peace until they yielded to sexual embrace, and they very soon learned that the only way to live in a way to control their own person was to assume indifference to petting and kissing. If men were to control such emotions and live as though life had some elevated sentiment of affection as well as of the sexual passion they would find many a happy home with disagreeable wives. Women often think as men *ought* to understand them that what often is the result of ignorance, is a total indifference to their wife's desires, so long as their own inclinations are gratified.

Parents wrong their children by urging or commanding them to kiss people that are disagreeable to them. Men make their children and wives kiss corpses at funerals of near relatives when they loath the idea, but dare not refuse to obey when told to do so in a low and meaning tone. Kissing at meeting and parting in this country is so common that but few have considered the matter until they have lived half a life time and observed that a great part of it is only *endured* by one of the party, and is often disgusting, although from fear of offending, the real emotions are suppressed. Whoever by reason of superior strength would kiss another without the perfect assent of the second party, would, if under no fear of the consequences, take the basest advantages of womanhood, disregarding the most sacred of individual rights of person, under all circumstances in life.

And whoever ignores such individual rights sets himself down as a tyrant, whether the ruling motives of such a person are guided by ignorance or by selfishness. It is a crime upon the physical but a still greater one upon the soul, that must ever call forth hatred that may not be loud, but a silent hatred that is deep and bitter.

The old years of a man's life who does not acknowledge a wife's right of perfect control of her person under all circumstances, will be a loveless one, if not a wretched one; unblessed by the pure kiss of affection.

CHAPTER VII.

Hymens.

The idea about hymens that once broken are certain signs of maidenly purity, originated with brutal men, who assumed the marital privileges as *rights*, and instead of treating wives tenderly and gaining their confidence, and waiting until their own nature called for the sexual relation through their love of motherhood, and thus lubricating the vagina, and relaxing the muscular tissues at the entrance, have by brute force accomplished copulation, breaking blood vessels at the entrance of the vagina, and so injuring the uterus by such savageness that the whole woman nature so revolts that the menses flow as a temporary protection to her.

Precisely the same result follows at all periods in woman's life, even after she has borne children. Indeed, the vagina has been known to contract more tightly but an hour after repeated copulative acts, than it was before the first act after marriage. The whole system seems to spend its power to protect against such excess, in its efforts to effectually close the vagina, to prevent more injury to the whole nerve system, that is sure to follow, no matter how willing in mind, or even anxious a woman may be to yield to men's demands, for the sake of an expected retaining of his affection, or for other reasons.

This condition has confounded men, and made them think that women were designedly unaccommodating not only, but that they could assume the role of the virgin at will, and seem never to have copulated, and so they lose confidence in their having been maidenly pure.

The virgin wife who is compelled to yield to copulation before she is herself prepared for it by the natural lubrications, has her nerves so shocked that it frequently occurs that months pass before she is really willing to yield to the relation. There are instances where the relation is never desired, because of a disgust that women feel for husbands that never act as though wives had any rights but to yield to their demands, and so the relation instead of being a tender binding one, is an irritating, separating one, that fearfully injures his whole nervous system as well as hers. For a women cannot have an impaired nervous organization without a husband suffering in his nerves by his having contact with her.

His ignorance of the cause of many ailments that result from such relationships under such conditions, weigh nothing in preventing the effects.

Children are often born of mothers who have never had one sexual relation that has been other than a matter of toleration. The ovum when in a proper condition, meeting the matured spermatozoa the work of conception must result when such germ and sperm cells meet. So great is the affinity of an ovum and a spermatozoa that conception has taken place with whatever of the hymen there ever was in a perfect condition, as the following will show. A couple married under circumstances not favorable to having children for a number of years. No effort was made to have perfect copulation, and not until there were unmistakable signs of accouchment, would either of the couple believe an *enceinte* condition possible.

The attending accoucher upon examination declared that the most perfect hymen existed, and the woman must certainly be afflicted with a tumor that was about to be expelled, with probably fatal results from hemorrhage. To the surprise of all a fine child was born after a few hours labor, thus greatly muddling the brains of those who are so sure of maidenly purity by physical signs. Few people ever expect to keep girls pure through other motives than fear of results and exposures; but those who have no higher and nobler restraints, are unfitted for desirable motherhood, reliable wives, and the permanency of the friendship of pure marriage.

Men with their greater physical strength, ought to despise the very idea of taking any advantage of women who know so little about their own nature, and so much less about the strength of men excited by tobacco, and stimulating drinks. A man is less guilty who commits a murder, than the one who takes from woman a consciousness of her womanly purity. And he had better be dead than to carry on his soul the marks of his own degredation, to say nothing of the remembrance of the degredation of his victims. This will be more fully explained in the chapter on the language of the nerves, where the matter of the evidence of a well marked hymen, (*which very seldom exists*,) will sink almost into nothingness when compared with the deep metaphysical truths that are of immensurable importance.

It has been the experience of girls that have been married before the age of puberty or very soon after, that the sexual relation before the body was matured, was at first exceedingly painful, and such are firm believers in the humbug hymen theory, which as we have stated is very seldom found to exist, although the story is generally believed by both men and women, and is kept up to frighten girls out of vice – with what success, the terrible condition of society attests, and ever will attest until better motives for chastity are taught.

CHAPTER VIII.

Seminal Weakness.

So common are the ideas that it is "seminal weakness for men to discharge semen when not cohabiting with women," that some really honest doctors have gone so far as to advertise themselves to "cure" the same. Others have made it a means to make money, when they well know that the occasional emissions of that character is but an effort of nature to relieve itself of a surplus, just as the throwing off of the ovum in woman every month, is an effort of nature to rid the system of the ovum or eggs that are matured and unused. If men are in healthy conditions this will occur every month, to correspond with the emitting of the ovum in women. Whenever it occurs oftener in either men or women, it is either because of weakness or of unnatural excitement. Tobacco, all kinds of intoxicating drinks, highly seasoned food, the vulgarity of women's fashionable dress that is ever appealing to the basest passions, cause a drain upon the system that is undermining the constitutions of the masses. This must continue so long as women follow the ever changing fashions, which are studies to excite men's passions and get their money. As soon as men fail to be attracted by one style; as soon as its exciting novelty begins to wane, another fashionable means of keeping up this passional excitement is presented. Not alone are the lookers on these fashions injured in mind, body and morals, but the women themselves are fearful sufferers in all these regards. So intimately are all the interests of life blended, that neither sex can suffer alone.

About an equal number of men and women are matured and the unperverted laws of nature are such that men and women respond to them equally when living properly. Nature is full of order; and the ovum and the spermatozoa must be thrown off to make room for the constantly maturing. From the age of puberty, until the change in life, the process of throwing off the ovum is one essential to health; these pass from the ovaries through the fallopian tubes to the uterus. It is important that the spermatozoa in men should pass off also, protected by albumen as they pass through the many feet of tubing in the testes. Although all semen that is largely composed of albumen does not contain spermatozoa, it is a fact that where there is no albuminous discharges, spermatozoa is never found, and such men can not become fathers, although they may be in good health. Instances have been cited to disprove this, but close investigation has proved the correctness of our position.

We know an instance of this kind. A woman who had been a mother when her first husband was living, married a man who was very anxious to have children. In consulting us she stated the difference in the seminal fluid of the two husbands, and when we informed her that he could not be a father, she expressed regrets on her husband's account. In less than a year we attended her in confinement. In about two years after she became a mother again. Another physician acknowledged the parentage and removed from the city where they resided. Several persons saw through the intrigues and kept watch of the parties, and knew of the doctor visiting the city in question in a clandestine manner, without her husband knowing of the same. Precisely nine months thereafter she became a mother again. The woman's husband knew nothing of the doctor's last visit, and was reconciled to the idea that he was the father of all three of the children.

Many cases of real seminal weakness are caused by masturbation, excessive copulation, and by shaving the beard. This last cause is a cause of masturbation, for the whole nerve system is excited by the shaving process. If the face was not shaved at all, the beard would not be so thick and harsh.

Men very readily understand the affect on the nerves of the eyes when a dull razor is used on the face, and they will learn to trace effect to cause and understand the irritability of the organs of sex.

The face is a tell-tale of the life, and the time is not distant when all who look may read for themselves and clearly understand what men have seminal weakness, and what are the causes, for every vice and every outrage on the great laws of existence have their own peculiar evidences.

Beautiful young women will not always marry seminally weak men to save such men's lives, for they will understand that their suitors have so destroyed their re-productive power, that they may not be able to ever become fathers for their children, and if they do, such children will be miserable specimens of humanity, both in body and mind.

It is a lamentable fact that there are but few young men to be found that are fit for marriage.

CHAPTER IX.

Barrenness.

There must be some defect in the mind of a human being that does not desire children. The unperverted sexual desires are filled with a love of posterity, and should not be exercised except for procreation.

It has been said that "the love of posterity is greater in woman than in man," but this must forever be an open question, since man's brain is generally so poisoned with tobacco and intoxicating drinks, that we know but little about what he would be without having indulged in the same. But there is a stronger reason why men do not love their children as devotedly as women aside from the mother suffering. A sexually promiscuous life destroys the finest and tenderest loves of life to a great extent. The man or woman whoever debases the procreating functions by sexual variety or change, or who indulges for selfish reasons without desires for posterity, lose the power to become the parents of children of the finest minds, bodies and morals. And although they may not be idiotic, or may not be born hermaphrodites, yet they are liable to be enfeebled in body, dull of perception, or without the power to leave their posterity to the world – in a word they are barren. All stages and modifications of evils result from an abuse, or an improper use of the organs of generation. They should not be used at all until mind and body are mature, and then there will be a strength of character, strength of body and mind imparted to posterity that will be superior to both parents.

If bodies are mature before those in temperate climates are between 25 and 30 years old, the minds are not, it matters not how well they are educated, and no person should marry until the mind is mature as well as the body. Time alone can bring maturity that enables parents to give to children constitutions and capabilities of mind that are superior to themselves, or even equals with them. It is true that superior advantages of children to-day leads some to think that their children are an improvement on themselves, but had they had the same advantages in their youth, they would now readily see that the contrast is very great regarding the deterioration of their posterity.

The love of offspring implanted in the soul of those unable to become mothers, has caused many barren women to apply to us for a remedy, and to explain the cause of barrenness. We have seldom seen deeper looks of despair on woman's face than when she repeated the assertion that "there is no hope in the case." Men do not understand the depth of woman's love of posterity. So great is this that women of all ages, from before the age of puberty, until long after the ordinary possible age to bear children, dream of having infants of their own in their arms, and sometimes of twins and triplets. Few, if any men have any idea of the love of motherhood that is expressed by girls to each other, and many an illegitimate child that is forced from the mother's presence, for fear of publicity, would be kept regardless of consequences to her, if she were allowed to exercise her maternal rights. A most marked and deeply affecting instance of the love of children occurred in the central part of New York. A woman of nearly thirty years of age became a mother who was never married. The father left the country before the birth. A few years after she became the mother of another child, at which occurrence all sympathy for her was extinct. When the children were about half grown she was summoned as a witness on some neighborhood difference, and the opposing counsel questioned her in regard to her two illegitimate children of different fathers for the purpose of damaging her evidence because of her character.

She replied that the love of the father in the hopes of having his offspring was so great that she was ready to bear all disgrace for the sake of having his child that she loved so dearly, that she made an opportunity to have another child, so as to have one to love in her old age if the first should die.

The judge on the bench asked her why she did not marry if she thought so much of children? She replied that she had never had a chance to marry.

There was not a dry eye in the court, when they understood that woman's love of motherhood, and the judge in open court asked her if she would marry him. And at the close of the court they were accordingly married. Very few women are understood by men, only as some peculiar circumstances bring their real characters to light. This results from a false idea of modesty that men make for women to abide by, and then in their egotism treat women as though they knew all about them, better than they know themselves. How much men lose in the great work of soul and body elevation, men will never know until women make their own standard of what is *modest* and *right*. The one is in reality synonymous with the other. Ignorance and false modesty always accompany each other. The motive and not the words or acts are truly modest or otherwise. Whatever any one person in the world ought to know about the human body or its possibilities, organic or functional, all should know, for knowledge that is gained correctly is but the birthright of humanity. At this point we make an assertion that was never made before, that every woman, as well as every man, has a right to know before marriage whether that life partner is capable of parentage. Science has been so developed that this can be ascertained to a certainty, and thus prevent all of the disappointments and separations resulting from barrenness. There are many causes in both men and women. There are instances of barrenness, where the only cause has been the harshness of husbands on wedding nights. The nerves of the vagina were so shocked and partially paralyzed that they never recovered the magnetic power sufficiently to foster the life of the spermatozoa until the conception was perfected.

We have discovered that some women have such a cartilagineous osuteri, that the spermatozoa lose all of their vitality before they are able to pass over such an unmagnetic place before arriving into the body of the uterus where the minute placenta is formed, with the ovum in it, awaiting the spermatozoon. Our microscopic experiments have proved that one or more minute placentæ are formed every month in the uterus while a woman is able to bear children. It is through the fine magnetic attraction of the spermatozoa for the ovum that bring the former, or *sperm* cells, to unite with the latter, or *germ* cells. How great this attraction is will be seen in another chapter, where a case is related of conception without perfect copulation.

Another cause of barrenness, is because of an elongation of the labia of the osuteri, making the osuteri so gross and unmagnetic, that the spermatozoa cannot pass into the uterus because of the repulsion. Another cause is that the osuteri is so small that the menstrual fluid is forced through this orifice causing great pain and consequent inflammation, rendering conception impossible, because of the heat of the inflammation so soon destroying the spermatozoa. Another reason is, that the expulsive pains so injure or destroy the minute placenta, that when the inflammation subsides there is no ovum or placenta in the uterus to receive the spermatozoa. Another reason is that the albuminous fluid given off every month to fill the neck of the uterus as soon as conception takes place is of such a vitiated character that the neck of the uterus cannot retain it. Although this last substance could be contained in less than half of a small thimble, it glues up the neck of the uterus to prevent air and other influences from interfering with the great and beautiful laws of fœtal developement.

Barrenness is sometimes caused from temperamental inharmonies, but wrongs are every day to be met where the parents had better have been barren than to have united such temperaments, that the power of longevity was lost in the children, or the general make-up was defective.

Most of the cases of barrenness in women, yield to medical or surgical treatment. But there are cases in men, that cannot be remedied, and it is a crime for such men to marry without the intended wife fully understanding that he is powerless to become a father. No man or woman whose respect is worth having, but would thank another for honestly revealing their true condition.

The temperamental conditions have a wonderful effect on barrenness in old age, as is seen in the following cases.

The noble Italian lady, Dianora Frescobalh, was the mother of fifty-two children.

There is a monument in Aberconway Church, to Nicholas Hooper, who was a forty-first child, and the father of twenty-seven children by one wife.

The wife of the coachman of Charles X. became *enceinte* when sixty-five years old.

Margaret Cribsowne, who died in 1763 at the age of 108 years, married her third husband at ninety-four years of age, who was at the time of marriage 105 years old. They had three children, all of ordinary height, but they never had any teeth; their hair was gray, complexions withered, and had decrepit step.

In self-imposed barrenness, married men object to having children because of their trouble when young. Some from fear that they may be deformed, or that they may not be very clever, and no credit to themselves. Some because of a want of an understanding that maternity does not injure women in any sense as wives if all the laws are observed. Some because they are too penurious to pay the extra expenses that their wives would demand, or their own pride suggest. Some because they do not wish to have their wives ever in a condition where their own demands cannot be supplied, and where their wive's whole attention cannot be paid to them, for those who practice variety before marriage are tyrants *in* marriage, and generally continue their promiscuity to a greater or less extent, hoping by putting on a kind of rigidity of manners that they will convince their wives of their correctness of morals.

We would not do an injustice to men, for the same things holds true regarding women who practice a variety life, as is seen in some tribes of East India and in Africa, where the women have plurality of husbands.

The love of posterity is never as intense with variety people as with those who have always lived true lives.

The motives that call forth the love of posterity are many. The first and general one is that ever grasping to attain all that is within the possibilities of mortals, and to be considered equals with the rest of mankind.

Where honors and titles are inherited there is a desire to perpetuate that style of greatness, and it sometimes occurs that the most cruel of measures are resorted to for the accomplishment of such a purpose. The beautiful Josephine will ever be cited as an instance of this character.

A prevalent motive everywhere, is to have some one to care for them in old age, and no matter what are the examples of ingratitude of many children, a hope that theirs will be all they desire is ever indulged.

Few men can ever understand, and perhaps no man can, how deep is the love of posterity for the purpose of having something pure to pet and place their affections upon as the predominant motive, although they have all the other motives that men have also.

We have known cases where the maternal love was so great with women whose husbands were postponing for years their wives desired maternity, that they have been led to study regarding the fulfillment of such desire from another source.

We know of cases where widowers with children when looking for second wives, have protested against marrying women who were young enough to bear children.

Some young women have distinctly told such men that they desired children, and thus defeated the contemplated marriages.

There are men who become angry every time their wives become pregnant, and treat them as though they had committed some crime, and by such treatment compel them to actually commit a crime in producing abortion.

We know of a case where the maternal love was so great, that a wife was determined to have a second child, fearing that the first (about eight years of ago) might die and leave her childless. She succeeded in her plans for conception after a second month's trial, in taking the semen from the sheet and introducing it into the vagina. Her child was a well developed boy, with the exception of having part of the cranial bones entirely absent. It lived but a few hours.

Good men cannot form a clear conception of the base motives of some men regarding the tenderest interests of life, and they hurry their daughters into marriage with any sort of a man that has wealth or position, never thinking whether the man may be able to become a father of grand specimens of humanity or not, or whether his daughter may not be barren and she be an imposition on her husband. Deception on one side is as reprehensible as on the other.

CHAPTER X.

The Social Evil.

Rev. Dr. Muhlenberg in one of his sermons, gave a withering reproof to fashionable woman church goers as follows: – "One of the great inducements to women to ply an immoral trade, is a fondness for finery, copying their sisters in higher life, who, by their example of vain show in dress, have more to answer for in the matter than they suspect."

Nothing could be truer, and when once in the vortex, they find they can live easier and more idly than in other ways, not knowing that they will soon lose the mental power to concentrate their energies on anything that would be honorably supporting, unless endowed with an unusual amount of will power. They do not understand that there is anything to be thought of in the case but a loss of the respect of people, an avoidance of child-bearing, and precautionary measures against venereal diseases.

They do not know that their passions will not always hold out, and they know nothing about the fearful drain upon their nerve forces.

But one of the great motives in yielding in the first place, with the masses of unfortunate women, is a curiosity that is intensified with the inducements, and with the natural instincts of everything that has life.

We have failed to find any men speakers or writers that understand this, for the most abandoned will not acknowledge this to men who undertake to peer into their lives.

Men cannot deal with this question properly, because they do not understand women. The best of writers on this subject are full of false theories, and false conclusions that the mass of women who read the same assent to, because it is considered something quite creditable among women generally to speak of the sexual relation as simply a marital acquiesance on the part of women who are married, and of great passions on the part of any woman who is having such relations out of marriage.

The best of men writers, whose researches on these subjects have been great, will assert with all the assurance possible, that "women's passions are not as strong as men's." And they will bring what they term proof to bear them out in such assertions, but nothing could possibly be more radically false. On the other hand the sexual passions of women are stronger than those of men, but the early training of self control, make the habits of continence so strong that men mistake self control for weak passional natures.

There are times in every month of menstruating women that only the moral sentiments save them, this is a perversion of the love of posterity that a combination of causes have produced.

When the minute placenta is formed in the uterus and the ovum awaiting the arrival of the sperm cells to unite with the germ cells, there cannot be a louder call than is made with the nerves of the vagina, all intensified with menstrual flow that every month gives new power to the vaginal nerves. The very formation of woman ought to teach a scientific man that her excitement as a natural consequence would be far more intense than his. This is seen in the confessions of women whose husbands or lovers were using precautionary measures to prevent conception, and were not permitted to do so. It is seen in abundant cases where women marry men far beneath them, and some widows resort to all sorts of measures to gratify the sexual passions, and retain the respect of people by a chaste appearance if they can but gratify at all hazards.

The greater strength of women's passions as compared with men is seen in their willingness to take all risks of passing through the agonies of abortions that are often greater than those of full grown child bearing.

We must take human nature as we find it, and then try to make the world better by lessons of history, observation and experience.

Social evils are unregulated passions as well as perverted passions, and the want of local bathing, the use of condiments and of stimulants are fruitful causes of such perversion. The unhygienic style of woman's dress that compresses a portion of the body, and by its very length causes displacements of the uterine organs, and defective circulation of the blood through them and contiguous organs, keeps up an excited condition. It is estimated that seven tons of blood pass through the heart every twenty-four hours, and in doing this the blood is unnaturally heated in the organs of generation by the compression of the clothing around the waist and loins.

All the theories of shoulder straps and bodies on petticoats relieving this condition are very plausible in the minds of men physicians who never can know by actual experience, to how limited an extent is this true.

The ordinary length of women's clothing, arranged as best *it can be*, is detrimental to the organs of generation and much of the false reasoning on the subject has resulted from the ignorance of men doctors, who could not fully understand the subject *because* they are men. Not until women physicians experimented and traced cause to effect and effect to cause, was this subject understood.

The proper arrangement of woman's clothing (the reform dress) must become general, before there is any hope of mastering the social evil question. For while woman is kept unnaturally excited, or in a condition to be easily excited sexually, by the ordinary styles of her clothing, the social evil question will be one about which the brain will be muddled, and all efforts to reform by moral suasion, prayers, kindness, harshness, midnight meetings, houses of reformation, and other conceivable plans will bring but meagre and discouraging results.

The same effect of unequally arranged dress on the nerves of sensation, with the nervo-vital fluid is true, injuring women a thousand-fold worse than it is possible to injure men, because men have not the internal organs of generation that women have.

Both men and women must understand the chapters on The Language of the Nerves, and Pure Manhood, the necessity for daily local bathing and the avoidance of all stimulants, before the great problem of the cure of social evils are reached. And then both men and women must cultivate themselves in accordance with the highest ideas of both fatherhood and motherhood.

We are rejoiced to have an opportunity to quote Jules Favre of the Corpse Legislative: He says "The only way to solve the social evil problem, is to elevate the standard of morals for men to that of the purest women." That is most excellent, but he nor any other *man* can see to the very bottom of the evil or they would see that no *one* single effort or a single measure could do away with the monstrous evil.

There is so much to be said upon this subject, that full elaboration would be impossible in our limited space.

We must at this time enter our protest against the course of so-called "scientific men," who advise young men to "cohabit with women to improve their health." It would be no more monstrous to give such advice to young women than it is to young men.

The organs of generation are for the specific purpose of procreating, and if not used for that purpose the natural means of ridding the system of an unusual accumulation is taken by nature.

While marriage is favorable to health and longevity, because of many stimulants to exertion such as children and the accumulative interests consequent on marriage, we have abundant proof of the general good health of body and mind of those who have never married. Among such are the names of the following well known women:

Dr. Harriet K. Hunt, the first educated woman practitioner in America; Charlotte Cushman, the American theatrical star; Rosa Bonheur, France's greatest artist in animal painting; Florence Nightingale, England's most prominent army nurse, and Miss Burdet Coots, the great English philanthropist. The lives of these women prove what can be achieved by using the powers in other directions than those of sex merely, and letting the reproductive organs rest from excitement of indulgence. Woman individually, is the only one capable of judging when, how often, if ever, she is to take measures to become a mother as all men are free to decide what is of immeasurable importance to them.

Some of the greatest men that have ever lived have chosen never to marry, and have distinguished themselves by the use of brain power, instead of draining their systems through their organs of sex. Among these are Sir Isaac Newton; Gibson, the sculptor; Pitt, the statesman; Baron Von Humbolt, the scientist; Kent, the metaphysician, and Jacob Gremm, the philologist.

Unless there is a stay to the social evil, the time is not distant when the world will sink back into barbarism.

The few who put on their virtuous cloaks to shield themselves from a discussion of these subjects, preferring rather to ignore evils in their own circles and let the rest of the world take care of itself, are of but little use to us or the rest of humanity. Ignoring the evils of life is not the philosophical way of treating them. They should be discussed by the deepest metaphysicians, and all should be taught their existence and consequences, as the safe method of avoidance.

They *will* learn, it is impossible to prevent their gaining knowledge from the basest standpoints, and through the most vulgar kind of language. How much better to be taught correctly and fill the minds with correct ideas and the true uses of all things. Science knows no false modesty. Much of the social evil is far beyond the sphere of legislation, but can be reached and the wrongs thereof righted through knowledge in youth.

The effects of tobacco on the organs of generation are well known to the profession as excitants, and also as having an effect on the early decay of the generative functions of both sons and daughters, as well as parents. Dr. E. E. Phelps, Professor for many years in Dartmouth College; Dr. Napheys, the medical author; Dr. Pidduck of London; Dr. C. McDougal, Dr. Wells, Dr. Trall, Drs. Fowler, Dr. Gardner, Dr. Smith, and a host of others learned in the profession, are convinced of the social evils that are aggravated by the noxious weed – tobacco.

S. Weir Mitchell, M. D., of the Philadelphia Infirmary for Nervous Diseases, in a recent paper, says that "tobacco is of all causes the most potent in giving rise to general nervousness."

We hope the Doctor will give a learned essay upon the effects on wives of men who use the noxious poison by portraying at length how the lungs, the kidneys, the skin, and especially the prostate gland surrounding the urethra, gather up and throw out the poisons that are introduced into the system.

The social evil among the married prevails to an extent that is appalling. The very influence of sexual variety that the husband carries to his wife through his nerves in his sexual relation with her, impresses her with the idea of indulging in a variety also, and so the pure girl that he married with no other thought but of faithfulness to him, his own course of life has changed, and made her unable to resist a variety life. Her husband seduces young girls, and brings to her in his sexual relations with her the *spirit of seduction of the innocent*, and so she reasons that if there is something desirable in initiating young girls in sexual relations, that it must be equally so to initiate young men and so she pursues her course.

And just so long as men are unfaithful to themselves before or after marriage, will young men be seduced by married women. Such cases are increasing at a fearful rate, and will continue to increase until men who are stronger physically than women will refrain from degrading themselves by taking on the vile magnetism of illicit intercourse that once imbibed is ever after a part of the man, as much as his hand, and is a part of the inheritance of posterity.

Popular ignorance on these points will not affect the great laws, and while we have been able to make some discoveries and application of laws and principles of the science of life, we should consider *silence* upon such important matters a crime of great magnitude, when we contemplate that millions are living, and billions unborn that are to be benefited by such knowledge.

Both men and women suffer aside from the usual diseases of body and mind, who are actors in the social evil wrongs. Among the same are two that are fearful results, the prolapsus of the scrotum in man, and the terrible hemorrhages of the uterus in the change of woman's life. There are no reprieves from the prison of the soul. And no remitting of the penalties of outraged nature.

Even in animal life there are marked instances of the great law. *Somewhere* there is a rebellion against such wrongs in the shape of a mare having but two legs; a heifer having an extra foot growing from the shoulder; a calf having six feet, etc.

The magnetic power is the life, and to illustrate how poisoning is the variety touch, we relate the instances of the deaths of two of Barnum's choicest ponies.

A woman so degarded that not even the lowest attachés of Barnum's shows would associate with her sexually, was hired by them for a pony. The animal was fixed in a frame, but as soon as she was touched, he fell back dead. The same experiment was tried with another woman and another pony by these men, with the same result. These women submitted to the degradation to get their bread, and for the pittance paid, Barnum lost his valuable ponies.

Will men *never* see that in a thousand ways their oppression of women are visited upon themselves? The above case is but a financial retribution while the following is a physical one of a *poignant* character:

One of the young queens in the South Sea Islands married a prince who died while in the first act of coition. In due course of time the next brother married her with the same result. The third brother, according to the custom of every brother marrying his brother's widow until an heir was born, reluctantly married her, knowing that both his brothers had died from the effect of having the head of the penis entirely severed. He was cautious, and declared she had a little knife concealed inside of her, and as his mutilated condition was testimony in the case, she was killed and examination revealed the attachment to the uterus of three small boncs with sharp edges.

Nature has strange freaks in her efforts to enforce her law of the rights of woman to her own person; we say freaks, because we have not yet delved into the mysteries that envelop unusual cases.

There are instances where the daughters born from marital rape, have inherited such a power of vagina resistance, that the coition grasp in orgasm has caused a man the most excruciating pain. There are two instances in this city that are known to be such. One is a case of a woman in good social position, who has all the fierceness of passion of the father and the resistance of the mother, making her just the character she is.

No man ever has but one sexual relation with her and considers himself fortunate to be able to escape alive. It is utterly beyond her power to control in any degree the muscular tissues of the vagina, and the bruised condition of her victims are occasions of apologies and regrets.

The woman has property, and when she fails to win a victim through ordinary arts, she pays a consideration for whoever she can get, but no amount of money can make a second purchase.

The very atmosphere is filled with wrongs of man to woman of more or less aggravated character. Women are oppressed because they will not sink into the immoralities of the age, or even sanction the same. Woman is denied legislative justice because she has so much logic that she cannot see any reason why she has not as good a right to help to make and to administer laws that govern both men and women as men have, and *because she dares to dress in as time saving, health saving, strength saving and money saving manner as man.*

One class of men oppress because woman lives up to the purest ideas of the grandeur of earth life, while another class oppress woman because she goes to the extreme of immoralities. The question might arise which class of men are the better of the two?

An eye witness informed us of an instance of the latter that all men ought to know of. Sixteen men in one evening cohabited with one woman, and after the same, without one of them having given the degraded woman a penny, took a large dog and, with one accord, compelled her to submit to another degradation!!! While grand and cultured women are oppressed in high places, the very atmosphere is filled with oppression that is meted out to other women by men of lower grades, in ways that would shock the former oppressors. Thus the sentiment of oppression carries with it no safety valve. The very sentiment preached, lived or even cherished will return to your daughters through men of degraded habits, to sting like a viper, although you may have sung them as a bird before your reverses of station and of fortune.

It is a hard matter to decide where the greater crime exists, whether in debasing a pure and true soul with brilliant attainments, or taking advantage of one with little mind and meager attainments. Who shall decide which injures society the more? No canvas is of sufficient dimensions to delineate the features of these cases. But in the great future the canvases will be unrolled to view. Let imagination paint its own picture to every man according to life. One such will be related here:

A young girl is the victim of a promising young man. He deserts her and she sinks lower and lower until she is a filthy blear-eyed monster, sinking out of life in a below stairs den, from which she is boxed up and sent to "potter's field." The brilliant young man has so covered his various conquests that he has been called respectable all through life. He has wealth, position, a fine family, and finally dies in his palatial residence, and is conveyed to the family vault with public honors. Voice and press are loud in extolling his virtues, while he is taking up his quarters in the realm of the disembodied.

The first object that meets his eyes, grasps his hand, and speaks his name, is the degraded woman that is now one of the component parts of his "Hell." He starts in *consternation*, he tries to speak a *begone*, he attempts to wrench his hand from her grasp, but finds himself powerless. He then takes a retrospective view of his life and goes into all the labyrinths of labyrinths through which his victim and victim of victims has passed, and with every thought and shadow of a thought, comes home to him the dreadful realization that *he* has been the grand *mogul* of the pure creatures destiny before him. The company he sought in earth life, and robbed of their magnetic power, rush to him in spirit life, with all the bad magnetism that are far worse than a literal fire and brimstone.

A son of a wealthy and prominent gentleman in a northern city, who was boarding at a fashionable hotel, took a woman in bed with his wife who had been a friend of hers. The shock of misplaced confidence in both of them was so great, (and what of abuse was meted to the wife in other regards we may never know,) that wife became so demented that she almost entirely lost the power of speech, and scarcely knows enough to feed herself. This occurred several years since, and at last accounts she was still living and in the same condition.

How the mental and physical could be so affected, just what process of action on both through the nerves was the cause of the result, is a study for the metaphysician, and until it shall be solved, will come under the head of the "unknowables."

As the lower classes are so badly conditioned, we can only hope to right the wrongs of the social evils, through science in the *better* classes of society as regards wealth and general culture. Not better as regards morals, save that there is less of the positive brutality towards woman, and more of wooing into evil.

A case occurred in Washington as follows: A gentleman who was addressing a lady with the avowed intention of marriage, did, by positive force, succeed in violating her person. He married her soon after. But he so shocked her sense of the proprieties of life, the selfhood of woman and rights of woman to her own person, he so disgusted her with the sexual relation that she told him before marriage that she should *never* be party to such a relation again.

They have been living together for near twenty years, and no influence could be brought to bear to induce her to change her resolution. She has been uniformly kind and attentive to him except when the sexual relation has been suggested in any way, and then she has been endowed with superhuman power of resistance. He was not out of the borders of civilization and could not do as one of the Indian Agents did in Wisconsin a few years since, which was to hire two men to hold a squaw whom hc had repeatedly failed to violate alone. How long will it take to prove to white squaws that "men are women's protectors," and to dark squaws that the whites are a noble race sent by a great government to "civilize them."

How many prayers will it take to wash the soul of social evils gathered up in earth life? With many gathered up in ignorance of their *permanence*, but gathered for eternity.

We have said many times in our lectures that much of the failure to do justly to woman was more a misfortune than a fault, because man does not understand woman, and never will while there is one iota of barbarism relics over woman, preventing the largest freedom in thought and act. Imperfect laws must ever exist until there is perfect freedom for all the governed to make full statements regarding cause and effect in thousands of matters that men have no conception of, and never have even thought deeply enough to think it *possible* that there is a side beyond man's possible comprehension.

Even as late as 1787, the subject was discussed regarding the complete evidence of rape.

The thought never occured to men judges or juries that a child or even a matured girl was ignorant of what an "emission" was, that she must swear to in order to *prove* rape.

The common law would not take penetration as sufficient evidence of *rape*, until the eyes of men were opened by the testimony of a woman who had borne several children that "she could not swear that emission had ever taken place."

(Forcible penetration whether in marriage rapes or in any other, at any time, more frequently than otherwise, causes more or less hemorrhage. In any case the vagina seeks to protect itself from the injury of friction by lubricating with the natural secretions, if possible, but if not able to do so then it is assisted by help from the uterus in an ill-timed menstrual discharge.)

There were no women on the dignified benches nor in the ignorant boxes, for the age was not blessed by Justice Esther Morriss, Lawyer Belva A. Lockwood, Jurymen Mrs. Amelia B. Post and Mrs. Editor Hayford, and a Law Journalist, Mira Bradwell.

Forced contact of the genital organs should be met with the severest penalities of rape, since such an act is but premonitory *to* and *with* carnal intentions, and is prevented only by some circumstances connected with the case, such as being frightened by other parties appearing, or impossibility of penetration without serious results, etc, etc.

Infants but two and three years of age are often raped, by men of all ages, not only for present gratification, but to familiarize girls of immature ages with carnal matters, and to excite, so that seduction may be easy in future. We could mention many instances of this kind of outrage, but one will suffice.

A case occurred in New Orleans, eight years since, where a young man of nineteen years of age took his employer's little daughter of three years and gave her venereal disease. The attending doctor gave the author a history of the treatment of the case with the minute vagina and urethra that made treatment so difficult and so uncertain regarding her future condition.

The only just way to deal with a man guilty of rape is to *castrate* him, for a man who has once been guilty in the face of all the influences against what is worse than murder, a term in prison will not make respectable.

The time is coming when a respectable lawyer will not defend such a man for filthy lucre – he or she will not draw up every point of law and twist it so as to defeat justice.

It is a lamentable fact that nearly every case of rape, gives a ruined victim to the world, for the vile magnetism that is imparted by the fiend, is so infused in the system of the victim that vice of the various grades is irresistible, (see the Language of the Nerves.) Let judges and attorneys hereafter look upon and talk up to juries the metaphysical injuries as no courts have ever heard before – let no lawyer plead an after life of an injured girl as a reason why there should be no verdict against him.

So long as children are begotten by force, so long as boys have the example that physical strength shall rule over women of any age or under any circumstances in life, will the outrage of rape be committed.

More children are begotten in marital rapes than in any other way. If the ovum is in a proper condition and is met by the spermatozoa conception must result, for the laws of conception cannot be controverted by anger or hatred on one side and outraged womanhood on the other.

The ordinary dress of women of all ages makes the facilities for rapes complete, and until the moral reform undersuits, and indeed the whole reform dress is worn, the best of girls and even women will be raped by certain classes of men.

The first step towards making the world better morally, is comprehended in not only a full knowledge of the effects of vice as seen in the Language of the Nerves, but in all womanhood being properly protected by dress in its best style.

The ordinary dress of woman by debilitating her body causes her mind to be also weakened. Woman is, *if not in absolute misery from dress*, so uncomfortable that she cannot think gravely and deeply. If a man has but a sliver in his finger, he cannot write a fine article or do himself justice in a speech. That is as nothing compared with the enervating effects and miseries of woman caused by dress.

In order to have a sound moralist, one able to cope with life as it is and leave pure examples as well as precepts, the dress question is of practicable importance.

How much of immorality is directly chargeable to woman's dress, we cannot pretend to elaborate in this work. This much we will affirm, that there will be scarcely any perceptible difference in the tone of morals – difference for the better, until both immature and mature woman is protected by dress, as no women *are* who dress in the ordinary styles. This is so well known that it needs no mention, only to remind the better class of men, that while there are all around us women dressed so that the facilities of vice are perfect, we can expect nothing better than street rapes occasionally and parlor rapes without number.

We cannot too strongly impress upon the fathers of daughters their duty in seeing that their little girls are instructed in regard to the certainty of protecting themselves against rapes, by grabbing the testicles. So sensitive are they that a man is at once weakened and made powerless to injure woman.

A case occured in Pennsylvania, where a young girl learned that her seducer was about to marry. When she saw him again he renewed his immoral attentions to her with a response from her hands in the shape of actually fracturing the muscles of the penis. The best of medical attention was procured but he was forever crippled and disabled, but the injury to the testicles is as effective a protection and much easier. And when women generally understand their power of protection, by knowing how sensitive is the scrotum, rapes will be fewer. But sexual wrongs will not cease until the reform dress becomes general. The underclothes are so constructed that a rape would be impossible.

REFORM UNDERDRESS.

The undersuits are perfect covering from head to feet. They are so arranged as to be a perfect protection. They are economical as regards amount of cloth and washing. One suit comprising drawers, chemise and cuffs. The stockings are drawn over the drawers, doing away with the necessity for any devices to hold up the stockings. Nothing has been invented in the shape of stockings suspenders that are not injurious in some way. It will be readily seen that there are no bands around the waist as is the case where drawers are worn in the usual way. No one's hips can support drawers or petticoat bands without injury to the kidneys and bladder in men, and to those organs in woman, besides the more serious effect of a pressure upon the internal organs of woman. They are directly over the fallopian tubes, ovaries and top of the uterus injuring by inflaming, as well as prolapsing.

All kinds and classes of evils show their own legitimate effects in a diversity of ways, unexpected as well as anticipated, for no evil stops with a single result. To such an extent is this true, that the most logical and metaphysical are filled with surprises regarding what were yesterday casual discoveries, and reliable evolutions of thought, and with expectations regarding what is to-day acknowledged to be buried as "unknowables." Years and ages elapsed before some features of the mighty predictions in regard to "the sins of the parents being visited upon children's children," were seen in their unmistakable truths, as antenatal results. But no mind can fully compass this prediction of the seers, or rather the philosophical metaphysicians of the past. Even to-day but few rush back to causes for lessons of prevention but blindly walk forth with their sophistry regarding cures, in the shape of prisons, asylums, almshouses, midnight meetings and reform schools.

An opportunity is afforded to illustrate the deep-rooted, and wide-branched antenatal evils both in China and America, since a hundred-thousand Chinese have come to our Western shores. Only about ten thousand of these are women. Fashion in China has made women helpless, and therefore crippled their morals by crippling their feet, and unfitting them to perform the active duties of life.

And so the home work is done by men. The outrageous crippling of women *all over* by dress, unfitting all American women for the duties of life, both among the rich and the servant classes, has made it imperative that men should take the places of house servants and maids of all work. This demand is supplied by the Chinamen. They perform all the household duties the same as a girl would do, and is it at all surprising that, being so constantly with women and girls of the family, (men with all the passions of men without much culture of brain) is it, we repeat, surprising that with only one China woman in the country to nine Chinamen, that such men should by both foul and fair means improve sexual opportunities, since a large number of even this small number of China women are used exclusively by American men? And these men, the husbands and fathers of their employers.

The American women before and since their residence in the far West, found it impossible to employ white girl labor without their husbands and sons having sexual commerce with them, and now the tables are unexpectedly turned, and husbands and fathers can no longer expect purity at home, except where it is from *intelligence* and not from ignorance and protective exclusion. Men's wives all over the country are ripe for *anything* since their husbands, *through the language of the nerves*, and in so many ways have proved their own course in life, and unwittingly paved the way for their wives and daughters to walk therein.

As true as the needle points to the pole, is the condition of the women of the country ebbing with billow swiftness to the heartless shoals of sexual license.

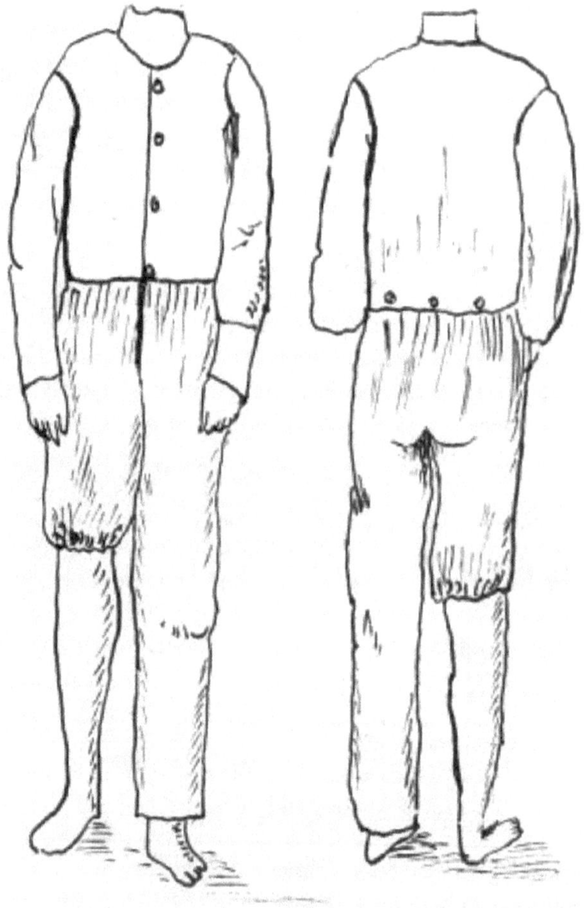

Reform Undersuit.

WOMAN'S DRESS.

The question of dress and the social evil is so great that we can but mention the same in this work. We quote from men and women as follows:

Here I wish to call attention to another point of practical utility – the relation of dress to prostitution. Long ago I observed that in peasant life, where dress was loose and simple, illegal prostitution was nearly unknown. In cities, where cost in cut and quality of dress are extreme, the greatest proportion of prostitutes to the whole population is found. Investigation has even proven that the excess of costume and adornment exhibited is matched by excess proportionate in social vice and intemperance generally. It is found that of abandoned women not over one in twenty are so from choice, not over one-fifth from real necessity, and the majority are so from a desire to dress as richly as the wealthy when their earnings are insufficient. Dress and the fatigue of laboring in its perplexities is the first inducement.

T. W. ORGAN, M. D.,
Ohio.

That woman should be the victim to customs so demoralizing and destructive to the highest good of all is the misfortune of her sex, the curse of the race. How intelligent aspiring women can consent to drape themselves in costumes that are a badge of servitude and an emblem of imbecility is a problem unsolved. To philanthropic minds, no subjects seeking the general welfare appeals for aid with more reason than this of substituting comfort and freedom for torture and tyranny in dress.

Considering how it cripples the physical and dwarfs the mental faculties, how æsthetic culture and soul aspiration are defeated, we find pressing incentives to earnest effort for its overthrow.

Brave souls with persistent energy consecrate their lives to the service of humanity.

S. L. O. ALLEN,
South Newbury, Ohio.

I sympathize with all who cry and sigh for deliverance from the fickle yet persistent goddess – Fashion, who subjugates nearly all the women of our land. It astonishes me that they so easily yield, when their freedom needs but general revolt. How *can* a man think his daughter equal to his son when she finds satisfaction in bonnets, sleeves and skirts that forbid achievements, and he is intent on vast interests?

Women have always been slaves, and are, if not wholly on the chattel principle, they consent to be so shackled and feebled by fashion, that the few who know what they want have not mind-force to put on the *means* of *power*, the *emblems* of *liberty*, and take *both* as fast as able.

Of all the difficulties with which she now contends, none is more serious in direct and remote bearings than the dress imposes. The great thing in the way of deliverance is that fashion makes her dress not only the symbol of her sex, but of inferiority because of sex. I care not so much that sex be shown by her dress, as that it thereby compels her to suffer disadvantage in the use of her powers.

J. C. JACKSON, M. D.,
Dansville, N. Y.

ORGANS OF CHEST, ABDOMEN AND PELVIS.

1. Lungs.
2. Heart.
3. Diaphragm.
4. Spleen.
5. Stomach and part of liver.
6. Intestines.
7. Uterus.
8. Vagina.
9. Bladder.
10. Anus.
11. Spine.

The first principle to be observed in dress, is perfect freedom of motion for every muscle. There can be no restraints without injury, not only to the particular part, but to every part, through the law of sympathy.

There should be such an equal distribution of clothing, that the blood may circulate freely. This cannot be the case without an equal temperature, for the blood is expelled by cold to respond to the invitation of heat. This is also true regarding the circulation of the nervo-magnetic vital fluid, which is expended so largel\

y in transporting the ordinary clothing of women.

The man who loads his beast of burden with utterly useless gearing, would be considered idiotic or insane; but what shall we say of him who oppresses woman because she relieves herself of utterly useless weights and locomotion obstructors?

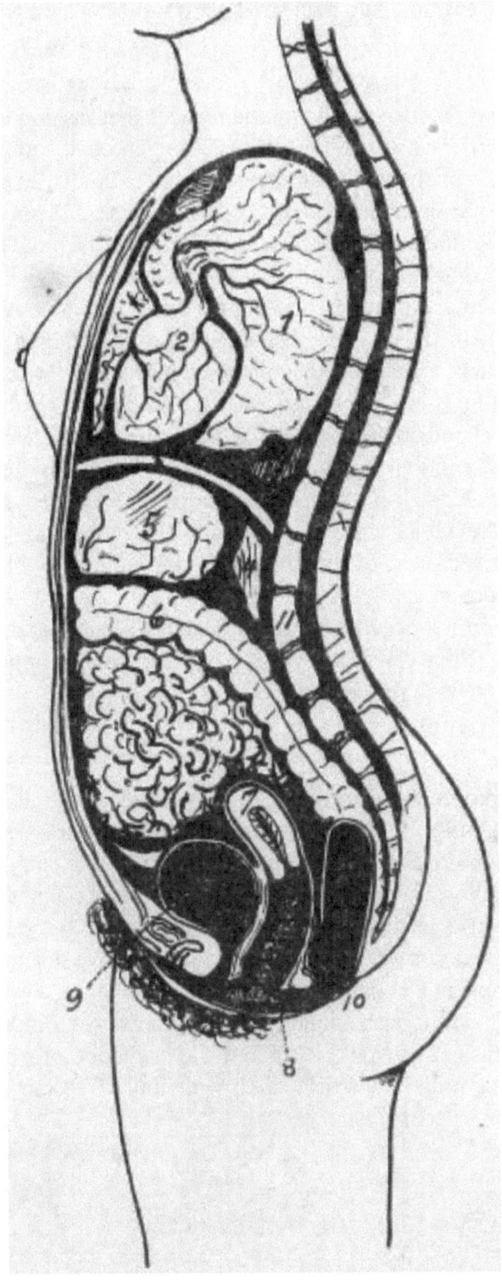

Organs of Chest, Abdomen, and Pelvis.

Would that I could encourage weak, deluded women to be true to themselves, abandon slavery to fashion, and gain strength to fulfil life's duties joyously!

MRS. S. E. MICHENER,
California.

Men and women while acknowledging the ravages that fashion makes on health, insist that the style we substitute must be beautiful, and that garments clothing the legs separately are homely and unattractive, though exceedingly convenient. They do not reject the most deforming device of fashion. The difficulty is plainly here: long habit and transmitted tendency have so accustomed the mind to follow the frequent changes of fashion that it readily assumes that the last style is preferable, and accepting without comparing and choosing for itself, individuality is silenced and weakened, and only the false notion that drapery alone is feminine, speaks in taste. Conceding the point of a general chain of consistency, all that is required to make a natural dress beautiful is *use*. If long use can make the caricatures that licentiousness and avarice have palmed on the ages appear beautiful, have no fears that something comforting, strengthening, liberating and rejoicing will not prove beautifying.

While bodies are caged in the petticoat badge of dependence and inferiority, minds and souls are subject to evil, psychologizing wills and cannot command themselves; whereas crowns of strength, joy and sufficiency, with choice of place in the exercise of power await the Unbound Woman.

Fearing to put forth endeavors because all cannot see and approve the purpose involved, because children accustomed to wading cannot appreciate walking, would be cowardice withering to my spirit.

MARY E. TILLOTTSON,
Vineland, N. J.

Woman having no proper physical training or scientific advantages, no highly remunerative employment or official trust, they are, as a rule, untaught, unskilled, unenterprising; hence have thought more of adorning the body than of high culture. To captivate the superior sex, win approval and companionship, has seemed the aim, dress the means.

Fashion and goods speculators see their chance and make both dupes and fortunes by millions, reckless of the ruin. Deploring the grave dilemma, I gladly hail every earnest movement among women, however difficult, to correct the bad taste, pernicious example and foolish stupidity seen in the wasteful profusion and absolute deformity of fashion. I would encourage the institution of a style for women, combining neatness, propriety, artistic skill, with entire freedom of choice and in accordance with the laws of health.

WILLIAM L. GARRISON,
Boston, Mass.

"My motto in dress is Utility, Comfort, Economy."

LUCRETIA MOTT,
Philadelphia.

I think the tyranny of fashion in dress the greatest obstacles to reform.

C. A. BARTOLL,
Boston, Mass.

I feel anxious that this dress movement, so well begun, should be carried out by American women, on American soil.

* * * * *

Popular opinion ever opposes reforms, and makes them move like ships against head-winds.

A. B. BRADFORD,
Enon Valley, Pa.

In view of the immense importance of rightly relating clothing to the law controlling these precious living temples, no more sacred theme can claim our care. Looking on humanity to-day, the most striking abuse of law is apparent in the burdens dragged by women in lieu of legitimate dress. A thorough, radical change in their style becomes at once a necessity.

WILLIAM S. FLANDERS,
Cornville, Me.

Leaden apathy or racking pain is far nearer the rule with us than the exception. It needs no argument to convince thoughtful observers that the most prolific cause of this is the pernicious modes of prevailing dress.

J. CHASE,
Vineland, N. J.

The woman whose dress shows she is human proves she is worthy of equity.

Women cannot grasp and shape their destiny till done through physical freedom, till feet are free as hands, legs as free as arms.

J. TREAT,
New York.

The styles of the civilized world, so called by the monster monarch, fickle fashion, are irrational life-destroying, mind-belittling, brain-heating, waist-compressing, ankle-wrenching, feet-pinching, back-breaking, lust-engendering, child and mother-murdering, race-degrading.

Women should see that asking rights is useless till they take the *right* to clothe themselves at least as comfortably as men.

J. M. ALLEN,
Massachusetts.

Preaching Freedom in Fetters.

What can be said of the many woman speakers advocating liberty, equality, spiritual elevation and moral reformation, yet pleading, with bodies legs and feet almost helplessly hampered? I view them with a sickening sense, pity them from the deeps of a sad soul and exclaim, poor, sick sisters! The most that you are doing is to burlesque your weak, coward selves! You fall before a Juggernaut that has no palliating merit! What is life without health? What value has freedom without power to use it?

S. MITCHELL,
Vineland, N. J.

When a dress prevails that gives full scope to all bodily powers, long depressed womanhood may reach normal endowment.

A. R. DAVIS,
Worcester, Mass.

RETROVERSION OF THE UTERUS.

In retroversion the uterus (4) presses against the rectum (6), preventing the feces from reaching the anus. While the top of the uterus presses against the rectum (6), the osuteri presses against the bladder (3) and the intestines (2) fall upon the uterus and all of its attachments. In this plate, in anteversion, will be seen the abnormal position of the pelvic organs of woman. Organs of chest, &c., is the normal condition, as demonstrated by Berta Von Hillern's power to walk. Were a corsetted, long dressed woman to attempt such physical culture, worse abnormal conditions just mentioned would be the result, bad as are nearly all women at present.

1. Spine.
2. Intestines.
3. Bladder.
4. Retroverted Uterus.
5. Vagina.
6. Rectum.
7. Urethra.

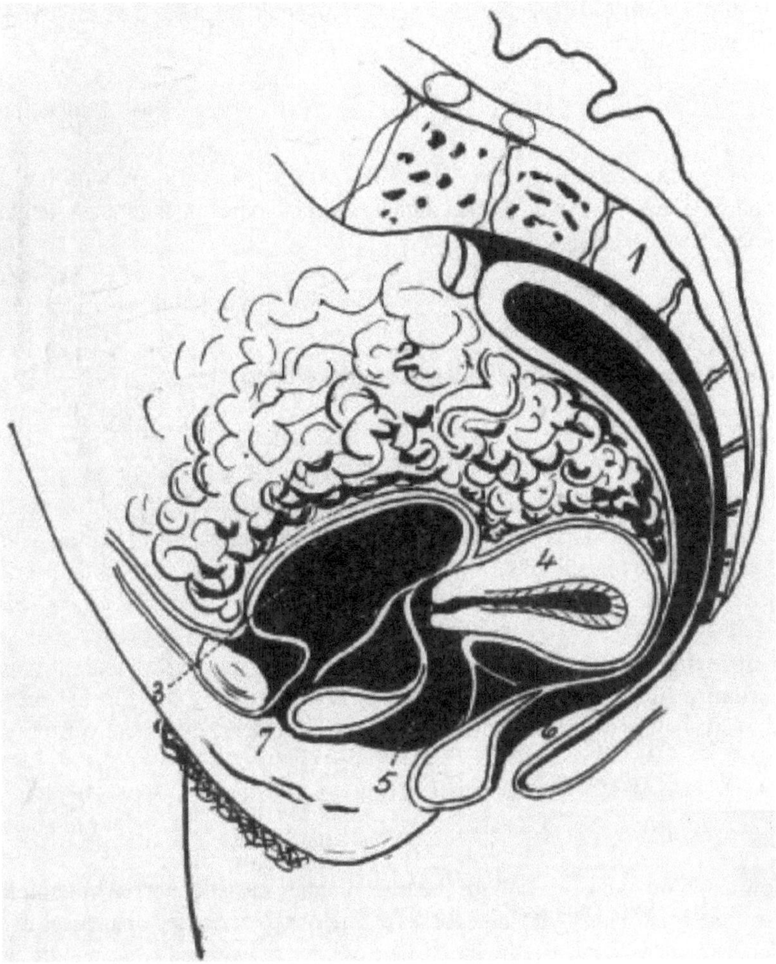

Retroversion of the Uterus.

Reformers aiming at a style to serve health and all the duties and high attainments of our manifold capacities are right, and should be abetted by all lovers of human welfare.

J. M. SPEAR,
Philadelphia.

To enlightened taste that is truly beautiful which is in harmony with law and immutable order. Whatever dwarfs human powers comes of ignorance, tends to weakness and woe, and is deformity.

D. M. ALLEN,
South Newburg, Ohio.

I cannot express my admiration of woman's reformed dress.

E. M. HOWARD,
Ohio.

It is a sorry sight to see a specimen of elaborately dressed frailty, and know that in those lovely shoes are comfortless feet, in that coil of beautiful hair an aching head, and under exquisite folds and puffs all manner of pads, pains and miseries.

Two things seem needed to remedy abuses in dress. First and best, is *independence* in women. * *

A professional man whose wife wishes to wear a short dress fears it would compromise him in his profession. He makes her carry his fortune on her hips. A husband would look better saying, "my dear, dress comfortably if you can.

REV. S. C. BEACH,
Norton, Mass.

How can those who ever call for the freedom they have not persist in trampling on the more important rights they possess? Their style of dress embarrasses every motion, and makes a most aggravated slave of the ever-worried *body*, and through that the never free or full-grown mind. Healthful dress cannot well be unbecoming. Tight waists, draggling skirts, half-clothed legs, for a business woman, are worse than ludicrous – are suicidal.

S. L. TIBBALS,
Manchester, Va.

My dress is what is known as the American Costume. I have no thought of returning to the slavery and corruption of Fashion, but *do* expect to change my style when finding what is better. I have traveled much, and know the slights, cold shoulders, jeers, etc., that the ill-bred offer.

L. F. STEGMAN,
Allegan, Mich.

Merciless Fashion annually sacrifices millions of human beings on its murderous altar. A sound mind in a sound body, a free mind in a free body, mean something that ought to open women's eyes to the duties they owe themselves. Girls study physiology and are not taught to apply its lore or regard its many warnings. Their lives pay the penalty.

J. H. COOK,
Columbus, Kan.

The varied benefits and constant comforts of my dress are so great that no temptation to return to swaddling clothes has assailed me. And yet underlying this important change is a principle that should prompt us to persevere, if selfish aids should prove, as some have said, not compensatory. Abolishing the servile imitation of degrading customs, especially in dress, is among earth's imperative duties.

EMELINE A. PRESCOTT,
North Vassalboro', Maine.

Experience teaches me that a woman may wear the costume and gain respect by simply respecting herself.

C. FANNY ALLYN,
Stoneham, Mass.

I have made my own way in the world. Have succeeded in the vocations of teacher, merchant and farmer; traveled from Maine to Florida; met all shades of treatment, from profound respect and high encomium to low shouts of rabbles, and the hiss of well-dressed bipeds. Think I have never talked with a stranger who was prejudiced against the dress without making the path easier for the next one he may meet in the American Costume. Through all opposition the personal benefits of the reform have compensated; but had it been mainly sacrifice, the thought of working for the amelioration of woman and the elevation of humanity would still have been the beacon-star guiding me on amid all discouragements.

S. P. FOWLER,
Vineland, N. J.

The sympathies of my soul are with those laboring to convince weak women that they need not obey life-torturing fashion.

F. E. REECE,
Minnesota.

We should have liberty to experiment with the widest range of garments, and use any that are adapted to our taste, needs and employments, without private or public molestation. Until this can be done all discussions on the relative capacity of men and women are ill-timed and in bad taste.

OLIVIA SHEPHERD,
Vineland, N. J.

Yielding to usage and prejudice lulls conscience, and fearing gossip checks the course of knowledge. Woman aspires to high culture and pursuits, and seems not to know her slavery to dress forbids attainment.

L. E. JACKSON, M. D.,
Dansville, New York.

The laws of health, beauty, fitness, economy, convenience, comfort and decency are violated in most of women's present styles.

All know what is threatened if we call our brother a fool; but I call him who weds a fashionable woman in these times a fool, and risk consequences. His risk must surely be great as mine. Saying less, I should be unworthy to subscribe, – Friend of Humanity.

P. PILLSBURY,
Concord, N. H.

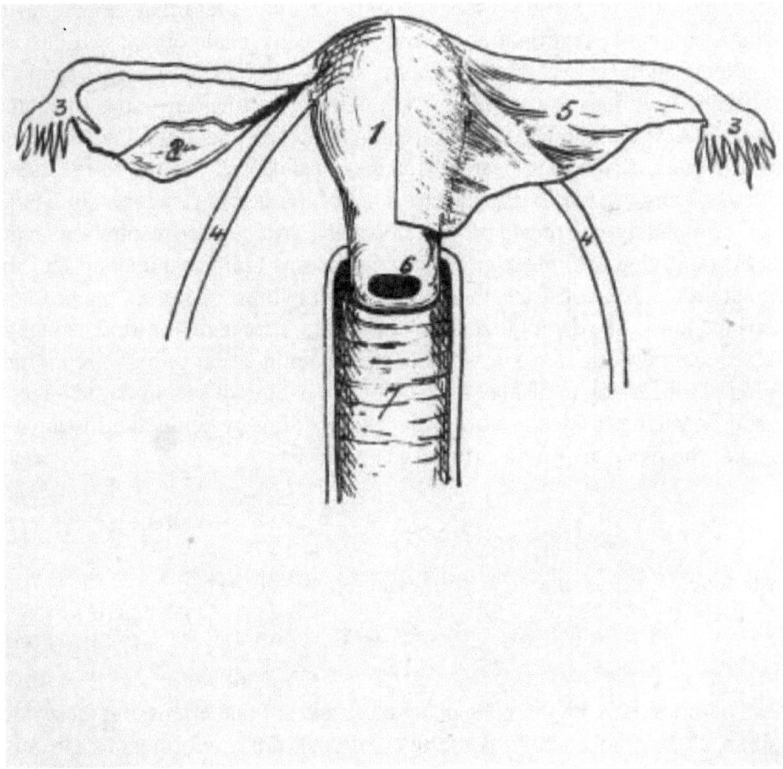

Uterine Organs.

For twenty-five years I have been teaching medical classes to trace most of society's maladies, especially those of women, to the dress that devitalizes the whole system, hence deteriorates the offspring, early made orphans. It has long been my custom to classify the four leading curses of civilization thus: 1st, alchol; 2d, tobacco; 3d, drugs; 4th, fashion. But the more familiar the subject becomes, the more I see of incurable cases, – traceable to corsets and draggling skirts, meretricious head-gear, and leg-beating flounces, – the surer I come to reverse the order and place fashions in dress at the head of the horrid category. No woman, dressed fashionably, can breath or walk normally. Without free respiration no pure blood flows, giving firm muscle to act and vigorous brain to think and feel. Just to the extent that she constricts the lungs, loads the hips, oppresses the head, and burdens the limbs, she demoralizes her whole nature, becomes morbid, demented, paralyzed and perverse. I see no hope of her attaining relief or higher conditions of any kind till ceasing to display in costume the badges of self-imposed degradation, and banishing the scare-crow whim that natural, hygienic dress is unwomanly, takes the free use of lungs, ribs, legs and feet.

R. T. Trall, M. D.
Florence, New Jersey.

Fashionable attire is ruinous to the sexual organs of women.

Dr. Sarah B. Chase,
New York City.

If space permitted, we could make many thousands of quotations, but these could not all speak so emphatically as the lives of such dress reformers as Dr. Susan Way Dodds, St. Louis, Mo.; Dr. Lydia Sayer Hasbrouck, Middletown, N. Y.; Dr. Lydia A. Strowbridge, Cortland, N. Y.; Dr. Ellen Baird Harman, Florence, N. J., and other physicians who are practical exponants of the vital principals so important to over-burdened women.

The doctor, whether man or woman, who does not advocate a reform costume for woman, clearly shows an ignorance of the causes of diseases and displacement in woman, not only, but fails to comprehend one of the chief causes of the deaths of 100,000 infants annually, the imbecility and diseases of boys as well as girls, besides the tendancy to insanity, and a long train of evils that one with large causality and metaphysical acumen is appalled at beholding.

Such an array of evils grow out of woman's ever changing, extravagant, licentious, debilitating, diseasing, immoral doll-baby dress, that fashion imposes upon women, that make the great mass of them perfect monomaniacs on dress, that appalls a practical exampler of modest, useful, economical, moral, healthful, common-sense costume.

Men who encourage this and women who talk about "reform schools" or reforms of any kind so arrayed and gewgawed, had better repeat the words of Edward Faxton until they can fully understand them: "*They who would reform others, must first reform themselves.*"

These diamond words are utterances so deep and comprehensive that those who do not heed them, are sure to find themselves in a position too ridiculous for common pity. But a little time will elapse before the world will see this truth in all its clearness.

Reforms of all kinds are so linked and interwoven that they must progress together; but in order to be permanent they must have the foundations secure. Such foundations are in health of body and mind, and *the ordinary costume of women disease both.* Not only do they have this effect on women and their children, both girls and boys, but husbands of such wives suffer also.

They are irritated in their sexual organs, and they seek other women for relief. The irritability is an effort to throw off impure elements, and the more the remedy in either variety or excuse is sought, the harder nature labors to throw off the deleterious elements gathered up, producing still greater irritability that is mistaken for strength of passion.

Every means is devised to satisfy this morbid state, and with shame for the depravity of human nature we record that in our own country not ordinary men, but so-called *gentlemen,* are guilty of using the rectum of their wives. This is for the double purpose of getting strong muscular contraction, and to prevent conception.

There is no language that can express the more than barbarous outrage of such acts. The agony that is experienced by woman until the sphineter anii is so expanded and lacerated that it has lost contractile power, cannot be expressed. Such is the construction of the rectum that large fœces can, without difficulty, be voided, but nothing of half the size can be introduced without extreme agony, not only, but after the inflammation subsides there is a tenderness and uncomfortableness besides an inability to control the fœcal discharge, necessitating them to wear a protector from exposure. They cannot sit down without being in misery. Their whole nerve system suffers from this most cruel tyranny. Cancer of the bowels finally results. But the men are not exempt from penalties for violation of law. The nearer the worn out, effete matter approaches the exit, the more poisonous it becomes and neither sitzbaths or *enema* can cleans the parts so but that much remains in the multitudinous folds.

This filthiness is absorbed by man and produces a depravity that he cannot throw off, besides urethral stricture caused by repulsion to the filthy unnaturalness of such contact.

The bare proposition from a husband to a wife for such a relationship ought to be a sufficient cause for divorce, but when it comes to compulsion, imprisonment for life ought to be the penalty.

Astonishing as it may seem to women, there are many men who actually believe that no rape of any kind can be committed on women. They have this idea from the illustration of Queen Elizabeth of England, who would not sign any death warrants because she believed that every woman could take care of herself. She did not realize in her protected position how brutal men would dare to be, and how much greater was man's physical strength.

Men will never have just laws until women physicians are in the great councils of the nation.

Nothing but the sternest sense of duty to helpless women could impell us to pen what is so revolting to every sense of decent humanity as is the shameful recital of outraged decency just related. Moral courage is carried to its greatest tension, but above all this a whisper of encouragement comes as we write through blinding tears, what we have been long agonizing over the necessity for writing, and struggling to get moral courage enough to carry out our convictions, that *ignoring evils can never remedy them.* The illogical and surface wise, but deeply ignorant, cannot see the necessity for arraying the evils of all classes before the broad light of day, and disgusting the beholders, little realizing that there is no effectual way of destroying the moths of corruption that eat out all grandeur of soul in the dark of ignorance and vice, and that sunlight of facts alone can do so.

We place evil on a pedestal, and array the results around it and behold the effect.

We call forth eternal principles and calmly discuss them. If silence could do the work, all christendom could not open our mouth, but as nothing but an *exposé* of the wrongs to woman and the wrongs to pure manhood can be rightened and prevented, all christendom can not close our mouth. Every wrong, no matter how base, has advocates attempting to justify the same not only, but to establish it as a right. It matters not how monstrous it may be. But of all the iniquities of the social evil we have yet to relate the following as the most heinous possible:

The idea has been disseminated that the "eating of semen by women and the sipping of the exundations of women by men, will promote health, prolong life, and promote beauty."

The public money might better be expended in teaching the monstrousness and results of baseness so vile that adjectives cannot be found sufficiently expressive to reach the case, instead of arresting for disseminating obscene matter.

Such degradation not only debases so that the whole expression of face is soon so hateful that one is repelled at a glance, but the brain is so injured that an incurable phase of insanity results.

What is thrown off by men and women have a certain mission and effect, and is then not only of no more use, but is a positive injury if retained. Nature makes no mistakes, and her laws cannot be infringed without penalties.

Nothing feeds the system that is taken into the stomach, only as it goes through the processes of digestion and assimilation, and instead of such disgusting uses of effete matter being beneficial to the organs of generation they are serious detriments.

It does seem that the depths of human depravity have been reached, and it is time that human beings realized that there is something better in life than making a study how to turn all the best of energies to licentiousness.

It is a great mystery to many, why men in high, lucrative and responsible positions cannot resist temptations to frauds, thefts, embezzlements, etc., but to us it is not so strange since it is well known that "wine, women and iniquities" have always been classed together.

The women who are the victims of such men, must dress fashionably in order to keep in their graces, and the men well know that large sums of money must be given women in order to have them dress well and live in a style becoming a mistress of theirs. It is necessary in order to cloak the true life of the woman, for the man to furnish means sufficient to have her be living on a seeming income. Thus the true relationship is covered up for a time, and calls seem to be those only of ordinary friendship in the position.

These women constantly living false lives of respectability, must of necessity be avaricious, since fashions are ever changing, and to dress as well as the wives, daughters or sisters of the men that support them, and in whose society they mingle, a large amount of money is necessary. The relationship sexual, with such women, so fills such men with the avarice that they imbibe from them through the magnetic influences of the relation, that such men are fit for any crimes to gain money. Men lose the moral power to resist evils when they take upon themselves the vile magnetisms of such women, who obtain a power over them that cannot be thrown off immediately. They lose the power of will, and no matter how much their reason may protest against their course, it is of no use when will is powerless.

We are not sure that it would not be a moral crime for any one to be silent who sees the causes and effect of human wrongs, and how government as well as individuals suffer because the true reasons have not been clearly set forth, and men given "line upon line, and precept upon precept" until the continued warnings shall be heeded.

PROLAPSUS UTERI.

1. Spine.
2. Intestines.
3. Bladder.
4. Prolapsed Uterus.

The uterus (4) is frequently prolapsed, so that the whole organ is outside of the vagina. The illustration before us shows that it is as nearly prolapsed as possible and not be outside of the body. The intestines (2) are also prolapsed. We have had a case where a portion of the same were outside and below the uterus.

See organs of chest, figure 9, that the bladder is nearly round in its natural condition. The shape see (3) in prolapsus uteri, and in retroversion, and in anteversion, that other organs are so pressed against it that it must yield its rotundity. In prolapsus all the organs of the pelvis are displaced. Few know that the ordinary style of woman's dress will produce this and all other weakness of women without any other cause.

This consummation of the basest of degradations is practiced not only by the fast but by husbands and their wives.

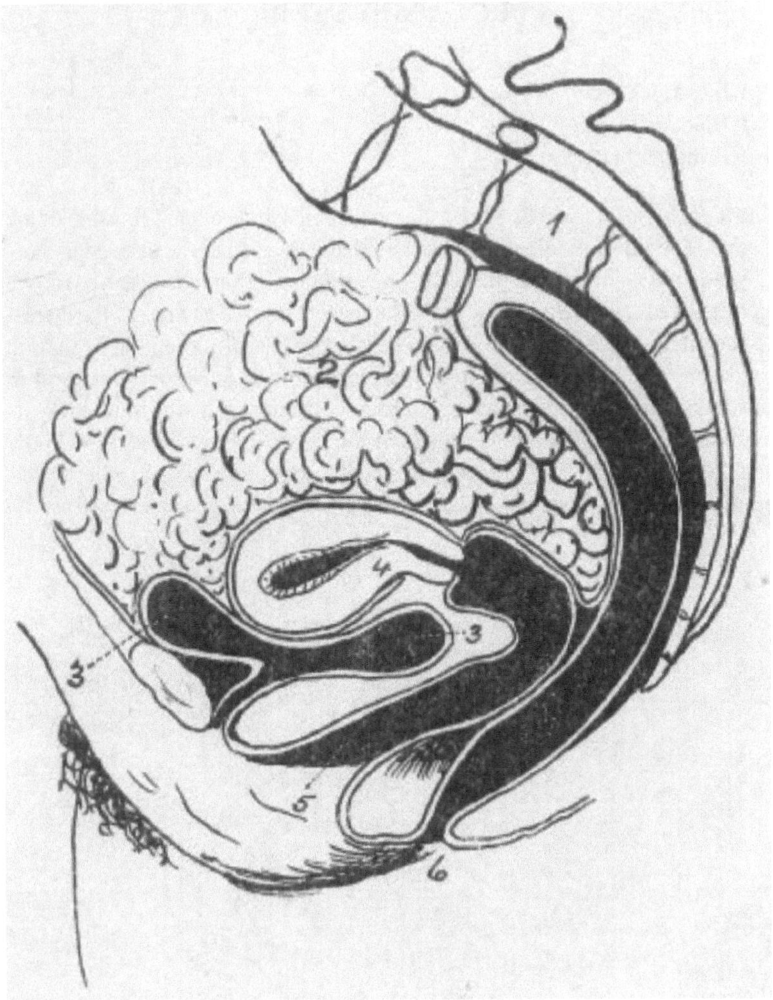

Anteversion of the Uterus.

PROLAPSUS UTERI.

1. Spine.
2. Intestines.
3. Bladder.
4. Prolapsed Uterus.

The uterus (4) is frequently prolapsed, so that the whole organ is outside of the vagina. The illustration before us shows that it is as nearly prolapsed as possible and not be outside of the body. The intestines (2) are also prolapsed. We have had a case where a portion of the same were outside and below the uterus.

See organs of chest, figure 9, that the bladder is nearly round in its natural condition. The shape see (3) in prolapsus uteri, and in retroversion, and in anteversion, that other organs are so pressed against it that it must yield its rotundity. In prolapsus all the organs of the pelvis are displaced. Few know that the ordinary style of woman's dress will produce this and all other weakness of women without any other cause.

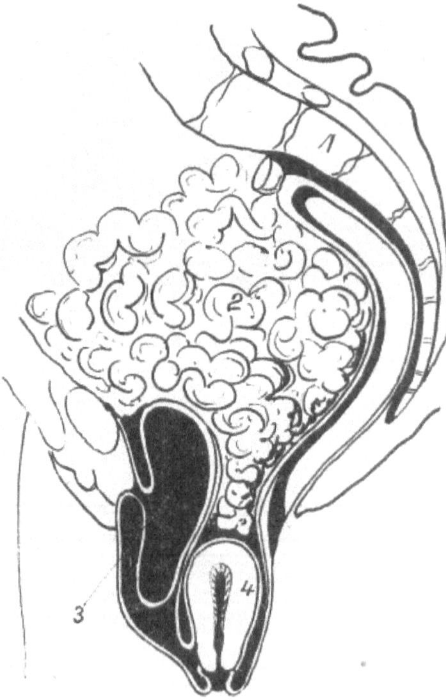

Prolapsus Uteri.

MASTURBATION.

There has never been a religious sect that has inaugurated the all-important law of protection to the unborn as have the Mormons. If all the evils with which they have been charged were true, they would weigh but little in comparison with the great and important ideas that they have established regarding the perfect protection of the *enceinte* woman from sexual abuse. All the strength of mind and body go to build up the child in utero, instead of enfeebling it by any sexual relation. Children born with such antenatal conditions have so much better nerves, and better control of their organs of sex, that they will have no desire to practice masturbation, to be polygamists, or sensualists. A large number of Mormons are not polygamists in practice, and do not use tobacco or any intoxicating drinks, and so we must look to the Mormons for a better race of people. Purity of manhood must come from the Mormons in greater numbers than from any other church unless there is a radical change in the churches, by advising the selfhood of women in the marriage relation to be sustained by their church creeds. Then will masturbation be lessened, and with a knowledge of its effects soon cease altogether.

The world was shocked when Fowler & Wells sent forth the truths to the world regarding the practice of masturbation being so great among the young.

Many people were quite angry because of the sweeping assertions made by these doctors, but close observation proved that all was true. The great injury to body and mind from this cause cannot be computed. The wrecks in insane asylums all over the country, the loss of general health, the inability to be stable, and a long category of evil results are now clearly to be discerned. All of which result from the utter ignorance of the subject. Tobacco, intoxicating drinks, pepper, and the heating and dragging of the mother's clothing all effect the boy in utero so that an effort for relief is made by masturbation.

The boys of to-day have more to contend with because of their antenatal condition than is apparent to those who have had but little thought upon the subject, for they are born with an inflamed prostate gland: this is situated around the urethra and in masturbation, (long before puberty,) gives forth a discharge. After puberty it frequently occurs that no amount of sexual variety or excess will prevent men from masturbation. This is sometimes practiced in the beds of their wives. This is more frequent after middle life than at any other time. Nature takes away the power of sexual gratification from men at a certain age. The time varies, and men who do not understand this law, rush to physicians for remedies. Excesses in sexual commerce and masturbation both leave old men with an irritable condition of the organs of sex, owing to an inflamed and enlarged prostate gland. The old man must pay for his iniquities in other ways than those usually considered.

Not only are the boys addicted to this practice as a result of the causes just mentioned, but one has only to visit the teachers of schools of every grade and age, where girls are sent, to be convinced to what an extent the wrongs of parents are visited upon daughters as well as sons.

No one can practice this vice without the sure marks of the same being left in the face.

In a certain country the making of rubber male organs for the purpose of facilitating girls in masturbation, is a lucrative business. The cost of manufacturing is about thirty cents, and they retail at from two to three dollars. They are of different sizes, and girls of various ages are taught by their companions their uses. When one size is outgrown, a larger size is purchased. They are kept at fancy shops attended by women, who ask their lady customers "what number of the Ladies' Companion they wish to have done up with their bundle." When the lady begins to talk about the magazines of that name, she is informed that "the 'Companion' is in a box."

This kind of masturbation, like all other ways of secret vice, sooner or later leads to sexual relations.

The effects of this vice on men are numerous. The most usual are consumption, insanity, softening of the brain and disease of the cuticle, and while all these are the effect on women, there is also an elongation of the clitoris, and a formation of warty excrescences on the vulva. Men or women who are addicted to this vice, cannot become parents of either a superior mental or physical type of humanity, because of loss of power. Such a person cannot be a desirable husband or wife, because of the loss of magnetic power.

Nothing so destroys the ability to think deeply, logically, gradually and connectedly as does orgasm even in the natural way if frequent, but especially in this true when produced in other ways.

The Oneida community learned this, and soon incorporated the idea in their religious teachings, and would have deserved the name of "Perfectionists," if they had lived up to their ideas, and not substituted promiscuity under certain arrangements. Their infringement of the great law, that sexual relation should not be had without emission, and that for posterity alone has aroused the thinker to decide that they have retrograded instead of advancing, for the long continued sexual excitement with suppressed orgasm is a serious injury to both body and mind.

Nature provides that the secretions of the relation should be properly mixed, one purpose of which is to sooth the nerves of both organs.

Their relationship is one of organized sensuality that does not fail to produce direful results on the minds and bodies of their participants, and but for the Onedia women wearing reform dresses, having an excellent diet, being systematic in exercise, and not being overworked, the bad results would be still more apparent.

The redeeming feature of the men, in never coercing women into sexual relationships has induced abused women to join the Onedia community. But we must forever condemn the double masturbation that sexual relation certainly is, when for licentious purpose alone, instead of for the procreation of humanity. But for women submitting to promiscuous sexual relations, they could not have their homes.

This we assert as a rule. Their submitting will make secret vice in their children a certain result, for such an excitement of the organs of sex cannot fail to produce their legitimate results in posterity.

It is well for the world that all kinds of experiments to evade the great and beautiful law of monogamic purity are being tested in a free country in an unrestrained manner under the law of religious liberty, for it is only through all of these experiences that those incapable of metaphysical depth can see the great laws of beauty and harmony as exemplified in the grandeur of a life free from all the objectionable features that such experiments have disclosed.

All kinds of vices and outrageous ways of human beings has caused some geniuses to invent remedies for relief from results in the shape of supporters, pessaries, trusses, uterine elevators, suspension bandages, etc., etc. But not until 1870 was the perfection of an equal to the Spanish inquisition patented by the United States. No doubt the inventor's intentions were good, as the following will show:

"My invention is a device for so covering up the sexual organs of a person addicted to the vice of masturbation, from his own touch and control, that he or she must refrain from the commission of the vicious and self-degrading act.

"It is well known to those who have charge of prisons, reform-schools, and the like, that the practice of masturbation becomes all but universal among those confined therein. It is also well known to physicians, and to some heads of families, that multitudes of children of both sexes injure their moral and physical natures for life by the practice of this vice.

"My invention is designed to put it into the power of those who have the control of all such persons to entirely prevent the practice."

We well knew that it came from a *man*, and he not a physician, for no intelligent woman would have been guilty of sending forth such an instrument, and when there shall be a woman doctor as an examiner for all articles intended for the use of women, nothing so monstrous will ever be patented. We will go farther and say *cruel*.

Here is the description:

"A band encircling the body just above the hips, the band being locked together behind by a small padlock, or other suitable device, the key to which is to be carried by the person who has charge of the masturbator.

"In front this band is connected, by numerous strips, with the lower band which at the rear passes down, one end under the leg, and both ends are attached to the rear of the pouch which pouch is made somewhat bag-like for the purpose of containing the organs. The front part of the pouch is attached to the lower band in front of the person.

"These various parts – the upper and lower bands, the connecting strips, and the pouch – may be of cloth, leather, or metal, or, in fact, any other convenient material. If made of metal, the parts which bear against the body must be padded to prevent chafing and injury to the person.

"The pouch should (at least I so prefer it) be made of rubber or metal, and at the rear a small hole or spout is left for the discharge of urine.

"The apparatus must be so fitted to the body as to have the edges of the pouch fit close against the person, so that it will be impossible for the wearer to touch the confined organ.

"If the connecting strips are made of metal, they should be hinged or pivoted to both the upper and lower bands, so as to allow free movement of the body.

"In addition to its property as a protector, this device serves a useful purpose in sustaining the bowels, like a truss, or as furnishing the foundation for the attachment of shoulder-braces.

"It is recommended that all the parts be made as flexible as is consistent with the office they have to perform."

In the first place there is no necessity for such an inquisitorial device, for a reform dress will prevent seduction and rape. If only pants are made in the ordinary way of slash fronts, anything of the kind would be impossible, for the vagina is so far from the centre of the pants rape could not be committed.

The undersuit is so constructed that a second barrier would also be met, and a third also in the second suit that is worn, as muslin and flannel are both worn, made in the same way. If for the purpose of preventing masturbation, a straight jacket will remedy that – but for the device itself. If worn in the daytime, in order for it to be large enough to cover the parts, and snug enough to prevent the vice being still practiced, it would interfere not only with locomotion, but so heat the parts that it would excite and agonize, besides inflaming the parts covered, and no matter what amount of "padding," it would irritate all around the pouch. The undried urine would agonize the girl. As for the strips around the legs, all women who wear the ordinary supporters with only cotton strips complain of chafiing. As for the padlock behind, that would prevent laying on the back – the bands around the body would so press upon the hips and body as to prevent laying on either side. But that is not the worst feature. No one can lay down and be at all *comfortable* with *any* fastenings around them, besides the positive injury to all pelvic organs, and no one can endure anything as snug around them when laying down as when sitting or standing, and if loose enough to be endurable, it could not be a *preventive* to masturbation. Any bands of any kind around the body are injurious we repeat to impress the fact.

To *prevent* an inclination to masturbation is the object of the wise. Do away with tobacco, strong drink and petticoats in parents, and children will not desire to commit the deed.

Teach the children to eschew tobacco, strong drinks, pepper and petticoats, and they will not be victims of social evils of any grade if *Unmasked* is put into their hands at an early age.

Where is there a father that will not thank the hand that saved both his boys and his girls by giving them a knowledge of *all* the evils of the world, that they may be forewarned and forearmed in their young years, before they learned by sad experience?

Any government, whether national or local, that obtains revenues from vice of any kind, whether it be intoxicating drinks, tobacco or contagious disease acts, pay dearly for such oversight, such ignorance, such downright crime.

When there is proper legislation regarding the manufacture of a sufficient quantity of intoxicating beverages for the arts, and a penalty for further destruction of grain and fruit food – a penalty for the manufacture of tobacco, or putting it into the market without strychnine or something so disgusting that it will not be used for other than insect exterminators, than we may with a diffusion of knowledge regarding baneful effects, hope to be rid of such evils.

As for *contagious disease acts*, and the revenue derived from the same; the two evils just mentioned are the parents of the necessity for considering the question, by irritating the whole nerve system, and especially that which is a part of and connected with the organs of sex.

Such inherited irritability, and such still farther irritability by use themselves, or by sexual contact with those who do use the same, are causes that we are astonished at so few comprehending. As for the efficiency of such a vile measure as the infamous contagious disease act, instead of lessening venereal diseases, it is increased – first, by the appearance of a freedom from the same when it is gnawing the intricate folds of the vagina, and has extended into the uterus, where it is impossible to discover the true condition, as not even labor pains can relax the uterus without so much blood flowing, that the true condition cannot possibly be seen; second, by men rushing into vice because it is sanctioned by law, and they have full confidence in the examination protection. But the most infamous (*and we pause for lack of adjectives to express any pure woman's emotions*) of anything ever enacted by men, is that *poor, seduced, helpless woman is made the disease monger of man*, under the guise of his being free from disease of the most agonizing nature, and seeking her because he *is* thus free and afraid of contamination, when the real fact is, that by variety life he has become diseased and thinks to rid himself by giving it to her.

Nothing can partake of brimstone selfishness to so great a depth as such an act!!!

But there is not a shadow of truth in the efficacy of such sophistry. The true logic is borne out by facts, that the freer such cases are from any excitement the better in all regards.

But as long as men alone make the laws, they will not submit to an examination themselves, to see whether they are free from disease, and a liability to give it to women. If it is proper for men in the profession to examine prostitute women to see that they are free from disease for men's use, it is as proper that women in the profession be also salaried to examine men prostitutes to see if they are free from disease for women's use.

Now be startled with "holy horror" at such a proposition as this, but remember that it is only turning the tables in words but when they are turned in reality regarding all of the one-sided sex outrages, the beauty of tweedledee and tweedledum will be as apparent to men as it is now to women.

A few men are even now looking at this one-sided moral business and taking action in recognition of the necessity of purity in men. Messrs. Walter M'Larens, George Warr, and others in London have a *Social Purity Alliance*.

Pere Hyacinth, (Catholic;) Zoadook Kahn, Grand Rabbi of Paris; the Archbishop of Paris; Rev. Dr. Baur, (Episcopal,) of Germany; Rev. Mr. Cook and

Saunter de Bloumey, of Geneva; M. Leon Richer and Theodore Manod, of Paris; Joseph Nathan, Alphonso Favre, Salvantore Colonna and Prof. Darneth, of Rome; Orris Brusea, of Milan; Rev. George Butler, F. W. Benting and A. L. Bernistee, of Liverpool; Henry Richards, M. P., Sir Harcourt Johnson, Right Hon. James Stanfield, Edward Blackhouse, Dr. Nevins, Dr. Routh, Dr. Drydale, Dr. Carter, Dr. Carson, Prof. Stewart, Prof. Sheldon, all from various places in England, besides many others that represent all the principal religions, the Materialists and the Spirtualists.

It is to be hoped that the time is not distant when every community will have a Social Purity Alliance among men, where vices of all kinds will be discountenanced.

The grand men whose names we have just mentioned, give their culture, position, words and examples to the great work. They attended the Geneva Congress last year, and one and all were disgusted with any sort of contagious disease acts, or anything sanctioning manhood impurity.

It is to be regretted that none of our finely cultured American women who fully understand the basic principles of the foundation of all permanent reforms, (*a proper dress for women,*) were not present. One practical exponent of a moral reform costume, would have given a tone and turn to the proceedings that would have sent reform a score of years into the grand future.

Every living example of an emblematic dress of purity, is worth a million speeches from those women who preach reforms of any kind while slaves to an immoral, bedecked, befurbelowed, and petticoated costume. Immoral women are disgusted with the inconsistency of such women who urge them to leave a life that provides the same extravagance and show of dress. Such long dressed women are ever calling forth a presumption in the minds of those they are working to reform, that there is the same want of proper protection of the organs of sex, and that the same facilities for vice can be found. And just as long as the ordinary long dress is worn, will there be such a presumption and such a reality. Cleanliness is next to morality. The fanning-mill of even ankle drapery, causes an accumulation of dust that reaches and excites the one who wears the same.

The purity of woman generally cannot be assured until the immoral dressing is stopped, for it unfits woman in body for the duties of life by its weight, cumberousness and expense, in mind by the drain of noble energies in following the ever changing fashions.

It is not frequent that a reliable and permanent structure of grand morality is builded upon stays, petticoats, and their accompanying absurdities, and the sooner the good men of the world see this and understand that human perfections of body, mind and morals, need sterner stuff than sham "*grace in drapery,*" (which is but a fitting term for languor and helplessness,) the world will be better in all regards.

Let all men do what is possible to encourage a sentiment of beauty of mind and large understanding of brain and boots, instead of talking sweet nonsense and praising little feet.

We call upon our so-called "protectors" to do their duty against the tyrant fashion.

When this is done women will need no protection from other tyrants. This monster one that sips vitality and virtue is the only one worth mention to be protected from, for all others will meekly bow when the tyrant fashion is destroyed.

Women and their children will not then be suicidists, but will gladly live as long as they can to be properly developed for another state of existence, and will not be constantly longing for someting to quiet their nerves. Men for tobacco and whisky, and women for gum and candy.

OBSCENE PUBLICATIONS.

The law regarding "obscene matter being sent through the mails," is an eminently proper one. But in order to be effectual, the power to decide regarding the character of questionable publications should be in the hands of the scientific and morally pure. Of all that have been arrested, few have deserved to be, and instead of decreasing their sales, the very arrests have excited curiosity regarding them. Those making quotations from the Bible are the only exception. The officer that is so ignorant as not to be familiar with Bible history, until informed in a court of justice by those defending themselves in suits for sending obscene matter through the mails, ought to cut out the obscenity and make a raid on all the Bible houses in the United States, in order to be consistent.

We think the Bible should be read by every mature person, for the grandest lessons are learned of perverted human nature, and the results of such perversion on posterity. The same immoralities with men making slaves of women were practiced then as they are to-day, and it would seem that the lessons learned from the Bible ought to prevent crimes of the darkest hue, especially with those who believe in its divine origin, that it does not, proves more than many are willing to acknowledge, and were it not for the friends of about fifty of many of the ablest clergymen in this country, we should here publish their names as proof of the vilest of immoralities having been practiced by them, and in nearly all instances their victims were "lambs of the flock," from the clergymen standing on the highest pinnacle of pulpit oratory, to the meekest of the clerical profession. Something more than the ordinary religion was needed for such men. Something plainer than even Bible history. Are their histories obscene?

Not only do members of churches commit all the crimes on the Bible calendar but the expounders of the Bible do just as badly, even to the incest of daughters under the pretense at first, that "*all* fathers have such a duty to do or their daughters would die," and afterwards threaten them with certain murder if they reveal the same.

It is but a few years since such a case occurred in western N. Y. while the clergyman was officiating in all his clerical duties for about three years of the time.

In Herkimer county, N. Y., in 1868, a woman having an only daughter about seventeen years of age visited her friend at a distance, leaving her daughter to keep house for her father. She had been absent but a few hours when the father of the girl asked her if she knew why her mother had gone on the visit, and then informed her of the duty of every father; and how he hated to be obliged to perform his duty; and that her friend, who died a few weeks before, would have lived if her father had done so.

* * * * * * * * * *

When her mother returned, she was so weary with travel that she reclined on her daughter's bed in the most quiet part of the house. Soon after dark her daughter, wearied with an unusual day's house work, retired with her. Late in the evening the husband and father returned from a neighboring town where he had been delayed on some business. He came to the daughter's room and immediately comprehending the situation took hold of both his daughter's feet (as he supposed) to awaken her, but through mistake in one of the feet awakened the wife and mother.

We lectured in the town where this occurred, but we have considered such a history too obscene to go through the mails to feed perverted taste, but we should be derelict in duty if we omitted here to show the infamous means taken by fathers to lie their own daughters into harlotry!

In closing this chapter on Social Evil, we must impress men with the magnitude of their duty to women in every relation of life, not forgetting their protecting power in prisons, station-houses, poor-houses, asylums and hospitals. All of these are more or less under the actual surveillance of men, when the women are weak in mind, body or morals, and more frequently than otherwise in all three regards.

Opportunities are not wanting to make easy facilities for vice, and that they are sometimes improved by both the doctors, stewards and others is a fact that cannot be denied, and that is a disgrace to civilization, since there are enough competent women doctors and stewards to manage the women's departments in all the institutions of the United States.

It is the duty of men to so protect all the women needing any public charities, and all who are by them locked up for any cause whatsoever.

They are not assuredly protected *as* women, unless every possibility of immorality is removed by women occupying every position relating to them.

Men are reared with the one idea prominent, that "there is a necessity for sexual relation with all men, and that all sorts of means to gratify their passions are in a way honorable," and wrongs to women will always result with opportunities, until the language of the nerves is understood, and that there is no such "necessity with men" any more than there is with women. And when boys are taught, as girls are, to control their natural passions, they will do so as well, and when they become men they will from habit be as pure. There are occasional proofs of this. When there are more pure men we shall soon find all excuses for vice placed where they belong. One of the flimsiest to keep women in an absurdly unprotected dress, is that it is unhealthy for women to be covered. Such talk from doctors, who were either knaves or were ignoramuses, have many times come to our ears. The fact is that a great deal of suffering is caused by a want of such protection. That it is a trick of the lascivious to have the facilities for vice easy is too patent for further mention, save that hundreds of women who have worn the reform dress for over a score of years can testify in regard to such dress benefiting them in every respect.

We do not know as our duty is done without again referring to Queen Victoria's domain, and entering our protest against wrong wherever it exist.

We refer her to the following facts and ask her to read our chapters on the Language of the Nerves and Pure Manhood, with the hopes that the wrong mentioned will be righted in the following manner. Pay her common soldiers so that they can afford to marry; remove their restrictions on marriage; repeal the Contagious Disease Acts; make provisions for the honorable self-support of the hundreds of thousands of women that have been the victims.

So good a woman as the Queen will not fail to do what is for the best good of her people when conditions are properly placed before her.

The preventing only one soldier in ten marrying in the English army has caused the Government to pass *Contagious Disease Acts* to protect the soldiers. These were passed in 1866 and 1869. At the close of 1874, 245,727 examinations were made on healthy women and girls. If these had not submitted they would have been imprisoned.

"The National Association" for the repeal of the infamous acts sent an address to the friends of Morality and Justice in America, and were represented by Mr. Henry J. Wilson and Rev. J. P. Gledstone, about two years. Since Mr. Wm. Haen, chairman, and Frederic Charles Banks, secretary of the Association.

The native women in India have committed suicide rather than submit to examinotions by State surgeons under the English Government.

In Yokohama, under British government, brothels have numerals over the doors.

In Hong-Kong brothels are licensed by the English Government.

We are opposed to having laws to compel vaccination, for it matters not how many cows the virus has been cleansed by, as long as there is enough of the poison to inflame the arm there is enough to injure the system, in insidious ways, that can be understood by reading the *language of the nerves*. Better trust to the possibility of having one poison of small-pox in the system than to deliberately introduce what no one knows how many poisons it contains.

CHAPTER XI.

Hernia.

Seven-tenths of the men are afflicted with hernia. This is too grave a matter to pass over with a mere mention of the fact.

The *reasoner* will at once look for the *cause*, while the unfortunate sufferers are testing the remedies.

Since all ages and both sexes are sufferers, we are surprised that no more remote causes than the crying of infants, and the severe toil of adults should be mentioned.

Here is a telling illustration of the truth, that women cannot suffer without men being sufferers also. The ordinary style of woman's dress so debilitates the pelvic organs of woman, that they are more or less prolapsed, as also are her abdominal viscera, the bowels. The whole of the organs of generation in women are weakened by their clothing. No petticoats, corsets, whalebones or any fastenings around the waist can be worn without injury to woman's abdominal and pelvic viscera. Men could not wear the ordinary clothing of women without injury, but it would be far less injurious to them than to women, because they have not women's pelvic organs to prolapse, to displace or otherwise injure.

But while women dress in this way, their sons are injured through them, to such an extent that many are born with inguinal hernia. In some cases it does not appear until a year or two of age. In a large number of instances, the membraneous tissue over the bowels and the muscular tissue over them, are so weakened that hernia is the sure result, from over work, a misstep, or from even less causes. When men evolve out of their might of ignorant oppression of scientific women who are dressing hygienically and use their influence and money to further general enlightment and practice of the true object of clothing, their sons and grandsons will be free from the sure tendency to hernia and not until then; it matters not what they may think regarding an ignorant standard of "taste," that is made by equally ignorant courtesans and *adopted* by them, not as a *principle of dress*, for ever-changing fashions cannot be principles. A reform dress is an embodiment of a principle; and as "principles are eternal," men will have the satisfaction ere long, to find that principles cannot be destroyed by any sort of oppression, but the real patriots and the true philanthropists, will join with the philosophers in establishing the same.

Dr. Nonot, the leading man of the profession in Paris, wrote the author a letter, in which he speaks of the ordinary arrangement of woman's clothing being one of the most fruitful causes of the weaknesses and diseases peculiar to women.

Dr. Banning, the great American inventor of *uterine elevators*, is explicit regarding the mechanical displacing of the abdominal and pelvic vicera by dress.

Prof. Phelps, of Andover University, acknowledged to be one of the most learned in the profession, said to his class "that the women of America would ere long be obliged to doff petticoats and put on pants, as the ordinary dress was an injury to the reproductive organs of woman and her whole nerve system."

It requires a high order of moral courage for a scientific man to express himself on the subject, when we calmly look the facts in the face, that so large a number of the women are monomaniacs on dress!

The general question now before the American people is not a *monetary* one; it is an *invalid* one. But examine the cut where the location of the organs of generation are plainly seen, and it will not be difficult for even the average man to comprehend what we have said regarding the mechanical injury of ordinary dress. It needs but little causality to readily see how hernia is the result of causes mentioned.

While woman's generative organs are affected as men's cannot be, because they are essentially different, so women who have anteversion, retroversion, inversion and prolapsus of the uterus not only transmit these tendencies to their daughters, but their sons have weaknesses of the organs of sex. Thus prolapsus of the scrotum may be directly the result of sexual excess, but there must be a weakened condition *inherited* to produce such a result, as is also the case with other difficulties that do not result from contagion. The law of inheritance is observed as nearly as is possible with the difference of sex.

CHAPTER XII.

The Language of the Nerves

PART FIRST.

Men argue that as the male animals pursue and force the females to yield, therefore the law of force in the sexual relations is the natural one for men as well as animal males; and that "as the male in the animal creation is always the one to take the initiative step towards the copulative act," that the question is thus forever settled that it is best and right for men to pattern after brutes and beasts. As well might such reasoners tell us that as beasts live in woods and caves, it is the natural and therefore the best way for men to live.

But so long as male brutes and beasts pursue the *force* system in sexual relation, and not wait until invited by female brutes and beasts, they can never rise to a higher condition; for, while they so degrade the companion in their most intense nerve association, that associate gives back to them enough of the degradation of force in *attempted* resistance, to keep the males down to nearly or quite the same level with the females, and often below them.

It is an insult to the higher types of brutes to compare them sexually with average men, for there are few in the whole animal kingdom that have as frequent and excessive sexual relations as do men. Among the animal exceptions are sheep, and but for such relationship being limited to a short season, and entire rest the most part of the year, they would not long survive. Sheep-growers have found that 5,000 ewes have conceived in one such season from a single male. It is not surprising that sheep should be so wanting in intelligence when all of their vitality is expended in sexual relations, for the losses through this source are losses to the brain! The same elements that repair the wastes of the one are requisite for the other; and hence it follows that those who have the most power in either direction have the power to concentrate the greater part of such power to either the purely intellectual or to the sexual.

Habits of thought and habits of life are magistrates, and the reasoner will at once see how important it is in youth and young manhood to cultivate the intellectual and higher faculties, and let the magistracy be of an ennobling nature.

But to return. It is not a fact that in the animal kingdom the males are all tyrants and take the initiative steps in sex relations, for, where they are living in a natural condition, the relations of the highest types of animals are mutual, called forth by the female. When the males assume rights of force the females resist, and hence the quarrels. It is said no other cause of quarrels are known to exist between male and female animals. The supreme right of selfhood asserts itself even in animal motherhood abilities, and resists invasion upon its rights – feebly, perhaps, but resists.

The very desire for the copulative relation is one for the *result* of the relation – the offsprings; and yet the love itself is often as much in embryo as the offspring itself; so little is the subject understood, because so little thought upon. And yet no man or woman can love another truly without a love for the future offspring that the relation of husband and wife is to produce. There is something wanting in pure love devotion if that want and love of posterity is not felt, even if not expressed. The marriage relation from the first should and would be one of no false delicacy, but as a pure relation if both men and women were pure and true to themselves before marriage, reserving their emotions for the one who was to be the partner of all joys and sorrows through the dim vista of middle life and old age. Whatever else influences the youth of both sexes, neither sex should ever swerve from the one fixed purpose to love and cherish the future husband or wife, and never be guilty of act or deed that would destroy or lessen the confidence in sexual purity. The well-being and complete confidence and happiness of the marriage relation demands equal purity, and such demand cannot be disregarded with impunity. Cumulative wrongs before marriage tell the tale after marriage – perhaps not audibly, but tell it just as plainly to husband or wife. To illustrate, we see, feel, act, smell, taste and hear all through the nerves. All these modes of communication are double, except the mouth from which we send forth speech; and when that refuses to tell the truth there is no power to stop the little tell-tale nerves. And so when every energy of the whole system is concentrated through the most highly sensitive ganglion of nerves, the life story is told in the ears of the nerves they meet through the agency of the wonderful nervo-magnetic fluid; and, although the power to fully comprehend *just* what the life of the other has been may not be possessed by all, yet a sufficient comprehensive power will be experienced to fully insure perfect confidence or to convince of deception, and that of a nature that there is an object in the deceiver concealing forever.

PART SECOND.

If men were better informed in regard to women, they would understand how it is for their own physical and mental interest to respond to a wife's call, as the ruling power in all sexual relations. Men would never force, or even coax their wives to yield to them if the laws of the relation of the sexes were well understood with all the insidious results of force, or or even of coaxing. Such is the construction of the nerves of the vagina, that when they are not in a condition to bear friction, they are morbidly sensative, and if compelled to endure it, either by stronger physical power, or by persuasion, woman feels a repulsion to man through the shock to the sensitive nerves, and just as clearly as though he had struck her in anger. When man uses force to compel against the desire of woman, even if she is perfectly healthy, a poison is sent forth from the walls of the vagina that injures his whole system, and shortens his days. So great is this poison that it sometimes produces an elongation of the urethra, causing intense pain, and has been thought by those not understanding the cause to be a cancerous growth. Some are able to walk about when thus afflicted, but months elapse before restoration is possible.

The poison that produces this result, is an abnormal forcing of the natural secretions of the vagina, that are farther poisoned by the stinging nerves of the vagina that act on the nerves of the penis when in the highest and most susceptible condition possible to any part of the system, and when beyond his power to resist the influences that are sent with more than lightning speed all through his whole nerve system. It is in this way that the "copper blowing" is accomplished in England.

The angry wife holds a copper penny in her mouth and when the orgasm is perfected by the infamous husband who forces her to yield to him; she blows with nearly closed mouth and poisons him to death. These two kinds of poisoning can be readily understood when we realize that the poison of a snake is harmless, unless the snake is angry and throws its venom into an otherwise harmless secretion, (as its only means of defense.) Women unconsciously use the first poison spoken of as *their* only *means* of defence against repetitions of tyranny, and in aggravated cases, have used the "copper blowing" as a perpetual relief from a tyranny worse than death.

Nothing in life more aggravates and angers women than any advantage taken of the sexual relation, but men who complain of unappreciative and cross wives are generally utterly ignorant of the cause of the same, and often out of real spite to punish them for something, compel them to submit to the sexual relation, when they do not dare to strike them for fear of law finding the marks.

Men see that these marital rapes quiet their wives for a time through fear of repetition, not fully understanding that the very quiet is a debility that will effect themselves as soon as a repetition is resorted to, and as soon as nature has struggled sufficiently to assert her right of individuality in woman, she feels the same anger so intensified that she resolves to kill her tormentor as a sure means of getting rid of a vile man that torments outside of the redress of common law.

But if these men do not pay for such conduct by losing their lives, they pay dearly for such fiendish cruelty in their old years, by having helpless and loveless wives who lose all confidence in them and all interest in anything that relates to their comfort.

The same unhappy feelings and unrest of soul that they caused their wives, is taken back upon themselves by the very relationship that gives little else to such men than a fiendish gratification that never soothes and charms, but instead, exhausts and leaves about as pleasant emotions as the conquest of killing a snake. And the wife instead of being left tenderly as wives expect and have a right to expect to be, they are left with about the same emotions of indifference as a dead snake would be left, or as a savage leaves a white woman after his captive raping of a woman who has been an hour in his possession, too frightened to have the power to even attempt a hopeless resistance.

And yet with this terribly truthful picture before us, with the mass of men feeling that they have a right to demand of wives and compel obedience in sexual relations, we look upon men with a charity that only one who has gone into the metaphysics of social life is capable. For no woman has enlightened them upon the subject of *real* causes, and *unmistakable* effects, and no man has had the facilities to trace effect to cause and cause to effect as we have had, and no woman, save a professional one, could delve into social life with a full comprehension of causes and remedies.

The whole question of the essential part is settled by *woman always having supreme control of her person*, as regards an invasion by men.

The sexual relation should be for posterity, and as soon as this is accomplished, there should be no other relation until another child is desired. No woman properly balanced and with perfectly healthy sexual organs has a desire for such relationship, and if she submits to the same, the Language of the Nerves is such that the child in embryo is so taught sensuality that the coming man or woman is affected for life with such antenatal influences. The prospective mother begins to hate the embryonic child, as her maternal love is all clouded or destroyed by sensuality, and she begins to devise ways and means to *destroy*, instead of cherishing the little unseen. It matters little whether woman is a willing or unwilling victim of sensuality, whether as a wife or a promiscuous mistress, the love of posterity is destroyed, and the woman who fails to rid herself of her unwelcome charge, brings into existence a sensualist, a thief, a robber, a hermaphrodite, or at best an inharmonious specimen of humanity, that hates its parents for being compelled to have such an unwelcome existence. All through the period of its embryonic life the Language of the Nerves is constantly taught, and the sentiments pervade every cell of the poor little piece of infantile helplessness.

The truer one is to self, (other things being equal,) the deeper and grander the thoughts. Who can tell to what depths of unknown science the human mind is capable of evoluting, if the nervo-magnetic powers are not injured in utero, or by themselves in conscious existence. What grandeur of comprehension of the eternal principles of brain power the evolution of thought shall yet give to the world, depends on pure manhood and pure womanhood to demonstrate.

It is deplorable, that many of the deepest minds, the most metaphysical reasoners, the clearest logicians, the grandest scientists and the purest moralists among women, must look in vain for their equals in all these regards, and die without leaving to the world specimens of humanity that shall be superior to themselves and capable of delving into the grandeurs and sublimities that are now beyond conscious possibilities.

If through the evolution of our thoughts, as contained in this little volume, the women of the future, on both sides of the great waters, shall have better conditions, we shall feel that our earth life has been one of noble effort, that no amount of contumely from the degraded can rob of pure satisfaction.

Editorial Headnote

Walter Rivington, *The Medical Profession: Being the Essay to Which Was Awarded the First Carmichael Prize of £200 By the Council of the Royal College of Surgeons, Ireland* (Fannin & Co.: Dublin, 1879), pp. 134–138

Walter Rivington (1835–1897) was a surgeon and lecturer initially in anatomy, and then in surgery and operative surgery, at his alma mater, the London Hospital, from 1863 until retirement in 1890, when he became Consulting Surgeon. He also was Dean of the Medical School, where a successful campaign to encourage entrance scholarships characterised his reign. Between 1878 and 1883 he was Examiner in Anatomy at the Royal College of Surgeons and became a Council member representing the 'Reform Party' in 1891, President of the Hunterian Society in 1883, and acted as Secretary of the London Hospital Club from the late 1860s until his death. Rivington was also a member of the Standing Committee of the Convocation of the University of London and campaigned against any alteration in the constitution of the University, recommended by the Commission led by Lord Cowper. When in June 1896, he came up in a University Fellowship election against fellow surgeon Joseph Lister, who was in favour of reconstituting the University into a teaching body, Rivington won the vote.

Obituaries noted that Rivington was only a 'good general surgeon', but with no advances to his name. His bent, indeed, was 'literary rather than practical'. He was, as a consequence, thorough and exact in all his publications, showing 'a patient industry, an extreme accuracy, and a completeness which exhausted the subjects at the time they were written'.[1] Rivington won the Carmichael Prize twice – firstly, in 1879, excerpted here, and, secondly, in 1887. The Carmichael Prize, instigated from a £3000 bequest to the College of Surgeons in Ireland by Mr Richard Carmichael in 1866, was awarded every four years. It sought to, as Rivington noted in his Preface to the 1879 prize-winning entry, provide a 'plain and unvarnished account of the state of the Medical Profession', coupled with consideration of the hospitals and schools, the state and mode of examination of the varied awarding bodies.[2] When the prize was first awarded in 1868, the *Athenaeum* remarked upon the hope that it would be 'something more than a stimulant to literary amateurs and a source of gain to printers and paper-makers'.[3] Nearly twenty years later, when Rivington won the prize for an identically titled essay on *The Medical Profession*, the length of the essay had reached 1200 pages, as opposed to the 500 of the 1879 version. The *Dublin Journal of Medical Science* despaired at the pointlessness of the exercise, when a book weighing four pounds could win the top £200 'essay' prize, and the second, coming in at only two pounds, could be awarded £100.[4] For the *Dublin Journal*, essays were original compositions; the Carmichael Prize appeared to encourage rehashing of tired medical histories and student-level periodicals. More vitally, no one read them – neither the profession nor the layman, who could receive no enlightenment from these exercises. Rivington's winning the prize twice attracted the notice of the *British Medical Journal* which remarked similarly on the 'portentous sign of the volubility of the times' when essays could be over 1000 pages, and recommended judicious editing.[5] The *Lancet*, however, viewed these publications differently as 'quite valuable' reference books exploring the 'organisation and condition of the profession'. For this periodical, the prize secured a 'large and enlightened view of the questions which agitate and affect the profession', and Rivington characteristically did not omit anything from the Druids to the admission of the dentists.[6] Although lengthy and exhaustive, the *Lancet*'s viewpoint has prevailed. Rivington's contributions remain key documents for understanding the quotidian minutiae, the history of practise from the earliest times, and the day-to-day frustrations, including medical women, that exorcised the profession in the later nineteenth century.

Notes

1 'Rivington, Walter, (1835–1897), Plarr's Lives of the Fellows, at https://livesonline.rcseng.ac.uk/client/en_GB/lives/ [accessed 10 October 2023]; 'Obituary', *BMJ*, 1:1898 (15 May 1897), pp. 1255–1256.
2 Preface to Walter Rivington, *The Medical Profession: Being the Essay to Which Was Awarded the First Carmichael Prize of £200 By the Council of the Royal College of Surgeons, Ireland* (Dublin: Fannin & Co.,1879).
3 'Science', *Athenaeum*, 2127 (1 August 1868), pp. 149–151; on p. 150.
4 'The Carmichael Prize Essays, 1887', *Dublin Journal of Medical Science*, LXXXVII (1 May 1889), pp. 422–424.
5 *BMJ*, 1.1474 (30 March 1889), pp. 717–718.
6 'The Carmichael Essays for 1887', *Lancet*, 132:3408 (22 December 1888), p. 1240.

6

THE MEDICAL PROFESSION: BEING THE ESSAY TO WHICH WAS AWARDED THE FIRST CARMICHAEL PRIZE OF £200 BY THE COUNCIL OF THE ROYAL COLLEGE OF SURGEONS, IRELAND

Walter Rivington

Source: Walter Rivington, *The Medical Profession: Being the Essay to Which Was Awarded the First Carmichael Prize of £200 By the Council of the Royal College of Surgeons, Ireland* (Fannin & Co.: Dublin, 1879), pp. 134–138

Some account must now be given of amendments of the Medical Act.

The Medical Act of 1858 has been amended nine times; once in 1859, twice in 1860, once in 1862, once in 1868, once in 1873, once in 1875, and twice in 1876.

In 1859 an Act (22 Vic., c. 21) was passed for the purpose of extending the time of registration, to repeal Schedule D, and to correct some clerical errors and omissions in the Medical Act.

The first Act of 1860 (23 Vic., c. 7) extended the time for registration and permitted the registration of Licences in Surgery. The second Act (23 and 24 Vic., c. 66) related to the College of Physicians.

In 1862 the Medical Council was incorporated by the 25th and 26th Vic., c. 91. The exclusive right of publishing, printing, and selling "The British Pharmacopœia" is vested in the Council, and "The British Pharmacopœia" is to supersede all existing Pharmacopœias in the kingdom.

The Medical Act Amendment Act, 1868 (31 and 32 Vic., c. 29), or an "Act to amend the Law relating to Medical Practitioners in the Colonies," was directed to the amendment of the 31st section of the Medical Act.

In 1873 was passed "The University of London Act" (36 and 37 Vic., c. 55) – the enabling Act before alluded to. It enables the University to make a law prescribing that no person can become a graduate in medicine unless he has passed the conjoint examination. Such by-law must be approved by one of Her Majesty's

DOI: 10.4324/9781003265238-6

principal Secretaries of State, and the assent thus given may be revoked at any subsequent time.

In 1875 "The College of Surgeons Act" (38 and 39 Vic., c. 43) – the enabling Act – was passed.

In 1876 two important Acts affecting the Medical Act were passed.

The first (Mr. Gibson's Bill) is called "the Medical Practitioners Act, 1876" (39 and 40 Vic., c. 40). It provides (1) that all legally qualified practitioners in medicine and surgery shall be capable of election as surgeons to county infirmaries and hospitals in Ireland, and (2) that the qualification of Bachelor of Surgery from any University in the United Kingdom legally authorised to confer the same may be registered under the Medical Act.

The second was Russell Gurney's Act. It is called "An Act to Remove the Restrictions on the Granting of Qualifications on the ground of Sex" (39 and 40 Vic., c. 41), and enacts that the powers of the bodies entitled to grant qualifications for registration shall extend to the granting of any qualification for registration granted by such body to all persons without distinction of sex. The exercise of such powers is not rendered compulsory. Defective provision is made for the continued exclusion of women from the government of the Corporations.

The profane attempt of ambitious women to enter the sacred precincts of the medical profession has aroused the warmest feelings of antagonism within the charmed circle of regular male practitioners. True it is that there have been medical women from remote periods of antiquity. The professional mind appears to be unable to contemplate with calmness the near prospect of actually existing female doctors, although its equanimity would be undisturbed by any historic portrait. It is not that the arguments against women undertaking medical practice are overwhelmingly strong, and that the supporters of female practitioners are perversely blind to their cogency – for the arguments on the other side are not without force – but that there is something in the nature of the idea which carries away a certain section of the profession, and leads to the display of an antipathetic feeling unsurpassed in intensity by any which is called forth by any other professional topic. Many of the most estimable members of our profession perceive in the medical education and destination of women a horrible and vicious attempt of women deliberately to unsex themselves – in the acquisition of anatomical and physiological knowledge the gratification of a prurient and morbid curiosity and thirst after forbidden information – and in the performance of routine medical and surgical duties the assumption of offices which Nature intended entirely for the sterner sex. Hence the antagonists of medical women lose all patience over the topic, and are incapable of arguing it with any approach to calmness. Indeed, what is called strong argument is generally mere assertion and a warmer display of feeling than usual. The eminent physician who would rather follow his daughter to the grave than see her studying practical anatomy forgets that he is not obliged to bring up his daughter to the medical profession, and that the fact that he would not allow his daughter to be medically educated is no ground for preventing his neighbour from allowing his daughter to acquire knowledge and skill. Neither does it amount to anything but an exuberant outburst of feeling to say that if women are admitted to degrees at the London University, the opponent of the measure will do his best to prevent any young friends or pupils from taking the degrees of the University. It would be going too far in the opposite direction to charge the antagonists of medical women with trades unionism; it would be considered justly offensive and gratuitous, but this is a charge which unprofessional supporters of medical women might urge and have urged with some plausibility, because the effect is the same as if the trades union spirit actually prevailed. Without professing ourselves to be at all enthusiastic in favour of a medical career for women – for we think that by frame, temperament, and mental constitution, woman is not well adapted for medical, far less for surgical practice – we think that it is not for the members of our calling to do more than exercise a private influence against the destination of young women to the medical profession. Medical practitioners are excellently placed for supplying information concerning the nature of a medical student's career, the difficulties and dangers of the profession, and for tempering the enthusiasm which has not yet encountered stern realities. It is not, however, the office of our profession to lead the van of any public crusade against the admission of women into our own ranks. Such opposition is sure to be decried as akin to trades unionism, and it is difficult to refute the charge. We may solemnly aver that the opposition of our profession to the admission of women is disinterested, and is solely to prevent injudicious women from embarking on a course which must prove injurious to them. Unfortunately our protestations would be received by the public with incredulity. The Legislature has determined that the experiment shall be tried. By all means let it be tried. It is said that there is a demand for female medical services amongst members of their own sex and amongst children. Be it so. The experiment will determine the depth of the demand. Prior to the action of the Legislature it was our opinion that there was nothing, and could be nothing, very dreadful in opening the stores of medical knowledge to women. It is illogical to confound the painstaking acquirement of scientific terminology with the gratification of a prurient curiosity. There is no heat in knowledge or science, and there is a distinct advantage in women acquiring exact medical knowledge, and aiding in its diffusion, instead of remaining in the crass darkness of popular fallacies and delusions. There is much need for the spread of information on ordinary topics, such as on the proper food and proper clothing for children, which women with a sound medical training are well fitted to impart. Furthermore, it was our opinion that the question of medical women was a very small question, which had been elevated into importance by the violence of the opposition. To move heaven and earth, metaphorically speaking, to endeavour to exclude a few ladies from the medical profession never seemed either a wise or a dignified procedure. We say a few, because we feel convinced that the movement must always be of a limited character. Women's disabilities are too many to allow more than a few to adopt the medical profession as a livelihood. Woman is too heavily handicapped to compete with man in medical practice. Were it otherwise, what right should we have to hinder women from choosing a professional career? and if it be so, what necessity exists for the lords of creation to interfere? Yet such is the inconsistency of the opponents of medical women that, though they insist that a medical career is impossible for women on physical grounds and sexual grounds alone, yet they are unwilling to trust to natural obstacles, but desire to shelter the women or themselves behind legal disabilities. Surely this displays "a will most incorrect to heaven, a heart unfortified, a mind impatient, an understanding simple and unschooled." Happily the Legislature has broken down the barrier, and a few years will demonstrate how little vitality is possessed by the movement for the medical education of women, how small will be the response in the ranks of women themselves, and with what false fears and vague alarms the professional mind has been agitated.

Editorial Headnote

Emma Hosken Woodward, *Men, Women, and Progress* (London: Dulau and Co., 1885), pp. 119–141

Although now obscure and forgotten, Emma Hosken Woodward (1845–1884) was a briefly successful sensation novelist and writer on the 'Woman Question'. She was born in Cornwall and lived in Wales, with her first husband and three children. When both her husband and young son died of diphtheria over a period of two years, she returned to her mother's home with her remaining children.[1] She was married again in 1882 to Bernard Barham Woodward (1853–1930), writer, researcher, and librarian at the British Museum and then the Natural History Museum.[2] They lived in West Kensington Park, London, where Emma Hosken Woodward died on 16 July 1884.[3]

Hosken Woodward's brief foray into novel writing showed clear signs of her later ability to combine thoughtful conversation with narrative. *Married for Money*, her short one-volume first novel, appeared anonymously early in 1875, and was advertised frequently that year.[4] The *Athenaeum* reviewed it as a 'thrilling tale' 'diversified by intervals of learned conversation'.[5] Although published anonymously, the three-volume *Bitter to Sweet End*, a 'charming story', received a lengthy five-page report in the *New Monthly Magazine* of July 1877. Set in Wales, where the heroine is born in secrecy to an Italian mother who dies soon afterwards, Gladys is adopted by a farmer and his wife, but turns out to be the legitimate daughter of a local landowner. Various complicated and exciting events ensued, but they are well worked out, according to the *New Monthly* reviewer, ensuring that the work was of 'superior class to the run of modern novels', with a 'thoughtful, meditative, and wise spirit'. This 'undercurrent of philosophic morality' and ability to tell a good tale would stand Hosken Woodward in good stead for her final work on *Men, Women and Progress*.[6] The novel was one of the *Athenaeum*'s 'Books of the Week'. Although criticising its anonymity and tendency to overwrite and to focus too much on addressing readers and reviewers, the *Athenaeum* praised the 'considerable reading' both in Latin and in European languages of the author (the reviewer has decided she is a woman from the evidence within).[7] George Saintsbury, in the *Academy*, called the novel 'decidedly tolerable', but was annoyed by the self-awareness of her (also a good guess) 'disquisitions'.[8] It was to 'disquisitions' that Hosken Woodward would turn in her next production.

Although completed in June 1884, *Men, Women and Progress* did not appear until February 1885, and was priced at 7/6, three shillings cheaper than *Married for Money*.[9] As the 'editor', her thinly-disguised husband, 'B.B.W.', explained in the 'Preface', Emma Hosken Woodward had died after the book had been completed, but before it could be fully edited. 'B.B.W.' dedicated the volume to Hosken Woodward's daughters, Agnes Emily and Gwendoline Mary, in the hope that they would follow their mother's example in aiding the 'weak and helpless'. The conversational genre employed as a narrative device drew both on Hosken Woodward's skill at weaving ideas into fictional situations and upon a longstanding familiar format for explaining scientific and political theories, popularised earlier in the century by Jane Marcet (1769–1858). This style did not please the *Saturday Review*, which was bored by the book, calling it 'stoutish' and 'full of the dreadful woman question', especially when it was 'debated in long talks by people who sit down and spout at one another in cold blood'.[10] Topics such as 'Women's Rights and Men's Wrongs', education, employment, social problems, and suffrage proved far more attractive to periodicals focusing on women's rights. The *Women's Suffrage Journal* recommended it to voters and to legislators, advertising the book on its front cover.[11] As a former contributor to their journal on 'Women's Rights in 1739', the *Englishwoman's Review* extolled Hosken Woodward's considerable virtues. Unlike the *Saturday Review*, this periodical saw judicious and balanced debate, with 'hesitation and difficulties', rather than zealousness, characterising the majority of the conversational pieces on this 'many-sided question'.[12]

Only one edition was produced of *Men, Women and Progress*, but its European popularity can be indicated by the advent of a German translation in 1893. *Männer, Frauen und Fortschritt* was published by the Weimar house Weimarer Verlagsanstalt, a key producer of works on the 'Frauenfrage' ('Woman Question') in Germany.

Notes

1 T.J. Bassett, 'Author: Emma Hosken Woodward', *At the Circulating Library: A Database of Victorian Fiction, 1837–1901,* 25 June 2023, www.victorianresearch.org/atcl/show_author.php?aid=2579 (accessed 10 October 2023).
2 Obituary: Mr B.B. Woodward', *Times*, 30 October 1930, p. 19.
3 *Morning Post*, 19 July 1884, p. 1.
4 'Mr Samuel Tinsley's List of New and Forthcoming Works', *Athenaeum*, 2468 (February 1875), p. 239.
5 'Novels of the Week', *Athenaeum*, 2482 (22 May 1875), pp. 684–686; on p. 685.
6 *New Monthly Magazine*, 12:67 (July 1877), pp. 94–98.
7 *Athenaeum*, 2588 (2 June 1877), pp. 701–702.
8 *Academy*, 267 (16 June 1877), pp. 530–531; on p. 531.
9 *Times*, 27 February 1888, p. 12; *Bookseller*, CCXXVII (5 March 1885), p. 254.
10 'New Books and Reprints', *Saturday Review*, 59:1532 (7 March 1885), p. 328.
11 *Women's Suffrage Journal*, XVII:CCI (1 September 1886), p. 1.
12 *Englishwoman's Review*, XVI:CXLII (4 February 1885), pp. 51–55.

7

MEN, WOMEN, AND PROGRESS

Emma Hosken Woodward

Source: Emma Hosken Woodward, *Men, Women, and Progress* (London: Dulau and Co., 1885), pp. 119–141

CHAPTER VI.

THE EMPLOYMENT OF WOMEN (CONTINUED).

'I AM far from disagreeing with all the ideas which (as complimentary chairmen say at a public meeting) have found such able advocates,' said Sir Henry presently, resuming the discussion that had been momentarily interrupted, 'but I think after all it is only to be expected that, just or unjust, there should be great difficulties in the way of women's obtaining admission to the higher professions, seeing that on the one hand people will scarcely give them employment until they have proved their capacity, and it is difficult to know how they are to prove their capacity without getting employment.'

'The only course, I think,' said Madeline, 'is to quietly persevere; the more they do and do well the more they will be called upon to do, and the less opposition will they meet with from all sensible people; but I have seen something of how sadly paralysing in its effect (even upon those who feel that with a fair chance they could prove the contrary) is the common notion that a woman's work must be inferior; women naturally resent the injustice of being judged not by ability but by sex.'

'Their being weaker is a strange reason for making the battle of life harder,' said Mrs. Silverton; 'and it is singularly inconsistent to bring this fact forward as an objection only when high class or well-paid employments are in question, whereas women may toil in our factories, may work in the fields, may stand hour after hour and day after day over the wash-tub, a young girl may do the whole work of a large house full of lodgers and carry up long flights of stairs heavy loads that would tax even masculine muscles, and yet no one thinks she is here out of her proper sphere.'

DOI: 10.4324/9781003265238-7

'But,' replied Sir Henry, 'if you prohibit men from engaging in light employments such as you were speaking of just now, and most of which I grant might be more appropriately given up to your sex, I think in common fairness you should not claim free admission to all the occupations in which hitherto men exclusively have been engaged.'

'Before this question can be settled,' said Professor Wray, 'we shall have to define much more clearly than any one has yet done, what is a man's and what a woman's work.'

'What are your ideas upon the subject; I suppose even you draw a line somewhere?'

'It seems to me the only sensible conclusion is that such mechanical employments as involve the greatest physical labour should devolve exclusively upon men, the lighter, those which require most delicacy and finish, upon women, that each should do in fact without restriction what they are most capable of doing, while all intellectual work should be freely open to competition, without regard to sex. It is neither just nor generous that men should shrink from free and open competition and take advantage of their own political and civil power to frame enactments, shutting in the face of women, anxious to earn a living, the doors of all the most profitable professions.'

'It is curious to note the posts that have on rare occasions been filled by women,' said Madeline, 'not excepting the office of Grand Chamberlain, and that of Clerk of the Crown in the Court of Queen's Bench. There is a place in Norfolk, for instance, where a woman was once appointed parish clerk, because, it was said, that in a population of six hundred there was not a man who could read and write. Women, in exceptional cases, have been both soldiers and sailors, while I remember seeing it asserted in a note to De Quincey's works that many women, in order to obtain fair wages and freedom of labour, have from time to time, disguised in men's clothes, got their living as bricklayers, grooms, or even navvies.'

'One can scarcely be surprised at their undertaking even work so unsuitable as this,' said the Professor, 'when in most cases you find, as we were saying just now, remuneration apportioned to the sex of the worker rather than to the amount or quality of the work.'

'*A propos* of this,' said Madeline, 'a literary man told me a few months ago that he was going to publish a series of manuals on popular educational subjects, but, with a view to economy, he meant to manage the business of printing, binding, advertising, &c., himself, giving some publisher a commission for pushing the books and for allowing his name to appear upon the title-pages. "Do you think women-printers are to be trusted to do the work as thoroughly as men?" he asked. "Certainly," I replied. "You see," he went on, "we think of employing them, as no doubt they would do it for about half the money." "That seems rather unreasonable," I said, "and, under these circumstances, I could scarcely venture to guarantee the quality of the work, as you would probably obtain only second-rate hands, and then cite your experience as a proof of the inferiority of women-printers in general." '

'The natural result of women's field of labour being so limited,' said Professor Wray, 'is, that such occupations as *are* open to them soon become overcrowded, and though their pay is inadequate, they cannot say as a man would, "Unless you raise my wages I shall leave." The profession of teaching is one that is always supposed to be open to educated women, but, except for those who have been trained and certificated, the demand for governesses is still very far short of the supply, a glance down the columns of any daily paper is sufficient to show this.'

'I heard of a case not long ago,' said Mrs. Silverton, 'where, to an advertisement for a nursery governess who was to have no salary, as many as three hundred replies were received.'

'I remember also some time since,' said Madeline, 'a clergyman advertised at the same time for a governess for his own children and a mistress for the village school, and though any candidate for the former post, while expected to be a lady, was to receive a considerably smaller salary, for this he received scores of applications, for the latter not a single one.'

'I quite agree with you,' said Sir Henry, 'that the position of women of the better classes when reduced to poverty is very sad, but the parish schoolmistress, it is evident from your own account, has not much to complain of.'

'I am not so sure of that; it is the almost universal testimony of Government Inspectors, that women-teachers at least equal men in ability and success, and yet they cannot command the same salaries. I remember seeing in the *Athenæum*, not long since, two advertisments; a master and mistress were wanted for an important school in Newcastle, the most the latter could receive, including capitation-fees, was 150*l.* a-year, whilst the former might get 300*l.* besides a house, and yet she was no doubt expected to be equally capable. Even those women who, thanks to Mr. Fawcett, are holding superior appointments in the Post-Office Savings' Bank, are doing their work, I believe, for about one-third of the salary received by men of the same standing, and the same disproportion is to be found in every department of industry.'

'It is the old question of demand and supply, I suppose,' said Sir Henry.

'Exactly,' replied his sister, 'and so long as the supply of women-workers is so out of all proportion to the demand, so long is it the duty of every one who loves justice to do all they can to enlarge this sphere of work.'

'But, honestly,' replied her brother, 'you must acknowledge, I think, that though old time prejudices may be to blame, you do not generally, amongst men now-a-days, meet with any active opposition to women who are anxious to work in some hitherto untried field.'

'I know many men as unselfish as they are just,' said Madeline, 'who would scorn to do it, but I am afraid they are exceptions. Sir John Bennett was once mobbed, so I have understood, for advocating the general employment of women in watchmaking; a few years ago in Paris a firm of printers wished to employ some women-compositors, but the men banded themselves together to stop it, and the idea had to be abandoned; only a short time ago at Kidderminster again, although velvet-weaving in no way affects the carpet-weavers, there was a strike of the latter against the employment of female labour on looms for making velvet.'

'The attempt to employ women in London as jewel-burnishers,' said Professor Wray, 'promised to answer well, some girls earning as much as three and sixpence a-day, but their master was unwillingly obliged to dismiss them owing to the jealousy of his male *employés*. In the potteries for many years men were so jealous of the competition of women-labourers, that they brought the whole force of their trades union to prevent women from using the hand-rest, which was of the greatest service in producing both rapidity and precision of work.'

'But they were not gentlemen,' said Sir Henry, 'in any sense of the word; I had not such fellows as these in my mind.'

'The conduct of the medical students in Edinburgh towards the six ladies, who, in 1869 applied for admission there to the regular course of study for medical graduation, was,' said Mrs. Silverton, 'much more disgraceful than that of those "fellows" whom you are, I am glad to see, inclined to be indignant with, and yet I suppose they called themselves "gentlemen," and anything but trades unionists.'

'I cannot help thinking,' said Madeline, 'that such men as these must have a sort of latent consciousness that they are themselves below the average, else why should they be afraid of women's competing with them, since water does not find its own level more surely than mediocrity either in men or women?'

'And yet they have the audacity more often than not,' said Mrs. Silverton, 'to bring forward the plea of women's incompetence against furthering their efforts to obtain work.'

'But we must not forget,' said Sir Henry, 'that employment being on the whole a fixed quantity, if women take to the occupations of men, the result will be the lowering of men's gains, which are often small enough as it is for the support of a family.'

'I think,' said Madeline, 'some better reason for excluding women from any branch of work is required, than the wish to keep up the price of labour by diminishing the number of workers. It is scarcely creditable to those who have had the making of our laws for some hundreds of years, that any steady and industrious class of the community should still with all their efforts often be unable to support themselves.'

'Besides,' said Professor Wray, 'it is a true principle of political economy that those who have something should be, to a certain extent, taxed for the good of the whole community; and so far from employment being a fixed quantity, we usually find that any equalisation of property is accompanied by increased production and more general prosperity. You might just as well exclude from industrial pursuits any other body of citizens on account of age or political or religious views, instead of making employment as it does now, except in the case of women, depend upon qualifications which cannot be decided save upon fair trial; there need be no fear that women will monopolise what men can do better, work is always sure, sooner or later, to fall out of hands that are incompetent; but, as Miss Acton was saying, it is just those men who have only inferior work to offer who are most jealous of their rights.'

'But after all,' replied Sir Henry, 'it is the man who has the household to maintain, and if, by increasing the crowd of competitors who are choking up the avenues to the most remunerative employments, you reduce the husband and father's already scant means, his wife and daughters are the chief sufferers, since he can no longer support them.'

'If wife and daughters had all learnt a trade or profession they would be self-supporting, and though what each individual earned might seem comparatively small, on the whole the family would be more prosperous than with half its members doing nothing.'

'In that case you would impose a sort of tax upon bachelors.'

'They must find their level like other men, and if they cannot get profitable work in the old country, it is always open to them in their youth and strength and independence to emigrate, to build new towns, and cultivate new lands. They will find no lack of employment in the Colonies; in Queensland, for instance, male labour is so much in demand, that it has been found necessary to import South Sea Islanders to till the ground. It would do much to relieve the pressure in this country if Government were to offer greater inducements to both men and women to emigrate.'

'We very frequently hear complaints against the Government,' said Miss Wynter, 'and of its indifference to the interests of women, and yet many recent enactments seem to have been passed solely with a view to their advantage.'

'Never was there a piece of more short-sighted and mistaken kindness than that "Shop Hours Bill" and the "Factory Acts Amendment Bill," for I presume it is to these you refer,' said Professor Wray; 'there are no more grievous impediments to the employment of women extant. Why should full-grown reasonable people be treated as infants? Surely they have a right to a voice in the matter, but that is just what is denied them.* The policy of interference which animates many of our lawgivers allows women to stave off poverty by the help of vice, and suffers them to run the risk of starving from inability to obtain work, but having found something to do, they must not on any account be suffered to injure their health by long and exhausting tasks.'

'But you cannot deny that over-work is bad,' replied the old lady, 'especially for the wives and mothers of families.'

'It is, no doubt, but there are worse things than this; if one of two evils is inevitable, all we can do is to choose the least; the hardest earned pittance is better than nothing to the mother whose children's food and clothing depend perhaps upon her labour; if the supporters of these measures were prepared to maintain all these women (and there are many thousands) it would be a different matter, but as they are not asked to do this, and probable would not or could not if they were, they should think twice, it seems to me, before they put difficulties in the way of poor women earning such scanty subsistence as, even when free to make their own terms, is the best which in most instances falls to their lot. I am sure you will agree with me,' he said, turning to Miss Acton.

'Yes, I have often thought that this treating women of full age and fair intelligence as irresponsible beings, this refusing them freedom to regulate their own time, and make their own terms with employers, well-meant though it is, has worked injuriously by depriving women of free competition in those occupations which they have always shared with men. It is strange that the would-be friends of women-workers in the humbler classes cannot see that these artificial restrictions, instead of increasing their power of earning, their power of self-protection, force dependence upon them, put fresh difficulties in their way, and oppress instead of relieving them.'

'How is that?' asked Miss Wynter.

'The result of the "Nine Hours Bill" is just this, that it has led to many hundreds of women being dismissed from places where perhaps they were working ten hours a-day, but were kindly treated and receiving good wages, and has obliged them to take to a lower class of work (which, not coming under the Acts, involves perhaps twelve or more hours daily toil), while men are taken on in their place, or if they are retained it is to have their small salaries still further reduced. I know some firms of printers where, since the passing of these Acts, the women-hands have been all turned off; for, subject as printers are to press of work, they must be free to make special arrangements for extra time. In the smaller workshops, too, the busiest hour is after nine in the evening, so the owners are ready to pay considerably higher wages to men so that they may keep their shops open as long as they think fit and avoid the annoyance of constant visits from inspectors. Thus women's earnings are diminished, and the stamp of inferiority placed upon their labour by their would-be benefactors.'

'There is a grim irony,' said Mrs. Silverton, 'in providing that women are to have a certain length of time during the day for their meals, when the very fact of this prohibitory legislation is to limit their power of obtaining food; besides, if long hours are so bad for women that the State must put aside all considerations of personal liberty, and legislate for them as though they were children, why confine their restrictions only to shops where textile fabrics or wearing apparel are sold? It leaves untouched provision-shops, public-houses, restaurants, lodging-houses, and other places where women toil, not ten, but often as much as fifteen hours in the twenty-four; whilst the home-life of most labourers' wives proves conclusively the truth of the popular proverb that "a woman's work is never done." '

'I remember,' said Madeline, 'hearing not long ago of a workman who had been very active in his advocacy of placing restrictions upon the employments of women; his own wife was of a reticent and silent nature, but like the historical parrot, she probably thought the more, and one evening when the husband returned about supper-time he found her quietly reading a book of travels. "Where is my supper?" he asked, with some alarm. "I never knew you to miss getting it before." "I tell you how it is," she said, "you are always a-laying down the law that women shouldn't work but eight hours a-day, just because you don't want to have them in the factory, now I got your breakfast at six this morning and worked hard till two, and that's eight hours exactly, and why should I work longer than them?" This put the matter in quite a new light, the husband, it is said, reconsidered his position, and after talking over the subject with his wife whom he had never known to neglect her duty on any frivolous pretext, he finally withdrew his support from those who were advocating the interference of Government with the liberty of working women. It is strange, but I believe even some of those who recognise the want of a larger sphere of work for women, are yet short-sighted enough to believe in these Acts.'

'And so inflict upon them their crowning disability,' said Mrs. Silverton, like the generous Sultan, who, on the entreaties of his wives, was induced to allow them to walk abroad provided they wore strong shoes, and forthwith forbad all shoemakers under the severest penalties to supply them with the same.'

'Whichever way we look at it,' said the Professor, 'this interference is a great mistake; I hear that in many factories where women have still been retained, employers compensate themselves for the compulsory short hours by making the work harder while it lasts, so that the women are really more fatigued than under the old system. Plausible, too, as is the plea that the future health of the nation demands that women should be protected against their employers, it is clear that our legislators cannot think protection desirable from the labourers' point of view, or why, when it was proposed to make these restrictions apply only to married women, should they have refused to consider the same on the ground that it would prove a discouragement to marriage?'

'You allow that it would be desirable in many cases,' said Sir Henry, 'that the hours during which women labour should be shortened, but how is this to be done except by legislation?'

'By the combined action of the workers themselves; their labour like that of men should be free to regulate itself by the natural law of supply and demand; at least, the Government which takes upon itself to limit women's labour, ought in justice to prevent men doing the work of women, especially since it is the avowedly selfish object of a large number of working men to use these restrictions as a means for driving women out of their trade.'

'Whatever may have been the ulterior aims of their selfish constituents, I really believe the Members of Parliament who were most influential in the passing of these Acts,' said Madeline, 'were as well-meaning as those faithful Court physicians who, in their anxiety about the King's digestion, starved him to death.'

'They are, perhaps, political homœopathists,' said Sir Henry, 'who, at least by your account, have acted on the *similia similibus curantur* principle, and held fasting to be the best cure for starvation.'

'If you can afford,' said his sister, 'to ridicule the collective wits of those Members of Parliament whose paternal solicitude has done so much injury to its objects, I hope when you take your seat you will vote for giving women liberty to judge for themselves what they want and are able to do; but you have to obey laws, my dear boy, this afternoon, not to make them. I know you are getting chilly from keeping so unusually quiet, we will go into the drawing-room and have some tea, it is nearly five o'clock.'

'It seems a shame to go indoors this lovely afternoon, but if my medical adviser thinks it expedient I suppose I have nothing to do but to submit.'

'Your medical adviser! Oh, you mean Madeline; I am glad our conversation has had such a salutary effect that your royal highness is ready on the spot to promote a woman to the post of physician in ordinary; if Madeline only had a diploma what an advertisement you might be to her; I am glad, though, that you believe in women doctors, I did not expect to find you so orthodox.'

'If your friend were a type – you are not supposed to hear what we are saying, Miss Acton – I should; but even were I to declare myself ready to put as much faith in them as in doctors of my own sex it would not be saying much, for I am inclined to share Abernethy's opinion that "the fewer doctors, the fewer deaths, the less medicine, the less illness," and to agree with the old writer who solemnly warned his generation – "Trust not thy body to a physician. He'll make thy foolish bones go without flesh in a fortnight, and thy soul walk without a body a sennight after." '

'How very profane,' said Madeline, laughing; 'at this rate you will want to do away with doctors altogether.'

'No, I do not go so far as that, but I think our plan of making sickness instead of health a physician's gain a very bad one, the best of them are too much inclined to encourage *malades imaginaires* as it is.'

'Have you any improvement then to suggest?'

'Yes; if I had my way our "medicine-men" should be paid fixed salaries for watching over the health of the community, just as clergymen are for looking after its spiritual well-being. In some parts of China (they are a wise people) doctors are paid so long as their patients are well, as soon as they fall ill the payment ceases; it is astonishing how little sickness they have in those regions.'

'Are the inhabitants guaranteed against accident also?' asked Madeline, unable to repress a mischievous smile as she compared the speaker's 'prave orts' with the pitiable condition in which she had found him not many hours ago, 'for if not, it seems rather hard that the unfortunate doctors' income should be taxed for burns, bruises, and broken limbs, things they cannot by the utmost stretch of the imagination be made accountable for.'

'I've taken tea in, if you please, ma'am.'

' "'Tis the voice of the butler, I hear him complain," ' said Sir Henry, as momentarily forgetting his injured foot, he attempted, with his usual impetuosity, to rise; he fell back quickly again, however, with a smothered expression of pain which he attempted to hide by murmuring with closed eyes and affected accents, as though the whole matter was simply a jest, ' "Died without the aid of a regular practitioner, such instances of death are rare." ' This by way of retaliation for Madeline's last remark.

'We don't want an epitaph for you yet, please do not suggest such a melancholy topic,' exclaimed his sister, as with pretended indignation, but real solicitude, she flew to his side. 'Really, Harry, you are disgracefully careless to attempt to walk alone,' but his only answer was to sit up.

'Give me your shoulder, little tyrant,' he said, laughing at her alarmed expression, 'and I will show you that I am not so lame as my arguments yet. Fancy Miss

Acton defending men-doctors after the way in which, from all accounts, many of them have behaved to the ladies who are anxious to enter their profession,' he added, in short jerky sentences, as they hobbled through the low French window into the drawing-room.

'A stern sense of justice to which I cannot attain,' replied his sister; 'for myself,' she continued, as the rest of the party followed, 'I am not at all sure that I do not, for the reason you name, enjoy hearing you run down the doctors even though I know you are in fun; I am so angry at the mean way in which several of them have behaved in regard to the admission of women to medical degrees.'

'It is true,' said Professor Wray presently, as he handed the cups of tea which his hostess was pouring out, 'that there has been a spirit of trades unionism shown by a certain set which is anything but creditable to men of education, and so-called gentlemen, but there are many honourable exceptions to this rule; I have heard doctors myself acknowledge that with such aptitude as women show in attending the sick and curing slight ailments, there is no good reason for refusing them every chance to acquire the training which would substitute scientific knowledge for what at best must without it be a species of empiricism.'

'*A propos* of amateur doctoring, Miss Cobbe, in one of her Essays,' said Madeline, 'tells an amusing story about her grandmother, who, like many elderly women, had obtained no small reputation as an unlicensed practitioner. Asking an Irish labourer his name one day, he replied, "Och, and don't ye know me, my lady, and didn't yer ladyship give the dose to me wife, and she died the next day – Long life to yer ladyship!" There is though, joking apart, always a certain element of danger, as every one knows, in amateur practice, and seeing that many women are born with such instincts that they are bound to be either doctors or quacks, I think the country ought to congratulate itself on the opening of the London School of Medicine for Women, which, if it does not show that doctors are developing a more generous spirit, is at least a testimony to the gradual change in public opinion.'

'But whatever attitude the profession, as regards its male members, may ultimately assume,' said Mrs. Silverton, 'it will not read very creditably in the medical annals of the nineteenth century, that after so many years in which women have been knocking at the doors of the medical schools, entreating for a training which will enable them to lead useful, self-supporting lives, they have only just, in this country at least, succeeded in obtaining a fair chance.'

'This change shows, at any rate,' said Sir Henry, 'that the prejudices you complain of are gradually dying out.'

'And yet at the medical congress only the year before last, though some of the profession were in favour of admitting women-doctors, the majority were opposed, while one of our leading physicians went so far, I believe, as to say that if any lady-practitioners were admitted he would walk out of the room. This of course was enough, but could intolerance go further?'

'Now women have a school of their own,' said her brother, 'we shall hear less, I suspect, of this active opposition, which has been, I fancy, in a great measure due to a dislike of men and women studying medicine together.'

'This has often no doubt been made an ostensible motive, as has the assumed dread of women's incapacity, but the real source of most of the opposition has been, I am convinced, just an unworthy fear of rivalry, no more.'

'I know one doctor at least who had the grace to acknowledge as much,' said Professor Wray; 'in fact, he declared that if women were admitted without restriction to medical degrees, his diploma would be of next to no use to him; and as for the plea of its being unfitting for women to attempt the study of medicine with men for examiners and fellow-students, the commonest understanding should be able to grasp the fact that until they can get training institutions and licensing bodies of their own there is no other course open to them. Besides, I do not see how any sensible, right-minded person could consider *that* an insuperable obstacle; in Paris, at Zurich, the sitting side by side with men, where all were diligently engaged in the pursuit of science, does not seem to have been subversive of women's best qualities, their modesty and gentleness, ultra-prudery is never a good sign, the most corrupt are generally the most severe, which leads me to think that it is not the noblest members of the medical profession who have raised this cry as a plea for excluding women; the students who find amusement in questionable stories, or subjects not enjoined by the exigences of their profession, are likely to be loudest in their protest, because the presence of women in the schools would necessitate that tone of manly purity which ought to, but does not always, animate students of the art of healing, noble in itself though it is.'

'I quite agree with you in thinking,' said Sir Henry, 'that the profession of medicine is one eminently suited to women, but I doubt if as surgeons they are equally likely to succeed, from the mere fact of their wanting the physical strength necessary for many operations.'

'In this, as in everything else, science is superseding mere brute force; in these days of anæsthetics, it is skill rather than strength that is needed, and therefore I see no reason why women should not succeed equally well in this branch of the profession.'

'Perhaps; but I do not like the idea, somehow; it is true enough, I suppose, what, I think it was Lord Sherbrooke once said, that an Englishman shies at a new idea like a horse at a perambulator, we must get thoroughly accustomed to a thing before we can be brought to tolerate it; to be respectable, it must have existed a hundred years at least.'

'And yet I do not think the idea of women-doctors is so absolutely new,' said Madeline, 'it may be a revival, but it cannot be called an invention of the present age; for among the Gothic nations women commonly practised surgery, and is there not some mention of a woman-leech in the *Iliad?*'

'You mean "fair Agamede with golden hair," ' replied Sir Henry.

'And there is Agnodice, the Athenian lady,' said Professor Wray, 'who, for the benefit of her own sex, was so determined to study medicine that she disguised herself in men's clothes in order to attend the classes of the physician Hierophilus. Masculine jealousy, it seems, is no new thing either, for it is said her success was so great that she suffered much persecution at the hands of certain male doctors, who summoned her before the Areopagus, and accused her of violating the law which forbad the study of medicine to women and slaves. But it is half past five,' he added, looking at his watch, 'and if I am to get back by seven, I must tear myself away and not delay the walk to Rapparee Cove I have been promising myself all day; I wish,' turning to Sir Henry, 'that you could have come too, but of course that is out of the question.'

'Unfortunately, yes; but I can walk, I think, as far as the library door with you, if you will kindly lend me an arm. I must write a letter before dinner, and I shall never get away unless I go now. Perhaps you will give me some credit this time, Miss Acton,' he added, turning to her, 'for having been interested in our discussion when I tell you that, although my letter was rather an important one, I literally forgot it until this moment.'

'I really believe he is in earnest,' said Mrs. Silverton, as the door closed and the ladies were left alone, 'he has been so preternaturally patient and quiet for him all the afternoon; but auntie, I have been watching you while we were talking, and wondering, as you said nothing, whether you class women-doctors amongst the inventions to which you object, or whether you are inclined to tolerate them.'

'My dear, you know without asking, I am sure, which side I shall take; nothing I have heard yet has convinced me that women have a right to usurp the functions of a physician; their place in the sick-room is that of a nurse, and they ought to be content with this; why, there are hundreds of medical men now who cannot make a decent living.'

'Is no woman then to be allowed to earn a maintenance till every man in the world is provided for? But that is always the way, anything that offers no opportunity of earning either money or κυδος women are welcome to, they may be nurses and nearly break their backs in lifting heavy men in and out of bed, they may be in perpetual contact with the foulest diseases, and act as midwives to the poor, who cannot afford to pay heavy fees; but doctors – no, that is not to be thought of, it is quite unnatural and, in short, improper.'

'Well, I can only say it would make no difference to me,' exclaimed Mrs. Knagge, 'however many women-doctors there were in the world, I would not employ one on any account; I should have no faith in them.'

'I think,' replied Madeline, 'if you were only once attended by any of the women-doctors whom I am fortunate enough to know, you would change your mind as others have done; for although granting that the conditions of training and experience are about equal, there might not be much choice between the average woman and the average man in point of ordinary intelligence and skill, yet the very fact of women having had so many difficulties to overcome and the earnestness this has required and developed, must have, I think, raised them above the average practitioner of the other sex. There is no law to compel us to employ a woman-doctor if we do not like it, but on the other hand it is at least equally hard that those who from principle, or the nature of their complaint, prefer to consult one of their own sex, however much they may desire the services of a skilful medical woman, are, in nine cases out of ten, unable to obtain them. Many a valuable life has been sacrificed to the natural delicacy which, in certain cases, has made women shrink from employing the services of a man, or if she has, at the solicitation of her friends, at last given in, made her fail to tell him all the facts necessary for a complete diagnosis of her condition, where she would gladly have employed and spoken freely to one of her own sex.'

'I should say it was nothing but false modesty that,' replied Mrs. Knagge, 'which the sooner it is shaken out of a woman the better; the question of sex ought to be entirely ignored in such cases.'

'I should rather say that it is only custom and habit which have ever reconciled women to the idea of men attending them in sickness. Modesty is often spoke of as a characteristic peculiarly feminine, at any rate men are not, as a rule, more than their equals in natural delicacy and reserve, and yet how would *they* like to be arbitrarily prevented from employing physicians of their own sex? How would they feel at being compelled in all cases to reveal their physical ailments to a woman? How would they like to be the subjects of an object-lesson (as women are every day at our hospitals) to classes of young women-students?'

'Of course,' said Mrs. Silverton, 'if their nature revolts at the idea, ours must surely have a right to do so. But, Madeline, I did not know you felt so strongly on this subject before.'

'I did not at one time, in fact I had not thought much about this view of the question, but within the last two years I have seen something of what women will endure in trying to hide their suffering in certain diseases rather than submit to the anguish and shame of outraged modesty involved in male medical and surgical treatment. About a year ago I undertook to nurse a respectable young woman who seemed to be far gone in consumption, and after a time she confided to me that the real basis of her illness was a serious internal complaint, the symptoms of which, in remembrance of certain past experiences, she had hidden from the doctor, who, of course, working in the dark, could do her no good. I began to remonstrate, but she stopped me, covering her face and shuddering – "Oh, please miss, don't! I'm not afraid of pain, but I went to the hospital for it once, and if you knew you would not ask me to go through that again – I'd rather die twice over – I thought I should never hold up my head again." As she entered into further particulars I began to understand and appreciate her feelings. "But," I said, "if I can get you the services of a lady-doctor who is specially skilled in cases such as yours?" "I did not know there were any," she said, gratefully accepting my offer to move her out of the smoky town into purer air, and put her under the charge of my friend. I am glad to say that the treatment was quite successful, and she is now a strong woman, thanks to the medical knowledge of one of her own sex. I do not think any stronger argument than this is wanted to prove the necessity for women-physicians, this poor woman would, undoubtedly, have died, as many others have done, victims to their own reticence and – I cannot call it *false* – modesty; not only individuals but the medical profession and the whole human race would profit by the removal of every prejudice-constructed barrier against the free study and practice of medicine by women, who, seeing that they must have, when once prejudice is overcome, greater facilities for making observations and discoveries in this field than men, an increased and more widely-spread general knowledge of the diseases of their own sex must be the result.'

'But,' said Mrs. Knagge, 'when it was a question of men and women studying together, you insisted that the nobility and purity of science should raise the mind above any questions of sex.'

'True, where they are labouring earnestly together, their sole aim and idea being to fit themselves for the relief of their sad and suffering fellow-creatures, the question of sex would not, I should think, be very likely to intrude itself, though I am sure every one would agree that, where possible, separate schools are to be desired. But the case is scarcely parallel.'

'Certainly not. It has been often, and I think truly, asserted,' said Mrs. Silverton, 'that the medical man who cannot banish from his work all personal ideas of sex is unfit for his profession. But you cannot expect the patient, whose knowledge of and interest in her complaint is the reverse of scientific, to banish from her mind all personal sensations of bitterness, pain, or repugnance; as M. Dupré said, in lecturing at the London School of Medicine for Women, a wish so reasonable as that expressed by many girls and women to be attended by physicians of their own sex, ought at all risks to be complied with.'

'And yet I do not see,' said Miss Wynter, 'that there is such a very urgent demand for them; in fact, I have heard a great many women declare, as Mrs. Knagge did just now, that however many doctors of their own sex there were they would always employ a man from choice.'

'The force of habit, auntie, that is all,' said Mrs. Silverton. 'Most of them have never seen a cultivated and able woman-physician; she is, to the majority, a new experience; and we know what that means, when conventional prejudices are at stake. And yet, when I say "new," we ought to remember that until comparatively recent times women were attended, at least in their confinements, by members of their own sex; it is the presence of men at such times that is an innovation.'

'Professor Wray spoke just now,' said Madeline, 'of Agnodice, and of the study of medicine being prohibited to women and slaves; I thought at the time that there are several allusions in classical writers, showing how strictly limited was the attendance of male-physicians on women.'

'Men-midwives are a disgrace to civilisation,' said Mrs. Silverton, warmly; 'I can quite believe what a friend of mine told me not long ago in speaking of this subject; there is no prudery or mock-modesty about her whatever; in fact, she is one of the most natural and unaffected of women; and yet she declared that when her first child was born, the feelings of horror and repugnance she experienced at having to endure the presence and services of a man almost a stranger, at a time when it was especially necessary that her mind should be kept as calm and her spirits as cheerful as possible, if they did not endanger her life, at any rate retarded her recovery. Madam Romanoff, in her *Rites and Customs of the Græco-Russian Church*, says that child-birth in Russia is much less frequently fatal than with us, and I have often thought that this may be due less to the superior skill of the ladies who, according to the same authority, chiefly practise midwifery, than to the probability that the patients are, by the mere fact of being attended by one of their own sex, saved from much mental misery and disquietude.'

'I am glad,' said Madeline, after a moment's pause, 'it is beginning to be recognised, even in this country, that medical women are wanted; but when it comes to a question of India, there can be, I think, but one opinion. Where there are some fifty millions of native women who, debarred by national custom and religion from medical aid because they cannot obtain it from those of their own sex, suffer miserably and often perish in consequence, the case becomes urgent, and I am glad to see that it is beginning to be so recognised by Government.'

'That appeal, sent a year or two ago to the Queen by the Maharanee of Punna,' said Mrs. Silverton, 'has done much service in calling public attention to the condition of Indian women, and to the necessity which exists that there should be established in that country a medical branch of the public service, by whose means they may have the aid of physicians and surgeons of their own sex.'

'I remember seeing something about it in the *Times*,' said Miss Wynter; 'but I have almost forgotten the circumstance.'

' "Things happened in this wise," as the old story-books say; it being strictly forbidden, as you know in the East, that the inmates of a zenana should be seen by any man except their nearest relations, and the princess of whom I was speaking just now having for a long time suffered from a painful internal complaint, her husband, in great distress, sent two hundred miles to Miss Beilby, a medical missionary at Lucknow, to beg her assistance. She went, and the result of her skill and care was that the Maharanee ultimately recovered. Some time later, when Miss Beilby was on the point of returning to England, the princess sent for her, and solemnly entreated her to tell the Queen, the Prince and Princess of Wales, and the people of England, what Indian women suffer when they are sick. The Maharanee was convinced that if the Queen were only told of their condition she would feel for, and try to help them; so she begged Miss Beilby to write down her message lest it should be forgotten. "Write it small, Doctor Miss Sahiba," she said, giving her pen, ink, and paper, "for I want to put it in a locket, and you are to wear this locket until you see our great Queen, and you are to give it to her yourself; you are not to send it through another." Miss Beilby had some doubt whether she would be able to comply to the full with these conditions. But the Queen having heard something of the message, sent for her soon after her arrival in England, and I am glad to say expressed warm interest in the question, entrusting Miss Beilby with a personal message for the Maharanee, and saying she wished it to be generally known that she would sympathise with every movement made to relieve the suffering condition of Indian women.'

'That I am sure she would,' said Miss Wynter, 'but at the same time the Queen is one of the last to approve of women, as a rule, stepping out of their proper sphere.'

'That most ill-defined of terms,' said her niece, *sotto voce*.

'You recollect what she says,' the old lady went on, without heeding the interruption, 'in the first *Journal of Life in the Highlands*, "Albert grows daily fonder and fonder of politics and business, and I get daily to dislike them more and more; we women are not made for governing, and if we are good women we must dislike these masculine occupations." '

'If every utterance of the Queen were to be taken as divinely inspired,' said Mrs. Silverton, 'your argument, auntie, would be unanswerable, severe though it is upon some of the noblest of our sex.'

'I have heard that quoted before,' said Madeline, 'in opposition to the earnest desire of many good women for a wider sphere of usefulness; but I do not think it is fair to take an isolated expression of what was probably a momentary impatience at a hard-worked and no doubt very trying position, and to cite it as a proof of the Queen's deliberate opinion in regard to the incapacity of women for such high duties as she herself has fulfilled in a manner which sufficiently disproves any modest assumption of inferiority contained in the remark quoted.'

'Besides, I am sure, during her whole career,' said Mrs. Silverton, 'no one could have been more rightly jealous of her royal prerogative; had she really, as some have tried to prove, thought it unfitting that a woman should have public duties, she would long ago have made the mistake of resigning in favour of the Prince of Wales, who, man though he is, few sensible people would venture to say could, with all his well-deserved popularity, make a better sovereign than his mother. But I hear Fred's voice; please excuse me, I *must* go and see what sport they have had. By the way,' she added, stopping in the doorway, 'did I tell you the other day of that child in the Board School, who, in his reading-lesson, would persist in calling the patriarchs "partridges," and was put into disgrace by a pupil-teacher for making *game* of the prophets? But I must not loiter, it is, as even you will allow, auntie, quite within a woman's sphere to look after the furnishing of the dinner-table.'

'Quite right, my dear, quite right,' said the old lady, nodding her head approvingly, and then turning to thank Madeline, who had just picked up a long row of stitches in her knitting, and was now winding up the ball of wool, which, as though with a sense of fitness, while its owner was entangled in argument, had been busy entangling itself around the legs of sundry chairs and tables.

Source Endnote

* Throughout the Bill to consolidate the Factory Acts, children, young persons, and women are repeatedly put in the same category as people who are alike unfitted to be free-agents.

Editorial Headnote

'Physical Society', *Guy's Hospital Gazette* (5 December 1891), 290–292

Guy's Hospital Gazette was first published in 1872, and was the world's oldest hospital periodical. It is still in press today as *GKT Gazette*, and recently (in March 2023) celebrated its 150th anniversary, and has now incorporated St Thomas' and King's Hospitals, as well as those studying dentistry, to chronicle the life and work of students at these institutions.[1] The first edition of 2023 still covers topics which have been concerning students since the nineteenth century, such as 'science and research', 'arts and culture', and reports from various, especially sporting, societies still form part of the content. Letters from the student community remain key parts of the *Gazette*, allowing readers to reflect on the challenges and triumphs of their education and position in life as future professionals.[2] As the current editors note, they aim to continue providing a 'voice' for students of the institutions they represent.

When the *Gazette* was first established the content provided, on the surface, more of a day-to-day account of clinical procedures at Guy's Hospital. By November 1872, however, the *Gazette* was already gaining attention from its medical and lay seniors. As the *Lancet* remarked in a 'Medical Annotations' piece on 'Students' Journalism', good and evil could result from the prospect of articles written by and for students. On the one hand, it noted, a student periodical could publish 'the various proceedings of the school and hospital' and act 'in some degree also as a bond of union and good fellowship between the students'. On the other, 'discredit' could easily be brought upon an individual and consequently the school by injudicious remarks. The reputation of medical students in the nineteenth century had been poor; they were satirised in popular fiction and in the press alike. Recent examples of the behaviour of male medical students at the University of Edinburgh towards their aspiring female colleagues had appalled both the profession and the public as retrograde and embarrassing. A chance to mend perceptions had been dashed by reference in the *Guy's Hospital Gazette* to 'Garotting at Guy's'. What luck, mused the *Lancet*, that Guy's was not dependent on public subscription; otherwise, money could have been lost from the institution in thousands. The offending article described what the *Lancet* labelled as 'exceptional therapeutic measures' for impeding respiration, but instead of applying the 'golden rule' of sticking to precise technical language, the *Gazette* had revelled in the gory and sensational. Such an effect, sniffed the *Lancet*, was 'indiscrete, useless, childish, and vulgar'.[3] The *British Medical Journal* focused on a more positive aspect of the student periodical that month: the pride to be taken in academic achievement, now that examination results were published in the press, not only for the individual, but for 'the honour of the institution to which he has attached himself'.[4] Medical students' reputations were at stake, but also that of a whole profession desperate to prove its serious worth.

The lay press picked up on the treatment's 'benefit' to women, exemplified by coverage in the *Pall Mall Gazette*, which was excerpted from Cornwall to Kent, via the West Midlands and Ireland. An 'age of heroism', commented *Pall Mall* sarcastically and 'not without alarm', was still with us, despite the profession defending its much more civilised responses.[5] '"Heroic treatments"' had neither disappeared nor fallen out of favour in the light of scientific and technological developments.

From the 1890s, the *London (Royal Free Hospital) School of Medicine for Women Magazine*, a much younger publication than the *Gazette* (see Volumes III and IV), would have the chance to put Guy's students' attitude to women to the test in inter-collegiate competitions between their respective Debating Societies. Guy's, indeed, was a regular sparring partner, written about with relish in the London School of Medicine for Women's periodical. By 1898, the LSMW debaters would see a motion which won arguing that, far from 'garotting', to use the language of the *Guy's Hospital Gazette*, or restricting women's freedoms, they could not be given too much liberty.[6]

Notes

1 www.kcl.ac.uk/students/the-gkt-gazette-relaunches-on-its-150th-anniversary (accessed 10 October 2023).
2 www.kcl.ac.uk/lsm/assets/gazette-150th.pdf (accessed 10 October 2023).
3 'Students' Journalism', *Lancet*, 100:2570 (30 November 1872), p. 792.
4 'Pass and Pluck Lists', *BMJ*, 2:621 (23 November 1872), p. 500.
5 'Garotting at Guy's, *Pall Mall Gazette*, 21 November 1872, p. 5.
6 'Debating Society', *London (Royal Free Hospital) School of Medicine for Women Magazine*, 10 (May 1898), p. 424.

8

'PHYSICAL SOCIETY', *GUY'S HOSPITAL GAZETTE*

Source: 'Physical Society', *Guy's Hospital Gazette* (5 December 1891), pp. 290–292

Physical Society.

The first debate of the session took place on Saturday evening last in the smoking room of the club, when the chair was taken by Mr. Wakefield, and more than sixty members were present.

Mr. G. Mackeson moved: "That this meeting is of opinion that every facility should be given to woman to enter the medical profession." In introducing his resolution Mr. Mackeson said that only a few years ago it would have been received with scorn and derision, but that they now recognised the claims of woman to be allowed some means of maintaining herself independently of man, for the census returns had showed that the feminine sex was increasing with alarming rapidity, and that marriage for all of them was entirely out of the question.

They must first ask themselves the question why it was that woman had not hitherto taken an equal place with man in the great professions and businesses of the day. He thought "Education" was at the bottom of it. The state of slavery to which woman was consigned in the lower levels of human evolution, clearly tended to dwarf and narrow her mind, and even as she emerged from that condition of slavery she was still governed by man in numberless ways, which, although less brutal, were scarcely less effectual as mentally stunting influences.

Mr. Mackeson then traced woman's life throughout the various epochs of history, and quoted Sydney Smith, who, writing in 1810, said, "A century ago the prevailing taste in female education was for housewifery, now it is for accomplishments." This remark, he said, applied equally to-day as it had done at the beginning of the century. It had, however, assumed larger proportions – for the educational programme of the iniquitous Board School free education scheme provided for the fostering, not of housewifery, or mechanics and general labour work amongst the lower classes, but rather of accomplishments in the shape of French, chemistry and physiology, etc. – and what good it was to a man to know

DOI: 10.4324/9781003265238-8

the process of digestion his food underwent when he was not taught a trade by which to make his daily bread, he for his part could not see. In the upper classes, too, the ideal of female education was not that of *mental furnishing*, but rather of *mental decoration.*

The speaker then dwelt on the fact that woman, after having passed through various phases of life, had bred a class of her own sex who desired to be more than creatures of accomplishments, and further, that some of them had already entered the medical profession, and, working under great difficulties and against hostile criticism, had passed their examinations with credit, and were doing good work at home and abroad. Can they not, therefore, give women still greater facilities for entering this, the most noble, the most self-sacrificing, and the most ennobling of professions? Could they not offer her the hand of brotherhood, feeling sure that she could never take their place, but that she would do good work by carrying religion and *medicine* hand in hand into the wilds of Africa or the Buddhist plains of India, by attending women of high caste prejudices in India who would otherwise suffer untreated, or fall into the hands of a rascally Brahmin or other medicine fetish man, and by treating certain of her own sex whose idiosyncrasy it was to prefer her to a male medical adviser.

On precedent, at any rate, lady physicians ought, he said, to be encouraged, for Grecian historians spoke with praise of the women doctors at Athens. In particular he mentioned one Agnodice who had been the pioneer of female practitioners.

In conclusion, Mr. Mackeson mentioned various qualities in woman which would be of peculiar use to her in medical work. He also spoke of one or two objections which had been raised in the columns of medical journals – particularly the subject of marriage – and he stated that he believed female practitioners made up their minds that medicine and marriage were incompatible, and that if they contracted the latter they would have to give up practising the former.

He quoted the following verses to show that a doctor wife would be a very queer blessing.

I'm the queerest of husbands, tho wife I have chose
  The practice of physic pursues;
There are not many men would have dared to propose,
  Or be standing just now in my shoes.

We sit down to breakfast, when lo! an express
  Comes to summon the doctor away;
A man ne'er can brew tea without making a mess,
  And there's nought but discomfort all day.

At night 'tis still worse, for the surgery bell
  Every moment is given to ring,
And although very often it's only a sell,
  Yet it might be a serious thing.

Still there'll come certain duties as time toddles on,
That she can't well by proxy achieve,
And how busy so e'er, our small daughter or son,
She must stay at home to receive.

How she'll manage things then 'tis not easy to know,
Nor what with the babe I'm to do,
When mamma to a long consultation must go,
And his next feeding hour is at two.

Mr. DALDY opened the debate for the opposition. He said that Mr. Mackeson had said all that could be said for the motion; but he held that the inequality of the sexes was not determined by education, but rested upon the inherent inferiority of women, to which the experience of all ages bore witness no less than the rhymes quoted by the mover. The question must be decided by the answer to the question. Is it for the common good that women should be doctors? And the answer to this question was based on the principle that every member of a community should do the work for which he was most fitted; and the qualities necessary for medical work – nerve, endurance, and, he might add, secrecy – were the qualities of men rather than women. He accused the movers of class selfishness and want of chivalry. Brain power, he thought, could, like muscular power, be estimated by weight, and if so, women were clearly not the equals of men. Lady doctors could only come from a class of female prigs in frocks who lost the privileges of their sex. The strongest point in favour of the motion – the work for medical women in India – could be got rid of, he thought, by the gradual enlightenment of the people of India, and the decay of caste prejudices. A Rajah's wife, some years ago, had submitted to the treatment of a medical man, telling him her symptoms, and giving him her pulse to feel from behind a curtain; and her example would be followed in the future. The very idea of women in the profession made him shudder, and he could not conclude his case more fitly than by quoting against the motion the very lines with which the mover had thought to strengthen his case.

Mr. A. SALTER would not hear of one sex prescribing the sphere of work for the other. He quoted Lady Florence Dixey's opinion that no education was allowed to women but that of idiots – no ambition but that of getting married. The position of women was even more unsatisfactory in Germany, where they were relegated to the kitchen and the scullery. The contempt a German had for an English working man who could carry his baby to relieve its mother was, he thought with Mr. Herbert Spencer, most shameful. It was only in civilized races that women's brains weighed less than men's; among savages there was no such inequality, and he thought the cry of the incapability of women was the whine of a cowardly cur.

Mr. W. K. STEELE thought Lady Florence Dixey's opinions did not strengthen the case for the opposition. He liked to think of women as ministering angels, not as P.M. clerks. It was bad enough to have women as fellow candidates at a medical examination, but the prospect of lady examiners was worse still. He described the shock he had experienced on hearing a lady come in saying she was ravenously hungry, she had been dissecting all the morning. There was, too, the selfish argument; women as competitors would not be handicapped as men were by the calls of whist, football, tobacco, and all the pursuits and peccadilloes, without which men could not exist. He thought women in becoming doctors were treating nature with a pitchfork.

Mr. Davies thought women were really the equals of men, and in some cases he had found them their superiors, to his cost. He thought that if women were to practice medicine, there would not be so many cases of neglected cancer among women. A very good working arrangement would be for medical men to marry medical women, and the latter to take the night work. The capacity women showed for observing and dealing with details, in itself made them fit for medical work; and if their brains were too light, that defect would be got over by the exercise to which they would be submitted.

Mr. Harris quoted Sir Thomas More to show that in that authority's opinion women should be oducated to take part in important work, and referred to the vigorous mental training that he prescribed for his daughter. The attitude of men towards women on this question he compared to that of a terrier and a cat – gnarling, but afraid to enter the lists with her.

Mr. Parry thought that the virtues most prized in women as womanly would be threatened with extinction by the course in favour of which the mover had spoken.

Mr. Parkes found fault with the remarks made by Mr. Steele as not being direct argument. Women he thought could accustom themselves to what they would have to go through as doctors, as much as they had as nurses. Opponents of the motion had talked of throwing open the profession to the rank and file of women, as if it was at present in the hands of the rank and file of men. It was not proposed to admit women of the class from which costermongers came to the profession; but there were women, such as Miss Fawcett or Miss Ramsay, who were more than fitted to compete with men. What were the qualities in which women excelled? Were they not tact and sympathy, the very qualities most essential in medical practice, and the want of which was a common source of failure among medical men. He quoted Lady Dufferin in reply to those who said that even in India prejudices would be overcome and women doctors become unnecessary. He thought that 200 years at least would be required for Indian caste prejudice to be forgotten.

Mr. Roper gave arguments to prove the inferiority of women to men. In Art and Literature competition had been free between the sexes, but with a very one-sided result. He thought that the future of society should be taken into consideration in deciding the question, and then by reference to Galton's Law of Heredity he thought the decision could only be against the motion. Women's sphere of work necessitated their inferiority. He thought that from what the world had already seen of lady doctors, it was clear that the attractiveness of the fair sex would be jeopardized by their numbers being increased.

Mr. EASTES pointed out that there were objections to women entering other professions. A Florrie Atkins or a Julie Tar was impossible.

Mr. STEVENS said that the qualities women would show in this profession were to be inferred from those they displayed in the only position to which the world admitted them; and there, in love, they were conspicuous for endurance and perseverance.

Mr. LEATHES thought Mr. Mackeson's proviso, that the lady doctors should not marry, might weaken his case. As a matter of fact it was found that where women had independent occupations there they married youngest. At the same time, if the growth of the population was to be arrested by a reduction of the marriage rate, then this would best be done by giving women some other ambition in life than that of getting married. He thought that even if women were on the whole intellectually inferior to men, there were many who were fit to enter the profession, and at any rate a policy of Laissez-faire would be wise, and the question would then soon settle itself.

Mr. HORA thought that there were many of the simpler and less taxing duties of medical men that might wisely be put into the hands of women.

Mr. HALE pointed out that evils first introduced into the world by woman should by woman be cured.

Mr. HOVENDEN was anxious that other prospects than the solitary one of domestic happiness should be opened up for women.

Mr. COLEMAN said the growth of the population might be arrested by an increase of the death rate no less than by a decrease of the birth rate, and for this reason he would support the motion.

Mr MACKESON was then called upon to reply, and in a very earnest speech he combated the arguments raised against him, and spoke very sarcastically of Messrs. Daldy's and Roper's attempts at criticism. The resolution was then put to the vote, and carried amid much enthusiasm by 33 votes to 27.

Editorial Headnote

Arabella Kenealy, 'How Women Doctors are Made', *Ludgate*, IV (May 1897), 29–35

Arabella Kenealy (1859–1938) had a short life as a medical practitioner, but a much longer one as a prolific writer of fact and fiction; articles, and full-length works appeared alongside a large number of novels. She was educated from 1877 and the age of 18 at the London School of Medicine for Women, qualifying as a Licentiate of the King's and Queen's College of Physicians of Ireland (LKQCPI) in 1883, thus becoming the thirty-third woman to be placed on the Medical Register.[1] After rejections from the New Hospital for Women as House Surgeon and the turning down of her offer to minister to cholera victims in Egypt by the Foreign Office, Kenealy ended up practising in Watford from the late 1880s.[2] Early retirement from her profession in 1894 was due to complications stemming from severe diphtheria. By this point, she had already written one of her best-known novels, *Dr Janet of Harley Street* (1893), which was on its fourth edition before the year was out, and which also received an American printing a year later. The *Westminster Review* summed up *Dr Janet* with a reflection on its author as 'not an artist in the highest sense of the word [but] a clever woman'. It was a 'new novel of unconventional type', containing 'incidents of a very exciting nature', 'occasionally objectionable', but possessed of 'narrative power'.[3] Such a comment could as easily be applied to its author.

Kenealy wrote about most of the hotly-contested topics of the day in all of the genres to which she contributed. Opinions on, for example, degeneracy, syphilis, motherhood, corsets, surplus women, vivisection, the dangers of athleticism, and the horrors of feminism filled pages of prose from the 1890s onwards. As her *Times* obituary noted in 1938, despite having to retire from her professional duties due to ill health, she 'was never idle for long'.[4] Kenealy's strident and fluid style, frequently tinged alternatively with wit or melodramatic language, lent itself to every genre from the short story to correspondence with medical periodicals. One of her many controversial interventions came in the Autumn of 1895 when she sparked a flurry of letters to the *British Medical Journal* after a letter entitled 'A Question of Conscience' recommended non-intervention in a case of threatened abortion due to syphilis.[5] The debate lasted several weeks, and brought Kenealy a great deal of publicity both inside and outside the profession; not all of it positive, needless to say.

Although written at breakneck speed, Kenealy's novels were enormously popular, reaching numerous editions, and her work was translated into a number of languages during her lifetime, including Danish, Dutch, French, and Swedish. She was particularly prolific in the 1900s and 1910s, producing works such as

Charming Renée (1900); *Dr Smith of Queen Anne Street and Other Stories* (1907); *King Edward Intervenes* (1910); *The Mating of Anthea* (1911); *The Woman-Hunter* (1912); *The Painted Lady* (1913); and *The Way of the Lover* (1914). The *London Journal* reflected on what they saw as her medical sideline in 1893 in their 'Persons of Interest' series. Kenealy, noted the *London*, 'was said to have entered the medical profession with the express intention of bringing its resources to bear upon fiction'. Indeed, claimed the periodical, 'burying herself' in medical student life was regarded by her friends as 'a waste of time'. Yet, countered the lady herself, it was invaluable for the 'study of human life' and its, interestingly, 'suggestive phases'. 'Marked success in her profession' led to concerns that the 'novelist would be lost in the physician', but literary talent had evidently won out, to the delight of the *London Journal*.[6]

In similar fashion to her fictional works, Kenealy's focus, in her contemporary political interventions, was woman's place in the world. She was not a feminist, in spite of her training and experiences and, indeed, argued against votes for women. The 1900s did, however, witness an engagement with the health and welfare of women and girls. She edited, for example, *Beauty Through Hygiene: Common-Sense Ways to Health for Girls* and *The Mother's Manual: A Month-by-Month Guide for Young Mothers* (both 1905). Later years saw Kenealy's robust defence of eugenics in *A Study in Degeneracy* (1911), the anti-feminist *Feminism and Sex-Extinction* (1920), and a turn to the occult in her final years when *The Human Gyroscope* was published (1934).

Notes

1 'Women Physicians', *Englishwoman's Review*, CXXIV (15 August 1883), p. 375.

2 Minutes of the Managing Committee of the New Hospital for Women, Book II: May 1882–March 1895; 4 July 1883, H13/EGA/20, London Metropolitan Archives; *Englishwoman's Review* (15 August 1883), p. 375.

3 *Westminster Review*, CXXXIX (January to June 1893), p. 697.

4 'Miss Arabella Kenealy. Novelist and Writer on Medical Subjects', *Times*, 21 November 1938, p. 14.

5 'A Question of Conscience', *BMJ*, 2:1811 (14 September 1895), p. 682. Letters poured in between 21 September and 12 October, when Kenealy wrote back. The *BMJ* concluded Kenealy's letter with a succinct warning that '[t]his correspondence must now cease', *BMJ*, 2:1815 (12 October 1895), p. 934.

6 *London Journal*, 20:508 (9 September 1893), p. 191.

9

'HOW WOMEN DOCTORS ARE MADE'

Arabella Kenealy

Source: Arabella Kenealy, 'How Women Doctors are Made', *Ludgate*, IV (May 1897), pp. 29–35

HOW WOMEN-DOCTORS ARE MADE

Written by Arabella Kenealy, L.R.C.P. Illustrated with Photos

THE true physician, whether man or whether woman, is born – not made. For medicine is essentially an art rather than a science.

You may educate your student in such wise that he shall satisfy his examiners as to his sufficient knowledge of the body, its structure and its physiology; shall be learned in the nomenclature of disease; shall have the latest diagnostic methods at his finger-ends; the latest pharmacopœial remedies at the point of his prescribing pen; but when you have done these things and have supplied him with licence to practise, you will no more necessarily have gifted him with the faculty of healing than you will have made an artist of one without sense of form, colour, contrast and proportion, by teaching him to draw straight lines or curves, to distinguish pigments by their names and characteristics, or to comprehend the rules of perspective.

Medicines must above all things be mixed "with brains, sir," and that with a very particular brand of brain. For example, there are in the pharmacopœia some score of iron preparations wherewith to recruit the blood corpuscles of the anæmic. Each is excellent in its way, but its way being the particular case to which it is suited, the onus of applying or of misapplying that excellence rests on its prescriber. And in this matter experience, unless read with special sight, goes for but little. "I found that form of iron act exceptionally well last week," the manufactured physician muses; "I will try it in this case." He does, to find it fail, because the very element whereby it succeeded in the former is in the latter case missing – and that element is the patient's idiosyncrasy, the thing most obvious and significant to the true physician.

I encountered in my student days a very striking example of the relative values of the natural and of the manufactured doctor. It fell to my lot to act as "clinical clerk" for consecutive terms of three months to two of our senior physicians. The

DOI: 10.4324/9781003265238-9

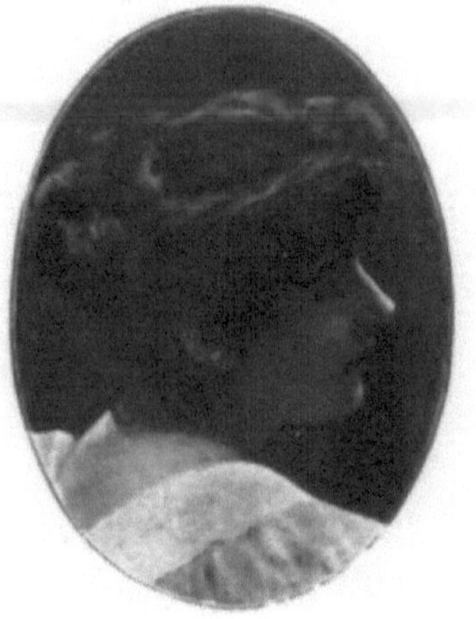

DR. ARABELLA KENEALY
Photo by Alice Hughes

one was the somewhat old-fashioned type of family practitioner, kindly, shrewd, perceptive and intuitive, with a fund of human sympathy and a grasp of character. The other belonged to a later school, a man of books and laboratories, scientific, logical and learned; a person of importance in the academic world, and one especially esteemed for his knowledge of therapeutics. The practice of the two men offered a striking contrast to me, young enough to weigh and find wanting my superiors in years and office. From the one I learned my optimism, from the other a hopeless pessimism of treatment. The rule-of-thumb man, as I have heard him called, though his practice was in reality of the very highest order, would muse upon the patient for some fraction of a minute with half-closed, far-seeing eyes, then seize a pen and impulsively dash off a prescription. More often than not he would be unable to offer to us inquiring students any very substantial reason for his selection of a particular drug. But that selection almost invariably turned out to be the right one. He was the most signally successful prescriber it has been my good-fortune to meet. His hospital rounds were a series of inspiriting successes. Gratitude and smiles from relieved patients greeted us all down the wards and in the out-patient room. A true type of the natural physician, he was gifted with some special sense which enabled him, as it were, to dive into the patient's physiological arcana, and detect the thing lacking.

My other senior, painstaking, conscientious and scientific, on all occasions supplied his students with excellent reason for his most excellent prescriptions. The most recent theories and results in therapeutics he discoursed for our instruction; yet with all due respect to a man for whom I had the greatest regard, I was bound to confess that not once during the whole of my experience of him did he really succeed with a case. He mistook the art of medicine for a science, and so applied it. He treated the disease instead of treating the patient, and he failed to such extent that at the end of three months' "clerking" in his wards I was a mere agnostic in the creed of drugs.

And this experience of mine has been again and again confirmed. The successful doctor – that is, the doctor who most benefits his patients – is not the bookish, scientific man, any more than the successful pastor – the man who most helps and comforts his morally sick flock – is he learned in theologies and sacerdotal law.

Much may be blamed to our present methods of training, which keep the student's head for ever buried in books, cramming his brain cells with cut-and-dry facts, formulæ, fetiches, he will have forgotten, or will have unlearned, long before he will have acquired any knowledge worth calling such of the art of healing.

So long, however, as efficiency is judged by way of examinations, which, though valuable as a test of sincerity and industry, are the poorest possible tests of an individual's capacity as a doctor, so long will the medical schools demand from their students an academic excellence to the attainment of which their essentially medical faculties are subordinated.

Whether or not the special faculties which go to make the good physician belong equally to either sex, is a point I will not raise. It is not proposed to justify here the existence of medical women, but merely to touch briefly on the manner whereby this fact is accomplished. The history of the earlier days of the movement with the oppositions, disabilities and insults, and on the other hand the chivalries, encouragements and generosities accorded it, have been told sufficiently often. The question now before us – if question there be – is not whether we shall have medical women, but in what number shall we have them? To judge by the fact that fifty new students entered their names last October on the books of the London School of Medicine for Women, making a total of one hundred and fifty-nine students in various stages of evolution, and this in addition to the entries of the Women's Medical Colleges in Edinburgh and Glasgow, it would appear that the United Kingdom is answering the latter question very satisfactorily. For of those who have qualified and have subsequently set up in practice, almost all have attained an encouraging measure of success: some are taking rank with the first physicians of our time, while one notably has risen to such eminence as to be named among the most skilful surgical operators of our day – despite the oft-repeated cry that surgery is a branch wherein women will never excel. And all this without symptom whatsoever of that "unsexing" process whereof we have heard so much and have seen less in the ranks of medicine than in any other field of women's work.

As might be supposed, a number of women drift after qualification, or determine before it, to India and other countries, the disabilities of one race of women proving in this way another race of women's opportunity! Of twenty-three women who qualified last year, nine have gone abroad as missionaries, or in connection with missions; the Society for the Promotion of Christian Knowledge assisting, to the extent of £75 yearly for four years, any woman offering herself for work in connection with a Church Missionary Society, or under a Church Bishop among "Heathen or Mahommedan Peoples." The Zenana Medical Mission also assists intending missionaries in their medical training.

But the opportunities for professional work at home increase apace. In nearly all our large provincial towns are to be found medical women in good practice, and some of these are attached to important local hospitals. Year by year more posts, such as those of resident-physician, or surgeon, in large institutions, are open to them. One lady has just recently been appointed Lecturer to a Medical School for Women in Ludhiana in the northwest of India. Another has left to become assistant to an Englishman practising in Persia, he having applied to the Council of the Women's College for such an assistant. Perhaps one of the most notable signs of the times on this question may be found in the fact that Mrs. Garrett Anderson, M.D., one of the best known pioneers of the movement and Dean of the Women's Medical College, has accepted the invitation (by unanimous vote of the Council) to be President of the East Anglian Branch of the British Medical Association.

A visit to the very modest premises of the London School of Medicine for Women will give but little notion of the important work in progress there, a work which is slowly revolutionising the most conservative of all professions. For this London School of Medicine has outgrown its habitation, spurred by which

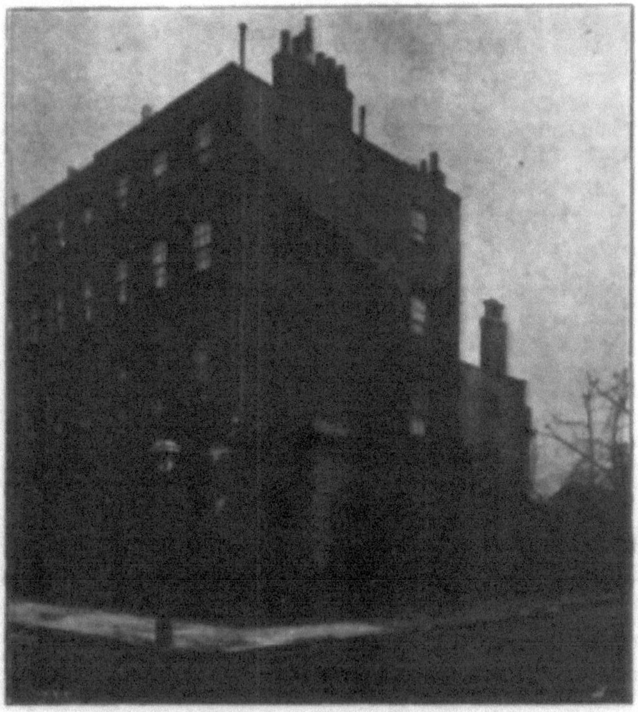

London School of Medicine for Women

Photo by Bolas and Co

necessity and the fact of the last entry of students having risen from the usual twenty-five or thirty to fifty, the Council has determined to build. To this end, however, additional funds are needed, and it would appear a very suitable celebration of the Diamond Jubilee of a Woman-Sovereign were some of her subjects to subscribe to the better accommodation of those Women Medical Students whose apparition has been by no means the least significant circumstance of her reign. For the present the College occupies a rambling old-fashioned corner house in Handel Street, Bloomsbury – a house with a high-walled garden and historic memories – one dignified in my days of studentship with a traditionary ghost. By this time, doubtless, that aristocratic shade has been shouldered out by shades of later date and lesser origin, whose frail tenements have subserved the needs of science, at the point of the dissecting-scalpel, but in those days the aura of an aristocratic vanished century still clung about the old house.

In the long, low, principal reception-room, opening by windows upon a verandahed terrace and thence into the garden, we drowsed on sleepy summer afternoons over fading botanical specimens, wherefrom we found it difficult to dissociate the impression of flowers. During the long six winter months this room was set with leaden tables, backless stools, and dank, methylated spirit-drenched chests. From early morning till late evening we occupied the backless stools on either side the leaden tables, following the course of muscles, veins and blood-vessels with studious knives. Beside us lay our open books, which we from time to time consulted; sometimes we asked questions one of another, or listened to the admonitions of our demonstrator. But for the most part we were a silent, intent group. Legends we heard of dissecting-room vagaries of masculine students, but they failed to inspire us.

We wore cotton over-alls, for the most part neat and pretty, and one coming suddenly upon us would maybe have caused a somewhat gruesome incongruity between ourselves and our tasks. Yet would it have been the most superficial of false sentiment, as superficial as that which shudders to see a woman dress an evil wound lest she should soil her pretty fingers. The kind of person whose pretty fingers will not stand good soap and water went out when women gave up wearing crape for dead canaries.

In the dining-room of the old house we committed to our note-books or to our memories the discourses of our lecturers, jotted down formulæ of chemical phenomena, packed our minds with the ten thousand and one circumstances of "foramina," "tuberosities," "grooves," and "surfaces," to be noted on bones for the future checkmating of wily examiners. In guest chambers opening upstairs upon a narrow corridor was our small pathological museum, its shelves adorned with bottled monstrosities, realities more gruesome far than wholesome normal ghosts; our materia-medica room, with its stores of sparkling crystals and its dried herbs. My lady's bedroom was our common room, the scene of teas and free discussion, her boudoir our library supplied with books whose titles she would either have been incompetent to read, or would have read with the affected shrug of her pretty shoulders, which it was in those days the fashion of her sex to turn on all things serious. On prize-days and at the annual Inaugural Addresses of our winter session, it may now be confessed, for other arrangements at present obtain, we assembled our company in the dissecting-room – that being our largest available room. The leaden tables and the tanks and student-stools were banished. In their places stood row on row of decorous chairs, drapings of red baize, and groups of palms and flowers. We all wore our prettiest gowns and holiday faces, and bowed abashed and with fluttering hearts to the distinguished personage who graciously presented us with our hardly-won prizes, or admonished us more or less severely upon the ways it behoved us, shouldering the burden of an onerous profession, to tread or to avoid. We loathed with a young and lofty loathing the well-dressed inquisitive personages who stared at us and our cherished pathological specimens through the pincenez of their curiosity, regarding both as something "odd" and allied, and inquired our ages and whether we had been baptised. But most of all the people we most hated were those who styled us "lady-doctors." They meant it kindly and in all respect, but we were trying so hard to be merely medical women!

However, we always enjoyed a sort of grim and secret satisfaction, remembering that these shocked conventional persons had sat for an hour on the identical spot where a leaden table or a tank of anatomical "horrors" had been and would be again to-morrow. Because they thought the flowers and baize and ourbest frocks "so very nice and womanly, you know," and "a female medical college" not the least bit shocking, with the exception perhaps of "those horrid little wretches in bottles upstairs!"

However, those who came to our Inaugural Addresses and our prize-givings were for the greater part our friends – the staunch and faithful who had borne the heat and burden of the day of opposition for us, who had supported the movement morally, actively and financially from its puny birth – and these were objects of our pride and veneration.

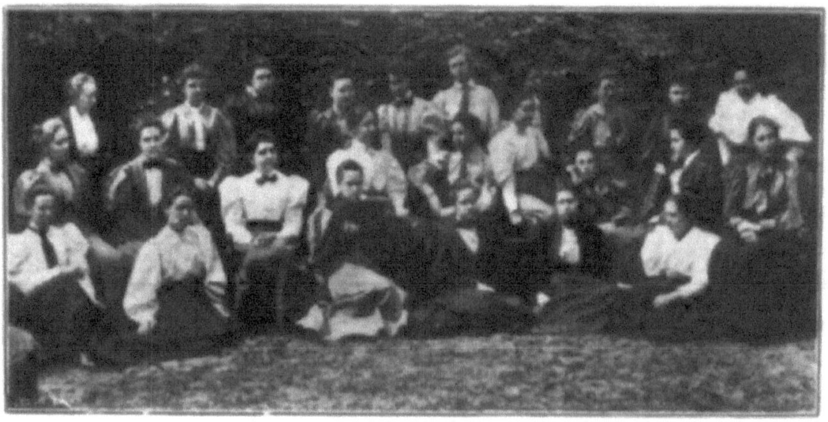

STUDENTS AT THE SCHOOL

Photo by W. S. Bradshaw and Sons

In our second year we made our first acquaintance with disease and hospital wards, attending the clinical and out-patient practice of the physicians and surgeons of the Royal Free Hospital, Gray's Inn Road – which most chivalrously opened its wards to women-students at a time when no other training ground in the United Kingdom was available to them.

Here we proudly recognised in the surgery, fractures or dislocations of those bones whose conformation in the dry we had so diligently studied; here with one end of our stethescope upon the patient's chest, and our ear laid to the other, we first learned to detect such small roughenings or other alteration of the heart-beats as show the working of its valves to be faulty; or the mucous bubbling, or other modified resonance indicative of lung-trouble. Here in the small theatre we shuddered over our first operation, and at its conclusion found our way into the court-yard for a reviving breath of air. We, however, punctiliously stopped short of fainting – for it was a point of honour with us to beat the record of our masculine counterpart who distinguishes himself notably in this direction. Here we learned from our seniors the arts of questioning patients, checking the confusing rush of eloquence wherewith the hospital-patient more especially enlarges on his symptoms, observing, marking, diagnosing, digesting and subsequently treating. Here we learned to look with eager interest for the effects of treatment, and of change of treatment, as the sufferers returned from week to week until dismissed "cured," or were taken as in-patients for more assiduous observation and attention. Thronging as hospital out-patients do in such large numbers, it is impossible to devote much time to each, consequently that time is efficiently economised and a habit of quick diagnosis acquired. With the exception of a certain number of male cases previously separated and reserved from them, the women-students see all the patients, male and female, presenting themselves at this large general hospital. It was at first regarded by many as an indecorum – to use no stronger term – that young women of a cultivated class and refined up-bringing should be permitted to "sound" the chests and bandage the limbs of an opposite sex; but in practice it turned out that the cultivation and refinement of their up-bringing, if it had done nothing more, had at least set them beyond the indelicacy of self-consciousness under circumstances to which self-consciousness did not belong. And the men, for the most part rough enough fellows of the artisan and labouring classes, have rarely been known to accept the situation other than with the most scrupulous courtesy.

A number of students whose homes are at a distance are accommodated (for there is no residence at the school) at a College Hall under the superintendence of a council, and in boarding-houses suitable managed.

In addition to the large experience afforded in general work, there are also at the Royal Free Hospital special departments for diseases of women, ophthalmic, dental and throat-and-ear practice, enabling the student, should she feel so inclined, to graft some speciality upon her general knowledge. Moreover, beside the years spent in daily attendance at the Royal Free, midwifery, fever and vaccination work have to be learned elsewhere. Practical midwifery is acquired by living in or

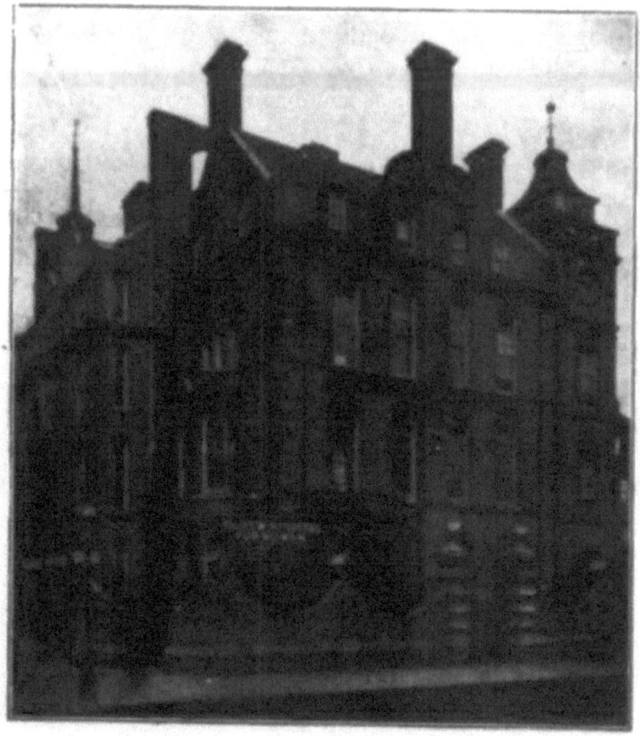

THE NEW HOSPITAL FOR WOMEN

Photo by Henry W. Reeves

near a Maternity Hospital over a period of three or six months, and taking cases under direction of the resident medical officers. These three or six months are weary months indeed, for the small persons to whose needs they are devoted are proverbial for topsyturvy notions with regard to time, choosing the most inconvenient hours wherein to enter upon life. If not resident in hospital, students lodge in the neighbourhood of the institution which they select for their maternity course. Under these circumstances the custom is to attach to the head of one's bed a bell with a rope hanging thereto and out of window, and this some hurried messenger from the hospital is bound to tug just at the moment when sound sleep has set in after a busy day. One learns to dress while waking, to fling on cloak and hat and arrive in the ward before one's eyes are fully opened, and even then not rarely to find herself too late, for hospital babies very frequently first see light in the cab which is bringing their mother to the wards, or within some minutes of arrival.

Fever work is done by three months' attendance in fever wards, and during this time the miseries of isolation are experienced, and the unsubstantiality of human friendship tried. For our dearest friends are liable to entreat us on no account under these circumstances to address a letter to them for fear of conveying some stray microbe with our news.

The device of vaccination is learned by weekly visits to a public vaccinating station, and here one acquires the fashion of a double-dyed treachery, cooing or ingeniously whistling in an infant's trusting face, while at the same time stabbing punctures in its plump and mottled arm. Here also we become acquainted with the fact that compulsory vaccination is by no means a popular measure.

There is in the Euston Road a most excellent hospital for the diseases of women and children. It contains some forty-two beds, and has a large out-patient department. It is manned exclusively by women surgeons and physicians, though on its consulting staff are eminent surgeons and physicians of the other sex.

Here women are eligible after qualification for resident house-surgeonships and clerkships, and here they have the opportunity of witnessing the latest and most complicated gynœcological operations conducted by operators of their own sex. Yet has the once styled "shrieking sisterhood" in reality shrieked so little that only the comparatively few are aware of the existence of this "New Hospital for Women" – a hospital whereto on its opening sufferers who had suffered for years in silence rather than seek masculine aid, gratefully flocked.

But old prejudices are disintegrating, times are changing – and the London School of Medicine for Women has its plans in hand for building. A block of laboratories is to occupy the east side of the old garden (and alas! the student's tennis court), leaving the present structure intact for its workers until these can be shifted to the new block. Then the old house, with its low reception rooms, its rambling corridors and crooks and corners, its memories and ghost will disappear with a past which strenuously denied the medical rights of women and raised the unanswerable suppose-a-cow-got-on-the-line species of argument.

Meanwhile the interested reader cannot do better than visit this romantic nursery of a great movement while it still retains evidence of its romantic childhood. If its humilities move him, then may he, like a fairy god-father recently conducted through its sombre walls by Miss Heaton, its kind and zealous assistant-secretary, testify his sympathy by a contribution toward the new building – a contribution which, in the case cited, reached the generous dimension of a thousand pounds.

I cannot better conclude than by an anecdote illustrative of a mode of thought adopted toward the movement by a member of the rising generation.

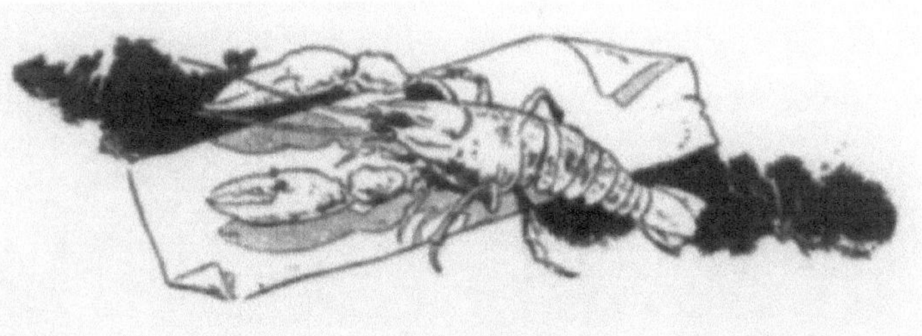

A small patient of mine who had first opened his eyes on the world in the presence of me as his professional adviser, and had retained my services subsequently during the ordeals of teething and whooping-cough, being questioned on reaching the age of articulacy as to his future calling, stood deliberating.

"Will you be a parson?" his interrogator assisted him. He shook his head emphatically.

"A soldier?" He was not so energetically sure, but he was sure.

"Will you be a doctor then?" was further asked. He gazed resentfully. The old Adam was in him. An insult had been done his dignity. "Why," he said loftily, "do you fink I'm a gell?"

Editorial Headnote

'Pioneer Women Doctors: Dr Elizabeth Blackwell, Dr Garrett Anderson, Dr Sophia Jex-Blake', in Edwin A. Pratt, *Pioneer Women in Victoria's Reign: Being Short Histories of Great Movements* (London: George Newnes, Limited, 1897), pp. 92–117

Born in Wolverhampton, Edwin A. Pratt (1854–1922) was an incredibly prolific writer, whose main publications spanned from the 1890s right up until his sudden death in late October 1922 at the age of 68. A former journalist, he began his career locally and early, becoming the sub-editor of the *Birmingham Mail* at the very young age of 19, followed by a stint in Manchester at that city's *Evening Mail*. Although he began as assistant editor, he became editor within three years. Pratt moved to London in the early 1890s, and became sub-editor on the *Times*, as well as contributing articles to the *Daily Telegraph*. Alongside his journalism, he published an array of books on economic, social, and industrial questions of the day; a move that was accelerated when he left his editorial position after a decade to concentrate on his longer investigations.[1] Always with an eye on current events, Pratt wrote full-length works covering, among many others, *Leading Points in South African History, 1486 to March 30, 1900* (1900); *American Railways* (1903); *The Organisation of Agriculture* (1904); *Trade Unionism and British Industry* (1904); *The Licensing Question* (1907); *The Rise of Rail Power in War and Conquest, 1833–1914* (1916); *The Christianizing of China* (1915); *British Railways and the Great War* (1921); and his final book explored *Scottish Canals and Waterways* (1922). Due to their global considerations and precise contemporary engagement, Pratt's writings were translated into other languages, including Swedish, Japanese, and Indian dialects.

Despite this ostensible focus on trade and industry, Pratt had a literary sideline in writings about women, and the last few years of the nineteenth century saw him publish three different books on key Victorian women. *Pioneer Women* (1897), excerpted here, was followed a year later by two biographies: *A Woman's Work for Women. Being the Aims, Efforts, and Aspirations of 'L.M.H' (Miss Louisa M. Hubbard)* and *Catherine Gladstone: Life, Good Works and Political Efforts* (both 1898). Pratt's journalistic background came into its own when synthesising enormous topics; a trait he would put later to good use in his writings on transport, for example.

Although, and unlike a number of his other works, *Pioneer Women* only achieved a single edition in 1897, it was a popular topic that spoke directly to the zeitgeist; something which explained its appeal to readers of the day. Indeed, its publication cannily coincided with Queen Victoria's Diamond Jubilee. This was a fact not lost on the press; as the *Morning Post* remarked: 'the time chosen for the appearance of his work could not be more appropriate'.[2] Priced at five shillings, it was a cheaper alternative to other larger considerations of the Queen's sixty-year reign. The *Bookman* included *Pioneer Women* in its 'Review of Jubilee Books', remarking on the need to wade through the flood of lives and surveys to secure only a dozen or so which provided 'literary and pictorial mementoes of the forthcoming commemoration, or a short cut to a general knowledge of the history of the last sixty years'. The periodical applauded the way in which Pratt dealt with this 'special department[] of energy' in a 'sensible' biographical format.[3] *Pioneer Women* appealed to a wide variety of reviewers, with topics ranging from employments, emigration, education, medical and nursing developments, Poor Law reform and philanthropic endeavour. It was labelled 'unpretentious' by the *Athenaeum*, a 'difficult task', because of the sheer vastness of the subject, but one accomplished with 'ability and conscientious care'.[4] While the *Saturday Review* lamented the focus on the middle classes (Pratt despised socialism) and that the topic could have been treated on a 'more adequate and scientific scale', they had missed Pratt's point.[5] As the *Englishwoman's Review* suggested, Pratt had, most vitally, given honour where it was due just in time as the loss of the pioneering generation was beginning to be felt.[6] In the year of Victoria's Diamond Jubilee what better treatment could be given to, as a German-language review made clear, 'how many areas of public life women in England occupy with the greatest success'? When a queen can build an empire, the reviewer, Theodor Barth, continued, women 'will probably also be able to supervise a school, preside over the administration of the poor or replace the male doctor'.[7] In *Pioneer Women*, Pratt recognised the value of pioneering women to society as a whole, as well as the momentous contemporaneity of a book which would also allow future generations to profit.

Notes

1 'Obituary', *Daily Telegraph*, 31 October 1922, p. 4; 'Death of Mr E.A. Pratt. An Authority on Railways', *Times*, 30 October 1922, p. 9.
2 *Morning Post*, 22 June 1897, p. 8.
3 'A Review of Jubilee Books', *Bookman*, 12.69 (June 1897), pp. 61–63; on p. 61; p. 63].
4 *Athenaeum*, 3630 (22 May 1897), p. 679; *Morning Post*, 22 June 1897, p. 8.
5 *Saturday Review*, 85:2203 (15 January 1888), p. 86.
6 *Englishwoman's Review*, CCXXXV (15 October 1897), pp. 273–274; on p. 273.
7 Theodor Barth, 'Das Regirungs-Jubilaum der Konigin Victoria', *Cosmopolis*, 6:18 (June 1897), pp. 833–842; on p. 840. My translation.

10

'PIONEER WOMEN DOCTORS: DR ELIZABETH BLACKWELL, DR GARRETT ANDERSON, DR SOPHIA JEX-BLAKE'

Edwin A. Pratt

Source: Edwin A. Pratt, 'Pioneer Women Doctors: Dr Elizabeth Blackwell, Dr Garrett Anderson, Dr Sophia Jex-Blake', in *Pioneer Women in Victoria's Reign: Being Short Histories of Great Movements* (London: George Newnes, Limited, 1897), pp. 92–117

CHAPTER IV.

PIONEER WOMEN DOCTORS: DR. ELIZABETH BLACKWELL, DR. GARRETT ANDERSON, DR. SOPHIA JEX-BLAKE.

In the earlier years of the Victorian era it seemed to be taken for granted that the profession of medicine was the exclusive prerogative of men, and should be carried on by them alone. It was not because the idea of women doctors was altogether unknown to the world, for in the Middle Ages women practitioners in medicine had a well-recognized position among both sexes, and were holders of academic medical degrees to which great value was attached; while early in the present century important positions were held by women doctors alike in Italy, France, and Germany. In England, however, it is only within the last few decades that they have been able to become accredited medical practitioners. The hostility towards them in that capacity dates at least as far back as the reign of Henry V., when a petition was presented praying "that no women use the practyse of fisyk under payne of long emprisonment." In fact, whereas in Italy, in the Middle Ages, medical women were not only allowed to take their degrees, but were treated with all honour, in England any woman who got to understand too much about the healing art was apt to be regarded as a witch, and dealt with accordingly. The one exception made in favour of women in this country was in regard to midwifery, which was entirely in their hands down to the sixteenth century, and mainly so to the middle of the eighteenth. It is not a little striking, too, that in the very year in which Miss Sophia Jex-Blake looked around for an opportunity to acquire a

DOI: 10.4324/9781003265238-10

medical degree, and saw nothing but closed doors in every direction, a Russian lady, Madame Kaschewarow, had the degree of M.D. conferred on her by the Medico-Chirurgical Academy at St. Petersburg, an event which created so much enthusiasm among the male students there that they not only greeted her with cheering which lasted several minutes, but placed her in a chair, and carried her in triumph through the hall. A comparison of this scene with the mobbing to which Miss Jex-Blake was subjected, later on, by some of the Edinburgh students, is not very flattering to our *amour propre.*

The result of the exclusion of women from the medical profession in Great Britain was twofold. In the first place it shut them out from what might be, for a number of them at least, a means of gaining a livelihood through honourable and remunerative work, and this in itself was an important consideration in an age when the necessity of securing a larger number of occupations for women was beginning to be more widely recognized. In the second place, there was the question whether women in large numbers were not being seriously prejudiced in their physical condition by their reluctance to consult male doctors with regard to certain of their ailments. On this point there was an abundance of testimony brought forward during the course of the agitation that arose, but suffice it here to say, by way of illustration, that in March, 1871, Dr. Mackenzie, of Inverness, wrote to the *Inverness Courier:* –

> "Having been a physician and surgeon for nearly fifty years, I state as a thoroughly well-known, undeniable fact that great numbers of women are sickly for life, and die, simply because they shrink from speaking of their ailments to men."

This statement was overwhelmingly confirmed by evidence adduced from many other quarters. In India matters were even worse, but here again a single illustration must suffice for present purposes. Writing to the Madras Government on April 16, 1872, Surgeon-General Balfour said: –

> "I estimate that of the 100,000,000 of women in India, at least two-thirds are, by their religious customs, debarred alike from receiving the visits of a medical man at their homes, and from attending for gratuitous advice at the public hospitals and dispensaries."

Yet, notwithstanding all this, the right of women to study and to practice medicine was only established by them here after a prolonged fight, carried on with indomitable perseverance against both the prejudices of centuries and powerful vested interests that were prepared to maintain a great injustice to women rather than tolerate their competition with men, although, as Mr. (now Sir James) Stansfeld remarked at the first distribution of prizes of the London School of Medicine for Women, in 1875, "trade unionism was none the more dignified when it appeared in the learned professions."

The history of the movement in this country dates back to May, 1856, when Miss Jessie Meriton White (Madame Mario) sent a letter to the Registrar of the University of London, asking if a woman could

> "become a candidate for a diploma in medicine if, on presenting herself for examination, she shall produce all the requisite certificates of character, capacity, and study, from one of the institutions recognized by the London University."

This request was duly considered, and in the following July the Senate passed a resolution declaring "that Miss J. M. White be informed that the Senate, acting upon the opinion of its legal adviser, does not consider itself empowered to admit females as candidates for degrees." Thus the first step was taken by Miss White; but as regards actual results the story to be told really centres around the lives of the three pioneers whose names appear at the head of this chapter.

DR. ELIZABETH BLACKWELL.

Amid the genial breezes of the seaside town of Hastings there still, happily, lives the actual leader of the movement for securing medical education and qualifications for women. An Englishwoman by birth, Miss Elizabeth Blackwell set the ball rolling in the United States, was herself the first qualified woman practitioner in America, was the first to be placed on the Medical Register of Great Britain, and was, also, the one by whose example Miss Elizabeth Garrett, afterwards Dr. Elizabeth Garrett Anderson, was led to follow in her footsteps, and become the pioneer in Great Britain.

Rock House, to which Dr. Blackwell retired some twelve or fifteen years ago, is a picturesquely situated abode built upon a rocky site which some one, at some time or other, has appropriated from the common land that rises above the town of Hastings. From the window of the cosy little sitting-room where Dr. Blackwell receives her visitors one looks down upon the harbour and the bay of Hastings, with a background of sea and cliffs – a picture that would be perfect but for the fact that what were once gardens at the base of the rock have now been utilized mainly for small house property. Yet, after justice has been done to the view, one is speedily absorbed in conversation with the hostess, who strikes one immediately as a person of strongly-marked individuality – a woman alike of ideas and ideals. These, too, are expressed with such force and clearness, and with a mental grasp so pronounced, that the question arises almost unconsciously to the lips, "Are you not still in practice?" The reply is in the negative, but the reason given is somewhat curious. Dr. Blackwell, it seems, has been in the habit of making not only a physiological but also a psychological study of her patients. She has diagnosed, as far as possible, the conditions of their inner selves as well as the ailments of their outer forms, believing, as she does, that the best work of a physician often refers to and influences mind quite as much as matter. But this addition of mental, or, as she calls it, "spiritual" treatment to the physical became too exhausting. "At seventy-six, you know," the doctor remarks, "it is too great a strain on one. There are younger practitioners in the field, and, as I have sufficient to live upon, I prefer now to leave them to do the doctoring, and occupy my own time with other things."

And these other things, one soon finds, ought to be quite enough to fill up all the time she can devote to them. One of her characteristics is, as she expresses it, to be always "a little way ahead of others" – a characteristic not altogether surprising in a pioneer! – and if at any time she finds that everybody agrees with her she concludes there must be something wrong. She thus forms a sort of minority *en permanence*. On various medical questions, which she freely discusses, she indulges in views that would certainly not be shared by the average orthodox practitioner of the opposite sex, looking at those questions from a man's rather than from a woman's standpoint. Then, as regards the general question of the present position of medicine, one learns that Dr. Blackwell is looking forward to a time when greater attention will be paid to discovering the actual causes of disease, rather than to various inoculations against disease; and when, too, discoveries will be made that will render less necessary the resort to heroic remedies in surgery, especially in the treatment of women. This is one of her ideals. Another is the advent of an epoch when the curative influence of sanitation will be even more fully recognized than it is at present; and still another is that while original research in physiology and biology should be promoted and encouraged, the experimentation on living animals should not be of such a nature as to cause pain. She recognizes "the right to kill," in the pursuit of legitimate investigation, but not "the right to torture." These views she seeks to carry out as one of the trustees and most active workers of the Leigh Browne Trust, which, among other things, has employed its income of £100 a year in sending a Commission to Paris, in 1890, to ascertain the working of Pasteur's method of inoculation; the publication of Dr. Carne Ross's pamphlet on the use of cinnamon in the treatment of cancer and other diseases; the publication, also, of "Biological Experimentation," by Sir B. W. Richardson, and other books and papers; and the giving in London of a series of "Humane Science" lectures in conjunction with the Humanitarian League, these lectures being all arranged by Dr. Blackwell herself.

Dr. Elizabeth Blackwell was born in 1821, at Bristol, and was the third daughter in a household of nine children. In 1832 the entire family emigrated to New York, which they succeeded in reaching after a passage that lasted seven weeks. Up to 1838 they lived in New York and Jersey City, but in that year the father, for business reasons, removed to Cincinnati, and there he died within a few months of his arrival, leaving a widow and nine children unprovided for. The three eldest daughters started a boarding-school as a means of supporting the household, and this was continued for four years until the elder brothers were able to earn sufficient to keep things going. Then Elizabeth began teaching on her own account, and she also took charge, for a short time, of a girls' district school.

How she came to turn her attention to medicine is told by herself in an exceedingly interesting little book, published in 1895, entitled "Pioneer Work in Opening the Medical Profession to Women: Autobiographical Sketches" (Long mans). She had, it seems, a positive antipathy to doctoring; but one of her lady friends was the victim of a painful disease, the delicate nature of which made the methods of treatment a constant suffering to her. This poor creature (who afterwards died from the complaint) said to her one day, "You are fond of study, and have health and leisure. Why not study medicine? If I could have been treated by a lady doctor my worst sufferings would have been spared me." The seed thus planted took deep root in Miss Blackwell's mind. She was in special want, too, of something to engross her thoughts. Inquiry showed, however, that there was then no way of her obtaining medical education, and the idea of such a thing was regarded by others as altogether impracticable. But the very prospect of overcoming difficulties and engaging in a "moral fight" on behalf of her sex had a great attraction for her, and after a time she resolved to conquer her natural aversions, and give herself up to the study of medicine. Yet first she must have money, and this very plucky woman took to teaching again with the express determination of hoarding every coin she could possibly save with the view of supporting herself later on.

So she taught by day and pored over her books by night, and then she began to look around for a medical school. Her applications to four medical colleges in Philadelphia to be received as a student were futile, and the dean of one of the smaller schools told her candidly, "You cannot expect us to furnish you with a stick to break our heads with." New York was also closed against her. Nothing daunted, and discarding the suggestion of some of her friends that she should put on the clothes of a man and go in disguise, she sent applications to a miscellaneous dozen of the smaller schools of the Northern States, a complete list of which she obtained, and, much to her joy, she received a letter in October, 1847, saying that her request would be complied with by the Medical School at Geneva, N.Y. It seems that when the authorities there received her application they resolved to let the male students decide on it, and to them, accordingly, it was referred. Some of them regarded the letter as a practical joke that was being played on them by the students at another school; but the final result was that they passed the following resolution: –

> "That one of the radical principles of a Republican Government is the universal education of both sexes; that to every branch of scientific education the door should be open equally to all; that the application of Elizabeth Blackwell to become a member of our class meets our entire approbation, and in extending our unanimous invitation we pledge ourselves that no conduct of ours shall cause her to regret her attendance at this institution."

The pledge thus given was honourably adhered to. The boisterousness and excessive animal spirits which had previously been characteristic of the class ceased instantly that Miss Blackwell put in an appearance in the following November, and the thoroughly courteous, considerate, and gentlemanly treatment that she received from students and professors stands out in bold contrast to the experiences of Miss Sophia Jex-Blake and her companions at Edinburgh later on. By the authorities of the school the advent of Miss Blackwell was, apparently, welcomed, not because of any lofty ideas of justice to the sex, but because her presence there was "a good advertisement." Such, indeed, it was; for Geneva, N.Y., has thereby acquired a degree of lasting fame which it could hardly have obtained otherwise.

Singularly enough, the only rudeness that Miss Blackwell received was from members of her own sex, who, with shocked propriety, would glare at her as she passed, gather in their skirts from the risk of contamination with her own, and make her feel as generally uncomfortable as they possibly could.

After two years' study at Geneva Miss Blackwell was unanimously admitted to the hospital wards of the great Blockley almshouse, at Philadelphia, for the necessary hospital work, and then, returning to Geneva, she completed her studies, passed her examinations, and obtained her diploma in January, 1849.

Dr. Blackwell says on this point: –

> "The admission of a woman for the first time to a complete medical education and full equality in the privileges and responsibilities of the profession produced a widespread effect in America. The public press very generally recorded the event and expressed a favourable opinion of it."

Soon, too, a number of ladies were seeking for qualification, and it is interesting to learn that one of the first to follow Dr. Blackwell's example was her sister Emily.

In April, 1849, Dr. Elizabeth Blackwell came to England, visited the hospitals of Birmingham and London, and, after spending some months at La Maternité, in Paris, was received as a student at St. Bartholomew's, London, thus greatly increasing her knowledge of medical matters. One of her "most valued acquaintances" during the St. Bartholomew's days was Miss Florence Nightingale, then quite unknown to fame. Miss Nightingale, under the escort of a footman, would call upon her in her rooms in Thavies Inn, and there, as Dr. Blackwell put it, in recalling the fact, they would "toast their toes" in front of the fire, while they exchanged their views and discussed their plans in life. It is to these fireside talks and to the influence exercised on her mind by Miss Nightingale that Dr. Blackwell traces her great and life-long interest in the subject of sanitation, which Miss Nightingale herself had so very much at heart. In her book Dr. Blackwell speaks of sanitation as the "supreme goal of medicine, its foundation and its crown." In July, 1851, she returned to America, and settled in New York, where a series of lectures which she delivered on the physical education of girls was of great service in enabling her to get a practice together. In 1853 she founded a small dispensary in a poor quarter of New York – a modest institution that developed in 1857 into the "New York Infirmary for Women and Children" (the first to be conducted entirely by women doctors), and, later on, into the "New York Infirmary and College for Women."

These early days in New York must have been somewhat trying to Dr. Blackwell. A woman of decided force of character, she had previously replied to a doctor who had advised her not to go to Paris to study, as it was such a horrible place: "If the path of duty led me to hell, I would go there;" while in one of her letters from Geneva, N.Y., she wrote, "I live simply, trust in God, and mock at the devil." But the malicious stories circulated about her in New York, and the manifold petty annoyances to which she was subjected in her pioneer efforts, were somewhat wearisome, and led her to exclaim, "I should like a little fun now and then. Life is altogether too sober." But her ideas of "fun" went no further than adopting a little orphan emigrant girl as a companion,* while before long she had well established her position, and surmounted most of her troubles.

In August, 1858, she revisited England, and in the following year gave a series of three addresses in London, showing what was being done in medicine by women in the United States, and the reasons for that work. Concerning the first of these lectures, given on March 2, 1859, at Marylebone Hall, she says: –

> "The most important listener was the bright intelligent young lady whose interest in the study of medicine was then aroused, Miss Elizabeth Garrett, who became the pioneer of the medical movement in England, and, as Mrs. Garrett Anderson, lives to see the great success of her difficult and brave work."

The year 1859 was further memorable because it was then that, under the operation of the Medical Act of 1858, the name of Dr. Elizabeth Blackwell appeared on the British Medical Register as the first qualified woman medical practitioner in Great Britain. It is necessary to the right comprehension of the whole subsequent position that the effect of this Act should be clearly understood.

It is true that under the clauses of the Act of 1858 there was no actual disqualification of women from taking medical degrees. The idea of women ever wanting to become doctors had not, apparently, entered into the thoughts of the framers of the Act at all. But it was expressly laid down that no person should be entitled to registration as a medical practitioner who had not qualified by passing the examinations of one of the existing medical boards in Great Britain – *except* in the case of those who had already secured a foreign degree, and had practised prior to the passing of the Act. Thanks to this exception, Miss Blackwell was clearly entitled to ask that she should be registered. Her request for registration was duly complied with, and she was thus the first woman whose name appeared on the British Medical Register, though she did so, be it remembered, in virtue of a foreign and not a British degree.

With regard, however, to women who had not obtained a foreign medical degree prior to the passing of the Act, their position was altogether different. Although, as already stated, they were not excluded by the Act, there were two steps that were essential preliminaries to their being placed on the register, namely, education and examination. Thus the medical schools and the examining bodies were the arbiters of their fate, and in the early sixties the former would not educate them, and the latter would not examine them.

How this position came to be altered, thanks mainly to the gallant efforts of women themselves, will be shown later on; but for the moment it will suffice to say that for a period of eight years the name of Dr. Elizabeth Blackwell, the first lady doctor in the United States, stood alone on the British Medical Register as that of the only lady doctor entitled to practice medicine in this country.

In August, 1859, Dr. Blackwell returned to New York and resumed her practice there. In 1865 she assisted in the expansion of the Infirmary for Women into a recognized College, she herself taking the chair of Hygiene. During the early years of this College she had the pleasure, she writes, of welcoming Miss Jex-Blake, then on a visit to America, as a member of the first class.

By 1869 special medical schools for women had been established, with the sanction of the Legislature, in New York, Philadelphia, and Boston, and in a number of Colleges women were received in the ordinary classes. The movement had thus been well established in America, and Dr. Blackwell once more came back to England for the purpose, among other things, of giving a helping hand to those who were striving so valiantly here to establish the claims of women doctors, and in England she has lived ever since. She started a practice in London, gave addresses on various occasions on health subjects, and took a leading part in the founding, in 1871, of the National Health Society, for the diffusion of sanitary knowledge. Dr. Blackwell was also greatly interested in the establishment of the London School of Medicine for Women. She joined the governing body, and likewise became a lecturer on gynæcology. She still occupies the former position. But, oddly enough, the health of this vigorous champion of sanitation, as she had been since the fireside talks with Miss Nightingale, in 1851, broke down as the result of her living in an insanitary house in London. After several winters abroad, she finally had to abandon her plans in the Metropolis, and retire to Hastings, there to pass the remaining years of her honourable and well-spent life.

DR. ELIZABETH GARRETT ANDERSON.

We have seen already that among the audience at the lecture delivered at Marylebone Hall by Dr. Elizabeth Blackwell on March 2, 1859, was the "bright intelligent young lady" whose interest in the study of medicine was to be then aroused, and who was to become the pioneer of the medical movement in Great Britain. Miss Elizabeth Garrett, the young lady in question, was the daughter of Mr. Newson Garrett, of Aldeburgh, Suffolk, a gentleman who thoroughly sympathized with her aspirations, and endeavoured to forward them in every possible way. She herself was then about twenty-one, and she was led, as she wrote to Dr. Blackwell in 1861, to choose the medical profession "more from the strong conviction of its fitness for women than from any absorbing personal bias." She began in 1860 by entering as a probationary nurse at Middlesex Hospital, and devoted her spare time to the study of anatomy, chemistry, and materia medica. When the first three months had expired she got permission to go round the wards with the house doctors, instead of devoting herself to any special department. The male students were at first somewhat amused; but when they found what great progress she was making they petitioned for her exclusion. The result was that she had to leave Middlesex Hospital. The applications she made to several other medical schools for permission to enter as a student were in each case unsuccessful, though in one or two cases the adverse decision was the result of only a small majority of votes.

> "Those gentlemen who opposed," she wrote in 1862, "always urged as one ground for doing so that, as the examining bodies were not prepared to admit women to their examinations, the school could not educate a woman to be an illegal practitioner, and that by so doing they would incur the certain risk of injuring the school in the eyes of the public without really aiding women."

The difficulty as to hospital practice was surmounted in time, but there was still the further difficulty with regard to the examining bodies. The College of Surgeons stated positively that they would not in any way countenance the introduction of ladies into the medical profession. Application was made, also, to the London University for the admission of women, though in this instance the request was based on general grounds, the claims of governesses and other women who required a good education being urged in preference to any demand for special concessions in the interests of women desirous of medical qualifications. The Senate, however, declared that it saw no reason to doubt the validity of counsel's opinion as given in the case of Miss Jessie Meriton White in 1856, and it accordingly declined to grant the application. Thereupon Mr. Newson Garrett got up a memorial to the Senate, suggesting that in the new charter, then about to be applied for, there should be inserted a clause removing the technical legal objection which seemed to be all that stood in the way of the admission of women. When the vote was taken there were ten members in favour of this course being adopted, and ten against, one being neutral. The Chancellor gave his casting vote against the application, which was accordingly refused. The result was communicated to Mr. Garrett in an official letter, which further said: –

> "I think it well to add that this decision has not been the result of any indisposition to give encouragement to the higher education of the female sex, a very general concurrence having been expressed in the desire stated in your memorial that an opportunity should be afforded to women of testing their attainments in the more solid branches of learning. But it has been based on the conviction entertained by the majority of the Senate that it is not desirable that the constitution of this University should be modified for the sake of affording such opportunity."

Miss Garrett had, therefore, to seek elsewhere for an opportunity to obtain examination, and, as the final result of her inquiries, she found there was only one examining body which either could or would consent to receive her. This was the Society of Apothecaries. When she applied, in due course, to this body, the opinion of its counsel, Mr. (afterwards Lord) Hannen, was taken, and he advised that as the purpose of their charter was to enable them to regulate the trade of selling drugs, and as there was no legal ground for refusing to allow a woman to sell drugs, they could not refuse to admit a woman to the examination imposed on candidates for their licence. The Society thereupon informed Miss Garrett of its willingness to withdraw from the attitude of opposition it took up at first, and admit her to examination, also allowing her to complete her education privately, by means of teachers in recognized medical schools, when, on particular subjects, she was not admitted to the public classes. But the concession was not made in particularly good grace, for exceptionally heavy fees were demanded for the instruction, and there seems to have been an idea that when Miss Garrett calculated how much it would cost her to pay alike these fees and the charges for the private teaching, she would speedily abandon what was regarded as a mere whim. But Miss Garrett paid the fees, filled up, by means of private instruction, the schedule of lectures required, passed the examinations, and in the autumn of 1865 her name was placed on the British Medical Register as that of the first female practitioner qualified by virtue of an English diploma.

In 1867 four other ladies, desirous of following in Miss Garrett's footsteps, presented themselves before the Society of Apothecaries, and were admitted to and passed the preliminary examinations. Thereupon quite a little panic arose in the medical profession. Was the monopoly which men had so long held to be now broken down by women? There were two on the Register already, and if three others were admitted still more would follow, and "there was no knowing where the thing would stop!" So an agitation was set on foot, and the Society of Apothecaries decided that in future they would not recognize certificates for private studies. As it was by this time perfectly well understood that women would not be admitted to some of the public classes, and that the other examining bodies maintained their attitude of either inability or complete hostility, the effect of the new rule was, for the time being, to deprive the would-be women students of their last remaining chance.

Miss Garrett had to go to Paris for her M.D. degree, which she obtained there in 1870, after an examination in which she acquitted herself with brilliant success. In the following year she married Mr. J. G. S. Anderson, of the Orient line of steamships, but she continued her practice among women and children. She had by this time gained a well-recognized position in the medical world. In 1866 she opened St. Mary's Dispensary in Seymour Place, in order that poor women and children should have the option of being attended by a woman doctor. Of this dispensary Miss Garrett was the only medical officer for some years, but after a time she was joined by some ladies who had graduated at Zurich. There had been a certain amount of questioning in some quarters whether or not women really wanted to be attended by a doctor of their own sex, but these doubts were speedily set aside by the number of women who came to the little dispensary for advice. It was soon found necessary to convert the dispensary into a small hospital. This, in its turn, underwent various changes, of which the present outcome is the New Hospital for Women in the Euston Road, where all the medical and surgical work is done by women. To this hospital, which involves an expenditure of about £4000 a year, women now come from all parts of the country, and Dr. Garrett Anderson said of it, in an appeal for additional funds, published in *The Times* of December 11, 1896: –

> "The results of the work compare very favourably with those in any other hospital in London dealing with the same class of cases. The wards are always full, and there are usually thirty or more patients waiting for the chance of admission. It is difficult to see in what way a better test could have been applied, or a more decisive answer given to the questions as to the willingness of women to trust doctors of their own sex, or of the ability of women to carry out the more difficult class of medical work. I have the less hesitation in giving public testimony to the high quality of the work, both medical and surgical, done at the New Hospital, as, while enjoying constant opportunities of judging it, I have not for some years had any share in the doing of it."

Dr. Garrett Anderson was, up to the year 1892, senior physician of this Hospital, where she is still consultant physician, and Chairman of Committee. She is also Dean of the London School of Medicine for Women.[†] At Christmas, 1896, she accepted an invitation to become president of the East Anglian Branch of the British Medical Association for 1897.

In a pamphlet entitled "Pro Aris et Focis," written in 1869, by Fanny Aikin-Kortright – who expressed her belief that "no thinking woman had yet spoken plainly, disagreeing with so-called woman's rights" – there is a reference to Dr. Elizabeth Garrett and Dr. Mary Walker, of whom it is said: –

> "Both have gone through what we cannot but regard as a fiery ordeal; both have come forth from the flames, still womanly women, and neither, thank God, has attempted to prove her superiority by forsaking the Christian altar.
>
> "Miss Garrett possesses a superior mind as well as superior attainments, and her character appears to correspond to her intellectual qualities. She has a great calmness of demeanour, a large amount of firmness, usually a good deal of fairness and coolness in argument, a pleasant countenance, a decided but perfectly feminine manner, an attire at once apart from prevalent extravagance and affected eccentricity.
>
> "No one can take exception to this unobtrusive and refined woman practising among women and children, which she states to be her sole aim, provided her medical skill should prove equal to her general talents."

Then in an article published in the *Nineteenth Century* of July, 1877, Mr. (now Sir) James Stansfeld, M.P., paid his tribute to Dr. Elizabeth Garrett Anderson, of whom he wrote: –

> "The marked distinction with which she passed her examination in Paris is well known, and her equal distinction and success in the practice of her profession are matters both of general and professional recognition."

To this it may be added that the distinction and success thus gained by her contributed greatly to the growth of an eventually vigorous public conviction that women had a capacity for medicine and surgery, that their demand to be admitted to the profession was a reasonable one, and that they were conferring, thereby, a distinct and much-appreciated service on the members of their own sex.

DR. SOPHIA JEX-BLAKE.

We come now to the story of Dr. Sophia Jex-Blake, upon whom the brunt of the battle fell so far as the actual struggle in Great Britain was concerned. She had, as already stated, become acquainted with Dr. Elizabeth Blackwell, in New York, in connection with the classes opened at the Infirmary and College for Women in that city; and she herself told, in a speech delivered at the first annual meeting of the London School of Medicine for Women, in 1875, how –

> "during a visit to America, she had first acquired her interest in medical study from seeing the noble work done by medical women which men never would have had the opportunity of doing, and especially the work done by Dr. Lucy Sewall, whose professional knowledge and personal character made her the ideal of what a woman doctor should be."

When, however, in 1869, after her return from America, she looked around with the object of finding some opportunity by which she herself could enter the profession, she found every door closed against her at home; while, though she might have obtained a diploma in France, Switzerland, Italy, or America, it would not have secured registration here because, as already explained, the Medical Act of 1858 would not recognize any foreign licence or degree obtained subsequently to the passing of that Act.

Miss Jex-Blake applied, in the first instance, though unsuccessfully, to the University of London. Then, in March, 1869, she turned to the University of Edinburgh, and there, after a discussion lasting several months, she and four other ladies were allowed to matriculate and pay the fees, being registered in due form as students of medicine. This looked very promising, especially as all the University authorities had concurred in the arrangements made. But after the ladies had been studying for six months a powerful faction rose against them. Certain of the professors and students, finding, much to their surprise, that the ladies were really in earnest, and were, too, gaining honours and prizes even in competition with male students, began to show open hostility, and this became still more conspicuous when the ladies (who, in the meantime, had been joined by two others) applied to be allowed to study in the wards of the Royal Infirmary. Not only, too, were they subjected to a variety of petty annoyances, but the students presented a numerously-signed memorial against their admission to the Royal Infirmary, and succeeded, for a time, in obtaining their exclusion. On November 17, 1870, matters resolved themselves into a regular riot. As the ladies were walking together to Surgeons' Hall they saw a mob of students and others who had gathered together in front of the gates, which were deliberately slammed in the faces of the ladies as soon as the latter approached. One student, more gallant than the others, forced the gates open again, and admitted the ladies, who passed in with much howling and yelling on the part of the mob. Not satisfied with this behaviour, the rioters also thrust a sheep into the room which the ladies had entered. "Let it remain," said the professor, when he saw the animal; "it has more sense than those who sent it here." When the lecture was over a number of the more gentlemanly students formed a body-guard, in order to escort the ladies safely to their rooms, and for some days afterwards this body-guard – known as the "Irish Brigade," from the number of Irishmen in it – accompanied them to and from the Hall until the rowdies got tired of their proceedings. The appeal to admit women students to the Infirmary was afterwards brought before a meeting of the contributors to that institution, but was there rejected, one of the professors declaring that they were obliged to consider "the interests of the male students, whose feelings of delicacy were violated by the idea of the presence of women." Indeed, so much were these feelings of delicacy affected that when, on one occasion, Miss Jex-Blake rose to speak at a meeting, the students howled and yelled at her in the gallery, and pelted her with peas, leading Professor Blackie to remark to her, with his dry humour, "Well! ye can say now ye've fought with beasts at Ephesus." In the streets, too, the ladies were followed by the possessors of these "delicate feelings" and treated by them in such a way that one of them, Miss Pechey, felt compelled to send a letter to the *Scotsman* of July 14, 1871, in which she said: –

> "It will possibly strike some people as sufficiently extraordinary that a knot of young men find pleasure in following a woman through the streets, and should take advantage of her being alone to shout after her all the foulest epithets in their very voluminous vocabulary of abuse; yet such is the case . . . . If the wish of these students is to bar our progress, and frighten us from the prosecution of the work we have in hand, I venture to say that never was a greater mistake made. Each fresh insult is an additional incentive to finish the work begun. I began the study of medicine merely from personal motives; now I am also impelled by the desire to remove women from the care of such ruffians. I should be very sorry to see any poor girl under the care (?) of such men as those, for instance, who the other night followed me through the street using medical terms to make the disgusting purport of their language more intelligible to me. When a man can put his scientific knowledge to such degraded use, it seems to me that he cannot sink much lower."

Meanwhile the pros and cons. of the whole question were being actively discussed in Edinburgh, and, as the result of a meeting called by the Lord Provost, a "Committee for Securing a Medical Education to Women in Edinburgh" was formed in the early part of 1871. This Committee rendered most valuable help. Among other things it relieved the ladies of financial difficulties, and this in itself was of no slight advantage, considering that the funds raised for various purposes connected with the movement amounted to over £3000. It was also the means of securing the admission of women students to the Infirmary after they had been excluded from it for two years.

On the other hand, however, fresh trouble arose when the lecturers at Surgeons' Hall prohibited, in effect, the attendance of ladies at any of the ordinary classes, and when the University Court resolved – as it did in January, 1872 – that it would take no further steps to enable the ladies to pursue their studies with a view to a degree, though it was good enough to offer, instead, some "certificates of proficiency," which would not have been of the slightest practical value. An action of "declarator" was then brought with the object of compelling the University authorities to afford the ladies an opportunity of completing their studies; but it failed on the ground that an illegal act had been committed at the outset by the University Court in admitting the ladies at all. This judgment was given in June, 1873, and it not only saddled the ladies with the payment of £844 law expenses, but gave them the unpleasant assurance that the battle in Edinburgh was over, and that for the time being, at least, they had sustained a total defeat. They struggled on, making fresh attempts in other directions, until March, 1874, when they finally abandoned the unequal contest in Scotland, and came on to London.

Here, as it was hopeless to look for the admission of women students to the then existing schools, a project was pushed forward with much ardour by Miss Jex-Blake and others for the opening of a London School of Medicine for Women. The idea was that such a school should be officered by recognized lecturers from a number of different hospitals, and a spacious old-fashioned house of one story only, with rooms looking on to a large private garden, was taken for the purpose. Miss Jex-Blake worked with great energy in raising the funds and enlisting the help of influential persons, and she gained the support of, among others, Dr. Ainstie, to whom the establishment of the School, of which he became the first Dean, was really due, though he did not live to see the formal opening in October, 1874. Dr. Garrett Anderson, also, had by this time obtained an established place in the medical profession, and was able to exercise considerable influence in the development of the scheme. Dr. Elizabeth Blackwell, who had now finally left America, also entered heartily into the work of helping her sisters at home so far as the state of her health at that time would allow; while a Provisional Council was formed, consisting entirely of medical practitioners, who, as the report for 1875–76 states, "came to the aid of the women students in spite of an amount of opposition and obloquy which an outsider could hardly understand."

So the School was most pluckily opened, with a total of twenty-three students for the first year, although there were then no examinations open, and no opportunities for attendance at hospitals. It was imperatively required by the examining boards that all students should pursue the bedside study of disease in hospitals having not fewer than a hundred beds, if in London, and a distinct staff of medical and surgical officers. One hospital after another in the Metropolis was applied to, but almost all of those which had the requisite number of beds were already appropriated for the instruction of male students, and there was great unwillingness to extend their benefits to women as well.

In the early part of 1877 a crisis was reached in the affairs of the School. The prospect seemed so hopeless that the lecturers declared it was no use going on any longer. The summer course was abandoned, and the closing of the School was imminent, when the good news was received that the Royal Free Hospital, which had no male school, had agreed to receive lady students, an agreement to this effect being signed on June 12, 1877. Thereupon the apparently moribund School got a fresh lease of life, and it has gone on successfully ever since.

In the meantime much had been done to secure Legislative assistance, and as the final result of a good deal of discussion and negotiation, which need not be detailed here, a Bill, introduced by Mr. Russell Gurney, "enabling" all British examining bodies to extend their examinations and qualifications to women (some of them having pleaded that they could not legally do so), became law in 1876. Of this merely permissive Act the King and Queen's College of Physicians (Ireland) was the first to take advantage; and early in 1877 Dr. Jex-Blake, Dr. Edith Pechey (who had both already obtained their M.D. at Berne), and other ladies, were admitted to the British Register through that College. But for those ladies who had not already been "educated" the hospital difficulty was still a fatal stumbling-block until the Royal Free Hospital threw open its doors to women students. Happily the action of the Irish College on the one hand, and that of the Royal Free Hospital on the other, secured for the ladies a final triumph in the movement which they had carried on with such pertinacity for so long a period. As championed by Dr. Sophia Jex-Blake the campaign had lasted eight years, while seventeen had elasped since Dr. Garrett Anderson, inspired by Dr. Blackwell, began her own pioneer efforts.

One week after the agreement with the Royal Free Hospital the Senate of the University of London, by a majority of sixteen to eleven, decided on the admission of women to its medical examinations and degrees, and various other examining bodies followed suit later on.

Dr. Sophia Jex-Blake settled down in practice in Edinburgh in 1878, and started there, in that year a dispensary for women, which was so successful that in 1885 a small cottage hospital was opened in connection with it. In a letter to *The Times* of September 22, 1896, pleading for funds to enable her to establish in Edinburgh "a thoroughly good women's hospital, officered by medical women, and open to all those who desire to secure the services of physicians and surgeons of their own sex," she said: –

> "I have now been in practice for nearly twenty years, and during the whole of that time I have been receiving fresh evidence that there are a very large number of women, and especially of poor women, who will not accept the necessary treatment from a man, and who have, in many cases, endured years of continuous suffering before they had the opportunity of obtaining relief from their medical sisters."

She has also had the satisfaction of seeing an Edinburgh School of Medicine for Women established and specially recognized as qualifying for the University of Edinburgh, clinical instruction being given at the Royal Infirmary. Of this School Dr. Jex-Blake is Dean.

At the present time the medical examining bodies that admit women are (1) the University of London; (2) the Royal University of Ireland; (3) the Conjoint Colleges of Scotland; (4) the Conjoint Colleges of Ireland; (5) the Society of Apothecaries, London; (6) the Scotch Universities; and (7) the University of Durham. Strong efforts have been made to induce the Royal Colleges of Physicians and Surgeons, London, to open their examinations and diplomas to women, but these have not, so far, been successful. In a petition presented to these Colleges in 1895 it was stated, among other reasons for the desired concession: –

> "Many women, both in this country and abroad, hold appointments on the staff of Hospitals for Women and Children; some of these Hospitals are worked entirely by women, and cases of all kinds and of all degrees of severity are received. Public bodies like the General Post Office, the Metropolitan Asylums Board, and various County Councils have appointed women as assistant medical officers in the institutions under their control. The British Medical Association, the Medico-Psychological Association, the Society of Anæsthetics, and the Anatomical Society of Great Britain admit women as members. In short, the reception of women into the profession is going on steadily, and experience has proved that those evils have not resulted which it was feared might follow the admission of women to the study and practice of medicine, and that there is a demand for women as medical practitioners."

Up to December 1, 1896, no fewer than 299 women had obtained diplomas entitling them to have their names put on the British Medical Register as duly qualified practitioners.

The number of students in the London School of Medicine for Women at the end of 1896 was 159. Dr. Elizabeth Blackwell, Dr. Garrett Anderson, and Dr.

Sophia Jex-Blake are all on the governing body of this Institution, which is the largest of all the separate schools for women, and the only one in England. For more than twenty years, as Dr. Garrett Anderson wrote further in her letter to *The Times* of December 11, 1896, already referred to, the school has been carried on in various hired houses, and it is now proposed to pull these down and build good laboratories, library, lecture-rooms, etc., at a cost of £20,000. Towards this amount there was £8000 in hand. An additional £4000 was wanted (the remainder of the cost being converted into a sinking fund), and, in appealing for contributions, Dr. Garrett Anderson said: –

> "Is there no large-hearted man or woman who will make a beginning by endowing a bed at the New Hospital, or by building a laboratory at the school, giving to either his name, and thus linking his memory for many years with the history of one of the most striking social advances seen in the present generation?"

Source Endnotes

* And her faithful friend and helper the "little orphan emigrant girl" of the fifties has been ever since. With a merry laugh she tells the visitor to Rock House how, in the early days of her adoption, she became so accustomed to seeing women doctors around her that on one occasion, after a gentleman had been, she exclaimed, "Just fancy! they call a *man* 'Dr.!' "

† For the story of this School, see pages 113–115 [in the original].

Editorial Headnote

Isabel Thorne, *Sketch of the Foundation and Development of the London School of Medicine for Women* (London: Printed by G. Sharrow, 1905)

Isobel Thorne (1834–1910) began medical training, but she did not qualify as a doctor. Instead, she became one of the best-known administrators of medical women's education, as Honorary Secretary of the newly-established London School of Medicine for Women. She would go on to hold the post for over thirty years, seeing the school from its shaky starts to prosperity and renown. When Thorne died in 1910, her obituary in the *British Medical Journal* remarked upon her aptness for the position. 'Eminently and happily fitted' for such a post, Thorne was 'steadfast in purpose and possessed of sound judgment'; she had also the 'faculty of disarming hostility'. The writer noted that the 'great success of the school is due' to her 'long co-operation with it'.[1] Although she did not qualify as a medical woman, Isabel Thorne was, therefore, intimately bound up in the movement from the 1860s onwards, and it was apt that she was the one to write a brief history of the school.

Born in London, at 21 she married Joseph Thorne, who was a tea merchant in China. The couple lived in Shanghai initially and Thorne reflected frequently on experiences with male doctors called out for herself or her children who, while excellent with patients of their own sex, were less effective with those of the opposite. A lack of sympathy and understanding was exacerbated by inappropriate personnel, as she witnessed herself, in India or in China. Her first child, for example, was delivered in China by an old ship's surgeon. Further personal experience cemented this belief, when tragedy struck and the Thornes lost one of their children to illness.[2] After the family's return to Britain, in 1868 Thorne's medical studies began initially at the Ladies' Medical College in London, but were later tied up with that of Sophia Jex-Blake at the University of Edinburgh, where she joined a number of women eager to qualify, and who spent four years from 1869 trying to do so. The *Sketch*, here reproduced in full, detailed her frustrating battles with the University, as well as its culmination in the setting up of the London School of Medicine for Women in 1874. As Thorne revealed happily, her husband supported her ambitions every step of the way, despite her domestic responsibilities.

While this is her only full-length work, in her position as Honorary Secretary and in her support for medical women, Thorne's name appeared very regularly in the press, both in Britain and in India, appealing for funds or sympathy. This little volume does not appear to have been noticed much outside the *Magazine* of the London School of Medicine for Women in January 1906, where a brief and positive review is concluded with a long quotation from the end of the *Sketch*.[3] It was, however, reflected upon when looking back at the progress made by women in the profession after her death. In June 1913, for example, the *Pall Mall Gazette* used it to embody 'all the struggles and vicissitudes she, with other women, who late won distinction, had to pass through to gain the victory for future generations'.[4]

Isabel Thorne's daughter, the surgeon May Thorne (see Volume IV), took over as Honorary Secretary of the School on her mother's resignation in December 1907. A scholarship was established at the LSMW, and was first awarded in 1913.[5] In 2019, after a century and a half, Isabel Thorne was one of seven women to be awarded her M.B. degree by the University of Edinburgh.[6]

Notes

1 'Obituary', *BMJ*, 2:2598 (15 October 1910), p. 1198.
2 M.A. Crowther and M.W. Dupree, *Medical Lives in the Age of Surgical Revolution* (Cambridge: Cambridge University Press, 2007), p. 160.
3 *London (Royal Free Hospital) School of Medicine for Women Magazine*, 33 (January 1906), pp. 586–587.
4 'Women Doctors. How They Have Won Through by Quiet Perseverance', *Pall Mall Gazette*, 20 June 1913; in London School of Medicine for Women and Royal Free Hospital Press Cuttings, Volume IV: January 1904-August 1915, H72/SM/Y/02/004, London Metropolitan Archives.
5 N. McIntyre, *How British Women Became Doctors: The Story of the Royal Free Hospital and its Medical School* (n.p.: Wenrowave Press, 2014), p. 181; p. 183.
6 www.theguardian.com/uk-news/2019/jul/06/edinburgh-gives-female-medical-students-their-degrees-150-years-late (accessed 10 October 2023).

11

SKETCH OF THE FOUNDATION AND DEVELOPMENT OF THE LONDON SCHOOL OF MEDICINE FOR WOMEN

Isabel Thorne

Source: Isabel Thorne, *Sketch of the Foundation and Development of the London School of Medicine for Women* (London: Printed by G. Sharrow, 1905)

SKETCH OF THE FOUNDATION AND DEVELOPMENT OF THE LONDON SCHOOL OF MEDICINE FOR WOMEN

By Isabel Thorne, Honorary Secretary

PREPARATION for the medical profession is now so free from obstacles for women, that it is difficult for students at the School to realise the state of affairs existing 40 years ago; perhaps, therefore, a few of my own recollections may be of use to them.

The first allusion to the medical education of women that I remember was a newspaper paragraph which I read in Shanghai about the year 1858, relating that Miss Elizabeth Blackwell, English by birth but resident since childhood in America, had succeeded after much difficulty in obtaining the M.D. degree of the University of Geneva, U.S.A. This was the first case in modern times of a woman taking the same course of study in preparation for the Medical profession as that required of men, and it is therefore to Dr. Elizabeth Blackwell that all who value the medical education of women owe a deep debt of gratitude.

In Great Britain a Bill was brought into Parliament to regulate the practice of medicine, which was in a very chaotic state. This Bill was piloted through the House of Commons by the Rt. Hon. W. Cowper Temple, and became law in 1858. A General Medical Council was established to keep a register of duly qualified medical practitioners. Dr. Elizabeth Blackwell had practised in London some little time before the Register was compiled, and when she applied for her name to be included, it was found she could not be refused, and thus an important precedent

DOI: 10.4324/9781003265238-11

was established, a woman's name appearing in the very first register issued by the General Medical Council of Great Britain and Ireland.

Subsequently Miss Garrett – better known as Mrs. Garrett Anderson – decided to qualify herself for the examinations in Medicine of the Society of Apothecaries, London, the only British Examination then not absolutely impossible to women. When she presented herself as a candidate I believe a legal opinion was taken as to whether she could be refused on account of her sex, but as she had managed to comply with all the conditions laid down for candidates, the opinion was in the negative, and in 1865 Miss Garrett passed successfully all the tests required. The Society then made a rule that no certificates of instruction would be received by them unless issued from a recognised medical school. This rule prevented other women following Miss Garrett's example, as all British Medical Schools refused to receive them as students.

During a residence of some years in China I had necessarily to call in male medical practitioners, who, however excellent as attendants on men, were not so well qualified for the care of women and children, and on my return to England I welcomed the suggestion of my brother-in-law, Augustus Thorne, D.L., J.P., that I should join an institution for women recently established in Fitzroy Square, by Dr. James Edmunds, under the name of the Ladies' Medical College. Classes were held in Chemistry, Anatomy, Hygiene, and Midwifery. Except as regards the latter subject the teaching was of a very elementary character. Dr. James Murphy, formerly Lecturer on Midwifery at University College, gave the lectures he had delivered to his male students, so that they contained more thorough instruction. I took great interest in all the teaching and the little I learnt made me wish for more. My experience in connection with the Ladies' Medical College caused me to realise very forcibly the risk of imperfectly trained persons being expected by the public to undertake the duties of fully qualified practitioners, and the danger of their being called in to treat all the ills that flesh is heir to, because they were acquainted with the normal needs of childbirth, and could attend midwifery cases.

Miss Garrett had shown that the Society of Apothecaries was not quite impregnable, so with my brother-in-law's support I applied to the Society of Apothecaries for leave to present myself at the examination in Arts for admission to the L.S.A., and at last received permission on condition that if I satisfied the examiners it would give me no right to be a candidate at the subsequent medical examinations as it would have done in the case of a man.

I was the only woman up for the examination in April, 1868, and got through, but all further progress was barred as there was no medical School in Great Britain to which women were admitted. In the spring of 1869 I was on the point of starting for Paris where there was a possibility of medical classes being open to women, when I met Miss Jex Blake, who had made an attempt to obtain teaching in Edinburgh University but had been refused on the ground that it was not advisable for the University to make alterations "in the interests of one lady." I decided to join Miss Jex Blake, as also my friend Miss Chaplin, whom I had known at the Fitzroy Square College, Miss Pechey, and Mrs. de Lacy Evans, so that we were a band of five women instead of one.

A fresh application was made which was favourably received by the Senatus and the University Court, and it only remained that the assent of the General Council of the University should be given to allow of arrangements being made. The Autumnal Meeting of this Council took place a few days before the winter session, a week or so after the matriculation examination, by which alone medical students can gain entrance to the University. In order to avoid the loss of time – practically a year – which would have been occasioned by waiting for the decision of the Council before matriculating, we obtained a special permission through the kindness of the Dean of the Medical Faculty to present ourselves for Matriculation, with the understanding that should the vote of the Council be adverse the examination would be void. Fortunately the motion "That women be allowed to matriculate and to form separate classes," proposed by Professor Masson and seconded by Professor Hughes Bennett, was passed by a very large majority.

In accordance with this vote a minute was promulgated by the University Court, held November 10th, 1869, stating that "All women attending such classes shall be subject to all the regulations now or at any future time in force in the University as to the matriculation of students, their attendance at classes, examinations, or otherwise." Thus after months spent in making and considering proposals and counter proposals we thought we had at last attained our object, although the onus of arranging separate classes was thrown upon us, and we had to guarantee 100 guineas for each class.

As we had passed our matriculation examination, we paid our fees, and received cards which proclaimed in red letters that we were Cives Academiæ Edinensis, our troubles seemed to be over except that we could not obtain anatomical teaching. However, we fulfilled the academical requirements of the University by arranging for classes in Chemistry, under Professor Crum Brown, and Physiology, under Professor Hughes Bennett. We also attended the laboratory where our demonstrator was Mr., now the celebrated Professor Sir James Dewar, F.R.S. During the winter session two voluntary examinations were held. The questions were the same in both "sections of the class," as the two divisions of the male and female students were termed, and given at the same hour, under identical conditions, in different rooms. After the first examination, when it was found that one of us had taken so high a place in the Chemistry class list that it was possible she might win one of the Hope Scholarships, the first intimation was given that distinctions might be made between the men and women respecting the distribution of prizes, the professor remarking that in the event of a woman taking the highest place, some difficulty might occur and the matter would have to be referred to the Senatus.

As the result of the two examinations four-fifths of the women were in the honours list, Miss Pechey being prominent as the best student in Chemistry of the year, the two men above her with higher marks being in their second session. As Miss Pechey was third on the list the first Junior Hope Scholarship was fairly hers, and much astonishment and indignation were felt when the professor stated he had awarded the Scholarship to the man below Miss Pechey, on the ground that the women's class was not the class for which the Hope Scholarships were intended. And here I may be permitted to mention the circumstances under which these Scholarships were founded. Some forty years before, Dr. Hope, the then famous Professor of Chemistry of the University of Edinburgh, gave a series of lectures to ladies within the usual lecture room. This course was very popular and was largely attended by a fashionable audience, who however were not admitted by the ordinary entrance, but through a window in South College Street, which was converted into a temporary door for their use. The pecuniary result of this course of chemistry was so satisfactory that Dr. Hope was enabled to endow four scholarships for the four students who took the highest number of marks in the voluntary class competition, senior and junior.

The endowment having been made from funds raised by a ladies' class, it seemed specially appropriate that a woman student should take a position rendering her eligible for a share in it, but on Miss Pechey appealing to the Senatus against Professor Crum Brown's award, his decision was confirmed, though at the same time that body decided that the women should have the ordinary certificates of attendance. Both these votes were passed by a majority of one. The two conclusions appear contradictory, for if the women belonged to the ordinary class, Miss Pechey's claim to the scholarship seemed indisputable. As soon as the public became acquainted with the facts much sympathy was expressed with Miss Pechey. There was also some unnecessary outcry against Professor Crum Brown, who, whatever his conclusions, was never actuated by mean or unworthy motives.

This episode was the cause of much unpleasantness and bad feeling, and the probable reason we had so much difficulty in our subsequent connection with the University. Up to this time we had not met with active opposition, but our success in the examination lists was our undoing, and the agitation became so intense that the following lines graphically describe the state of affairs that existed in Edinburgh during the next few years:

THE SONG OF THE NEUTRAL.

"When can I again invite
Friends of mine to come and dine,
Without danger of a fight;
Without danger that the party
Change its tone from frank and hearty
To the angry tone of strife;
As the theme so quarrel rife,
Croppeth up amidst the talk
As weeds crop up across the walk,

Of the doctors and the ladies?
When Christison resigns his chair,
And Andrew Wood is with the blest,
When the doctors cease from troubling,
And the ladies are at rest!"

Scotsman, January 19th, 1872.

The death of Professor Sir James Simpson, the introducer of chloroform, deprived us of an influential friend both in and out of the University at a critical moment.

The difficulty of obtaining a separate class in all the subjects required for the University curriculum in consequence of the inability of some of the professors, and the unwillingness of others to devote a double amount of time and energy to their classes, seemed likely to prove so great an obstacle that Professor Masson brought forward a motion proposing that women might enter the ordinary classes subject to such exceptions as the University Court might think fit. Through an allusion to the mixed classes at the anatomical lectures at South Kensington, it was thought that Professor Masson intended the anatomical class should be one of those thrown open, which caused an erroneous impression as to the purport of his motion. It had always been considered necessary by the women and their friends that a separate class of Anatomy should be arranged for them and they were willing to pay heavily for it. The difficulty Professor Masson wished to obviate was, that under the existing plan there must be a separate class in each course, for which we had to canvass and make arrangements, causing an expenditure of time and trouble incompatible with study, while it was in the power of any unwilling professor to put an end to our work and progress by refusing to lecture to us. Professor Masson's motion was unfortunately not successful, so we had to arrange for our summer course as best we could.

The Professor of Botany had asked the sanction of the University Court for our admission to his ordinary class but had been refused. Professor Balfour therefore repeated his lectures and arranged a separate class which some of the members of the Edinburgh Ladies' Educational Association also attended.

The Professor of Natural History was too ill to give a second course of lectures, so we made use of the privilege of taking a certain number of classes in the extra Mural School and applied to Dr. Alleyne Nicholson who consulted his students and decided to invite us to his general class. A very instructive course of lectures was given, which included dredging in the Firth of Forth, and we much enjoyed our summer teaching. How long ago that session is, is recalled by the fact that I remember hearing the news of the outbreak of the Franco-Prussian War when at one of Dr. Alleyne Nicholson's lectures.

The difficulty of obtaining anatomical teaching pressed heavily all the summer. Professor Turner declined to arrange a separate class, or to allow one of his assistants to do so. We asked Dr. Handyside of Surgeons' Hall, the only recognised teacher in Anatomy outside the University, to give us a separate course; he declined, but invited us to join his ordinary class, which invitation we accepted as well as a similar invitation from Dr., now Sir Patrick Heron Watson, for surgery.

During October everything went smoothly, but after we had applied for admission to the Royal Infirmary for clinical instruction and been refused we were subjected to petty annoyances that culminated on November 18th, 1870, in an attempt to shut us out of Surgeons' Hall.

We were proceeding in the dusk of a November afternoon to the weekly class examination when we found a noisy crowd assembled round the entrance. On our approach the gates were closed and a loud yelling and hooting were set up by men inside and outside the grounds leading to the Hall. We stood for a few minutes surrounded by the hooting crowd of young men, unable to make our way to the classroom which stood a little way back from the road, when a male student rushed from the Hall and opened the gates from the inside. We availed ourselves immediately of this kind assistance, passed through the gates and made our way to the lecture theatre where we found most of the class had assembled and the examination was proceeding.

On hearing the noise that accompanied the rioters, Dr. Handyside went out and remonstrated with them. They were chiefly University students who had no right to be on the Hall premises. When he re-entered the Anatomical Theatre the examination went on again, until suddenly there was a loud noise in the passage and a pet sheep belonging to the Curator of the Museum, which usually grazed on the lawn outside, was thrust into the theatre amid yells and shouts from the men and the bleats of the frightened animal. Dr. Handyside ordered the door to be closed and the sheep to be let alone, "for," said he quietly, "the poor beast has more sense than those who pushed it in."

By the end of the examination the winter darkness had quite closed in and a crowd had again gathered round the gates. We were asked if we would leave by a private door but we felt that it would not do to be intimidated, and relying on the support of our class mates, who formed a sort of bodyguard around us, arming themselves, in default of other weapons, with osteological specimens, we passed through the mob unscathed except that our clothes were bespattered with the mud thrown at us.

As the demonstration was considered a failure another was attempted, but for several days our bodyguard escorted us to and fro, and the noisy young men, finding these attempts to deter us were useless, ceased this method of trying to drive us away and carried on a series of annoyances worthy only of schoolboys, and of sending anonymous letters fit only for the fire.

The treatment we had been subjected to caused great indignation, not only amongst our friends but also amongst those who had not hitherto sympathised with us. Some medical students called to express their disgust at the way we had been treated; the columns of the local papers were filled with correspondence on the subject; and even the *Times*, the *Daily News*, the *Spectator*, the *Saturday Review* had leaders about the "Septem contra Edinem," for by this time our numbers had increased from five to seven, spite of all the difficulties we were encountering.

After the failure of the attempt to keep us out of Surgeons' Hall, we were allowed to complete our attendance on the classes of Anatomy and Surgery without further molestation, though not without remark, as the local papers were full of allusions to what we were doing.

Some of us took prizes in the class examinations but there was no public presentation to any prize-holder, as neither the President of the College of Physicians nor of the College of Surgeons would take the chair as usual, because women were amongst the prize-holders.

The question of clinical instruction became increasingly important. At the annual meeting of the contributors to the Royal Infirmary, the Hospital where all students receive their qualifying clinical teaching, held in January, 1871, it was known that the Lord Provost would propose the election of six gentlemen favourable to the admission of women as students. In consequence party feeling ran high, and the gathering was so large that it was moved from the Municipal Council Chamber to St. Giles' Cathedral.

After a heated discussion the Lord Provost's resolution was lost by a majority of six votes, and thus all chance of our obtaining hospital teaching was at an end for at least a year. An allusion in Miss Jex Blake's speech to the presence of Professor Christison's class assistant in the mob of November 18th, gave rise to an action for libel, and for the rest of our stay in Edinburgh law proceedings, in which we were parties, were almost constantly going on.

As the agitation continued to increase, and our struggles for a medical education excited more and more interest, a committee was formed to support our efforts to obtain a qualifying course for women in Edinburgh. More than 500 members quickly joined this committee, many well-known and influential persons, including Duncan McLaren, Esq., M.P., and Mrs MacLaren, of Newington House, Edinburgh, and others resident all over the country. Miss Louisa Stevenson, now so well known and revered for her great help to the Education of Women and to the Nursing Profession, became the Honorary Secretary. From that time we were no longer a few isolated women struggling for our own object, but the pioneers of an important movement, strengthened by friends willing to help with money and wise counsel.

Such help was greatly needed, for at the end of two years we five who had begun the struggle found we could get no more qualifying teaching. Having already taken courses of Chemistry and Botany in the University, and of Natural History in the Extra Mural School, we were eligible for the First Professional Examination. Three of us applied for admission to the examination, paid the fees and received our tickets. We were working on steadily for it, as we had done since we entered the University nearly two years previously, when, ten days before the date of the examination, official notice was given that we should not be admitted to it. This was a great shock, but supported by legal opinions obtained by the Committee, we appealed to the Senatus of the University against this order and the day before the examination it was rescinded. We all passed, taking honours in more than one subject. A similar order against the admission of women to the

Preliminary Examination in Arts for the medical degree, issued the day before the examination, was also withdrawn on appeal.

We had been refused our third year matriculation tickets, but the Senatus, many members of which were our strongest supporters, overruled the action of the Medical Faculty, and declared that as long as the regulations for the admission of women remained on the Calendar of the University, they must be carried out.

These orders and counter-orders caused us much anxiety, and in addition to the distraction which necessarily resulted from the uncertainty as to admission to the examinations, we were frequently obliged to interview our supporters in the University in order to explain to them our position in regard to the questions affecting us on which they would have to vote.

The election of the Lord Rector in the autumn of 1871 again brought the question of the women students prominently forward. All the undergraduates of the University are electors, and the medical undergraduates were much exercised as to the opinions of the two candidates on the burning subject of the admission of women to the medical profession. Placards in black and red appeared on the walls of the city antagonistic to Sir William Stirling Maxwell because he was a supporter of Disraeli, who favoured women's suffrage, and Sir Roundell Palmer was telegraphed to for his opinion as to mixed classes. Sir William was elected Lord Rector and, as President of the University Court, voted in favour of maintaining the regulations respecting women medical students. This aroused the indignation of some of his youthful constituents, and at his Inaugural Address there was such an uproar that much of it was inaudible. A body of students marched from the University to Buccleuch Place, congregating round the house where several of us lived, making a great uproar, yelling and pulling at the bells until we found it was desirable to detach the clappers. Finding their efforts to annoy had no effect and some policemen arriving opportunely, the noisy crowd at last dispersed. Subsequently some of the more gentlemanly of the students apologised for the excesses of their fellcws.

In October, 1871, the Committee supporting us offered to find rooms for the delivery of lectures, and to guarantee the payment of any fee to the lecturers that the Senatus might fix, provided that the University would recognise these courses of instruction as qualifying for admission to the examinations for the medical degrees. After a long discussion the Senatus decided by a majority not to take any action in the matter, and yet on January 3rd, 1872, the University Court again confirmed the regulations for the admission of women to medical study. Thus we were admitted to the outer court of the castle, but entrance to the keep, without which admission to the outer court was useless, was barred. All attempts too, to obtain permission from the professors to allow their assistants to give qualifying courses of instruction failed, though the assistants themselves were in several cases willing to give the lectures.

To enable the women students who had joined since 1869 to make an Annus Medicus, Professor Hughes Bennett kindly repeated his course of Physiology, or the Institutes of Medicine as it was called, and Dr. Stevenson Macadam gave a course of Chemistry in the Extra Mural School. Some of the senior students availed themselves of the opportunity to repeat these subjects, but they were useless to them for graduation purposes. In January, 1872, the Infirmary question came up again. This time there was a majority of votes in favour of the election of managers willing to make arrangements for women students. Professor Masson then brought forward a statute to decree that the clinical advantages of the Infirmary should be available for all registered medical students, under such regulations as the managers might appoint. Finding themselves in a minority the opponents of this proposal left the hall in a body, and after the venerable Dr. Guthrie, in a brilliant speech, had supported the statute, it was passed unanimously.

No one who was present will forget the striking manner in which the much-respected doctor, so well known as a leader of thought in Edinburgh, uttered the peroration of his speech. Drawing himself up to his full height, which was above the average, crowned with his long grey hair, and pointing towards the door by which Professor Masson's opponents had just left, in a clear and resonant voice he repeated Tennyson's lines: –

"Ring out the old, ring in the new,
Ring out the false, ring in the true."

Enthusiastic cheers greeted the utterance and we thought our long struggle was at last over. But when we applied next day at the Infirmary for tickets of admission, we were told that the votes must undergo a scrutiny and the result be confirmed by another meeting before the statute could come into force.

On the scrutiny being made it was found that several firms had voted in the majority. The Lord Provost was then served with an interdict forbidding the inclusion of the votes of firms in the number, or as a correspondent to the *Scotsman* put the matter:

"Tae quash the votes o' thae merchant firms
That supported the ladies' men, sirs."

Litigation on this point continued until December, 1872, when at last the election of the Managers voted for on January 3rd, was declared to be valid. It was rather late in the year for there was barely a month remaining for those managers to hold office, their term expiring with the year. On December 23rd a motion was passed by the Board of Managers to admit us on condition that the attendances were separate from the male students, and that we went only to wards where our presence was invited. Thus we were able at last to begin a course of qualifying hospital instruction, though of a very limited character, and even this we owed only to the magnanimity of Dr. George W. Balfour and of Dr. Patrick Heron Watson. The former gave up three hours a week to our instruction in clinical medicine, and Dr. Watson his Sunday mornings to teach us clinical surgery. This is all we could obtain after our three years' struggle.

There were no attendances on casualties or out-patients, no pathological demonstrations, no surgical dresserships, no special departments of any kind; we had to be content with what our kind friends could give, which was limited to teaching on patients in their own wards, and we were allowed to take notes on a few cases in Dr. Balfour's wards. Very grateful were we for the facilities thus afforded us, and for our teachers' goodness in bestowing on us so much of their valuable time. We availed ourselves of every other opportunity for observation that presented itself, and through the kindness of Dr. Peel Ritchie, the senior students attended the practice of the Royal Dispensary for six months; Chalmer's Hospital, which was then a small general hospital; and the Poorhouse Infirmary, through the kindness of Dr. Nevin.

During the following two years we completed our attendance on all the subjects required for graduation, but in courses of instruction given outside the University. We hoped that ultimately the University would recognise these classes as we were unable to obtain any more within its walls, and we were careful that the teaching should be on the lines of qualifying instruction in the Extra Mural School, that is, that the teachers should be recognised by the University, the lectures should be of the prescribed number, and the fees of the same amount as at the University.

Doubts as to the validity of the regulation passed in 1869 was the next weapon made use of by our opponents. It was true that all the statutory authorities of the University, from the Chancellor to the Senatus, had authorised them, but this did not prevent the question of "ultra vires" being raised. The Lord Advocate of Scotland and Sheriff Fraser gave their opinion that the regulations were in order and that an action could be brought against the University if the means of studying medicine were not afforded to women. After placing several schemes before the Senatus, offering to pay all expenses in connection with them, all of which were rejected, we decided to act on the Lord Advocate's opinion and to bring an action of Declarator against the Senatus praying to have it declared that the Senatus was bound to enable us to complete our education and to allow us to present ourselves for our medical degrees.

The defence of this action was purely technical and decidedly peculiar. It was maintained that before the Universities Act of 1858 was passed, when the control of the University was taken from the Town Council of Edinburgh, that it was only a College and incompetent even to grant degrees to men. This did not please graduates who had taken degrees before 1858. The Lord Ordinary, Lord Gifford, before whom the action was first pleaded, gave his judgment that we were entitled to be admitted to the study of medicine in the University, subject to conditions. This judgment would have enabled the Senatus to make due arrangements had they so desired, but instead of doing so it was decided by a majority to appeal against the Lord Ordinary's judgment.

After the delay of about a year, during which time fresh questions and difficulties were constantly arising, the appeal was brought before the twelve Judges of the Inner House, presided over by the Justice General, a former Lord Rector of the University who, in that capacity, had helped to pass the regulations now in question.

The Lord Justice General accordingly gave no judgment. Five of the Justices gave judgment in favour of the legality of the regulations, seven against, and thus it was decided that legally the University had exceeded its powers in making them. We had therefore been attracted to Edinburgh, paid heavy fees, and had lost over four years' time by the action of the University, besides being involved in costly law expenses. The Committee, however, came forward most generously and relieved us of all law costs. In all nearly £2,000 were spent in legal expenses. In addition the fees to the lecturers had fallen heavily on our small band, specially during the first two years. After that our numbers had increased which lightened the expenses, as we shared them amongst us.

Apparently we had failed completely in the object of our sojourn at Edinburgh, but time has proved that actually we had accomplished a great work by preparing the way for subsequent efforts, and by rousing public attention to the question.

During all this time Mrs. Garrett Anderson, M.D., for she had meantime taken her degree in Paris, had been steadily working on in London, had founded the nucleus of the present New Hospital for Women, and proved that a woman can practise medicine with satisfaction to her patients and to her male medical colleagues. The struggle in Edinburgh, under Miss Jex Blake's leadership, showed that there were other women anxious to fit themselves for a medical career. Therefore, although I personally shall never hold a medical degree, notwithstanding that I was for four years a matriculated student of the University of Edinburgh, and passed its First Professional Examination with honours, I do not consider the time spent there was wasted, as it seems to me that it is greatly due to the struggle in Edinburgh that it is now possible for women to obtain in due course a fully qualifying medical education leading to a legal qualification, as I will now proceed to show by narrating the foundation and development of the London School of Medicine for Women.

After the decision of the Court of Appeal that the action of the University of Edinburgh had been "ultra vires," we had to decide what to do next. There was the choice between carrying our case to the House of Lords, or of abandoning our claim against the University and trying elsewhere. We decided on the latter course; some of our number went to Continental Universities, but Miss Jex Blake, I, and others preferred to see what could be effected in London. Our great object was to obtain admission to examinations, that if passed, would entitle us to be placed on the Medical Register. Amongst them Miss Jex Blake found an examination in Midwifery at the College of Surgeons, Eng. Two women applied as candidates, but rather than examine them the whole Board of Examiners resigned, and, I believe, was never re-appointed!

Mrs. Garrett Anderson, M.D., L.S.A., and Dr. Elizabeth Blackwell were at that time, 1874, the only women on the Medical Register.

Miss Jex-Blake soon succeeded in gathering together a band of sympathisers. Dr. Anstie, of King's College Hospital, entered into Mr. Norton's idea that if a full course of study were provided, the Lecturers being already recognised teachers at Metropolitan Schools, one or other of the nineteen Examining Boards would accept their certificates from female as well as male students. The following formed a Provisional Council to carry out this idea: –

Dr. Charlton Bastian, F.R.S.
Dr. Billing, F.R.S.
Dr. Elizabeth Blackwell.
Dr. Broadbent.
Dr. Thos. King Chambers.
Dr. Cheadle.
Mr. George Cowell.
Mr. Critchett.
Mrs. Garrett Anderson.
Mr. Ernest Hart.
Mr. Berkeley Hill.
Professor Huxley, F.R.S.
Dr. Hughlings Jackson.
Dr. Murie.
Mr. A. T. Norton.
Dr. J. F. Payne.
Dr. W. S. Playfair.
Mr. Rivington.
Dr. Burdon Sanderson.
Dr. P. H. Stokoe.
Dr. Octavius Sturges.

With such an array of influential names, a complete course of non-clinical study was soon arranged, but funds were needed to carry it on.

Mr. A. T. Norton, Miss Jex-Blake, Dr. T. King Chambers and I undertook to take charge of any moneys entrusted to us to found a School of Medicine for Women. Thirteen contributors, each giving a £100, came forward; they were, Mr. Andrew Coventry of Edinburgh, Mrs. Holland of Liverpool, Mrs. Jex-Blake of Brighton, Mr. Edward Pease of Darlington, Mr. J. Priestman of Newcastle, Mr. E. M. Smith of Shanghai, Miss S. Jex-Blake, Mr. Walter Thomson, Sir Francis Goldsmid, M.P., Mrs. Pennington, Mr. Augustus Thorne, Mr. Joseph Thorne, and myself. This sum of £1,300 enabled the Provisional Council to buy the lease of a quaint old house and garden in what was then called Henrietta Street.

The Edinburgh Committee kindly handed to the London Provisional Council apparatus that had been acquired for the teaching in Edinburgh.

The following Lecturers were next appointed: –

Anatomy, Mr. A. T. Norton, of St. Mary's Hospital.
Physiology, Mr. E. A. Schäfer, of University College.
Chemistry, Mr. Heaton, of Charing Cross Hospital.
Botany, Dr. P. H. Stokoe, of Guy's Hospital.

Materia Medica, Dr. OCTAVIUS STURGES, of Westminster Hospital.
Practice of Medicine, Dr. T. KING CHAMBERS, of St. Mary's Hospital.
Surgery, Mr. BERKELEY HILL, of University College Hospital.
Forensic Medicine, Dr. DUPRÉ,* F.R.S., of Westminster Hospital.
Ophthalmic Surgery, Mr. CRITCHETT, of St. Mary's Hospital.
Pathology { Dr. CHARLTON BASTIAN, of University College Hospital.
Dr. CHEADLE, of St. Mary's Hospital.
Comparative Anatomy, Dr. MURIE, of Middlesex Hospital.
Midwifery, Mrs. GARRETT ANDERSON, M.D.

All except Mrs. Garrett Anderson were teachers recognised by the Colleges of Physicians and Surgeons.

Dr. Anstie undertook to be the Dean, and the new School was entitled "The London School of Medicine for Women."

I have entered into these details in order that there may be a record of the conditions under which the School began, so that students may know to whom they are indebted for the foundation of what may fairly be called the Mother School of all British Medical Women, at a time when much courage was required for a medical man to declare himself a friend of the movement.

Just when the Provisional Council was completing the arrangements for a full course of instruction fulfilling the requirements of the Medical Examining Boards in regard to non-clinical teaching, a terrible event occurred. Dr. Anstie was suddenly taken ill and died of blood-poisoning. His energy was so great and his assistance so valuable that without him it seemed as if the project would collapse, but Mr. A. T. Norton nobly came forward and took the office of Dean. The classes were opened on the 12th of October, 1874, with the following fourteen students, twelve of whom had been students in Edinburgh:

1. Mrs. Thorne.
2. Miss Sophia Jex-Blake.
3. Miss Pechey.
4. Mrs. Marshall.
5. Miss Ker.
6. Miss Annie E. Clark.
7. Mrs. Foggo.
8. Miss Vinson.
9. Miss Rorison.
10. Miss Shove.
11. Miss Elizabeth Walker.
12. Miss Agnes McLaren.
13. Miss Waterston.
14. Miss Fanny Butler.

The new-comers were Miss Fanny Butler, the devoted medical missionary in Kashmir, to whose memory a scholarship has been founded, and Miss Waterston, so well known in South Africa. By the end of the summer session, 1875, the number of students reached twenty-three.

It may be interesting to later generations of students to know that the lectures on Chemistry were given in a room on the left-hand side of the garden entrance to the old building, which was also used for Practical Chemistry in the summer, and that Practical Anatomy was carried on in the room on the right, which in subsequent years was the students' Common Room.

On May 3rd, 1875, the Provisional Council handed over the institution to a body of Governors elected by the subscribers and themselves. They included some of the most distinguished men and women of the day, the Earl of Shaftesbury, Charles Darwin, Professor Huxley, the Dowager Lady Stanley of Alderley, etc., being of the number. A three years' curriculum of non-clinical study was arranged and a constitution drawn up which was accepted by the Governors. Thus the London School of Medicine for Women was fairly started. Its prospects, however, were gloomy. Applications were made to the London General Hospitals for the clinical instruction of the students, but without success, and all the Examining Boards refused to accept the certificates of attendence at the School, in spite of the teachers being already recognised. However, there were gleams of encouragement. Mr. Ernest Hart gave two scholarships of £50 a year each for three years, and a committee of ladies at Birmingham one of the same amount.

Amongst the Governors was the Rt. Hon. W. Cowper-Temple, M.P., who had carried through the Medical Act of 1858, which was the principal barrier to the admission of women to legal medical practice, as it required all practitioners to hold the licence or diploma of one or other of the Examing Boards enumerated in its Schedule. Mr. Cowper-Temple declared that the Medical Act was not intended to confine the practice of medicine to men, for in 1858 the question of women entering the profession had not arisen. In 1874 he brought in a Bill to remove doubts as to the powers of the Universities of Scotland to grant degrees to women, but its second reading was opposed by the University of Edinburgh, and so it was thrown ont. In 1875. Mr. Cowper-Temple introduced a Bill to admit women holding foreign medical degrees to registration, but this also failed.

In 1876 the Rt. Hon. Russell Gurney, M.P., Recorder for London, introduced a short permissive Bill giving British Medical Examining Boards power to admit women to their examinations. It expressly provided that the licence or diploma should give only the right to registration by the General Medical Council and should confer no vote in the government of the Corporation that granted it. This Bill became law, but for a while no Board acted upon it. The University of Edinburgh actually declined to allow the women who had been its matriculated students for four years, and had taken all the courses of study required by its regulations, to present themselves as candidates, on the ground that some of the teaching had been taken in the Edinburgh Extra-Mural School instead of in the University.

Thus when the three years' curriculum was completed in 1877, the thirty-four women who had taken it seemed as far off as ever from their goal. The contributions, amounting to £1,903 and the students' fees to £1,219, had all been spent in teaching and maintenance, so no classes were held in the summer session of 1877. But the darkest hour comes before the dawn and so it proved in this case; just when the outlook seemed most gloomy the King and Queens' College of Physicians (now the Royal College of Physicians, Ireland), decided to admit Dr. S. Jex-Blake, Dr. Edith Pechey, Mrs. Atkins, and some other ladies who held degrees from the Universities of Berne and Zurich to their final examination. They all passed the examination and received the licence of the College. They were then entitled to be registered by the General Medical Council of Great Britain and Ireland and to enter upon the legal practice of Medicine. This occurred in 1877 and these ladies were the first women to be so registered since Miss Garrett took the licence of the Society of Apothecaries, London, in 1865.

Thus two difficulties were overcome: the teaching at the School was recognised and a qualifying examination was open to women, but the want of clinical instruction still remained.

During the autumn of 1876 the Hon. Treasurer of the School, the Rt. Hon. J. Stansfeld, M.P., met abroad Mr. James Hopgood, Chairman of the Royal Free Hospital, to which no male students were attached, and interested him in the efforts that had been so fruitlessly made to provide women students with clinical teaching. Mr. Hopgood promised to use his influence. Prolonged negotiations took place, and at length an agreement was signed on the 12th June, 1877, by which the authorities bound themselves on certain conditions to admit the students of the School to the wards of the Royal Free Hospital.

In order to compensate the Hospital for possible loss of support consequent on its taking this new departure, the School agreed to pay annually 300 guineas to the General Funds of the Hospital and to hand over all fees received for clinical teaching for distribution to the four members of the Staff, at the same time guaranteeing that the amount should not be less than £400 a year. Thus the School undertook to pay in all £715 a year, and the Right Hon. James Stansfeld, M.P., Frederick Pennington, M.P., and Mr. J. G. S. Anderson, made themselves personally responsible for these amounts.

After registration, Dr. Sophia Jex-Blake decided to practise in Edinburgh, and at her and Dr. T. King Chambers' request, I allowed myself to be nominated for a newly constituted post, that of Honorary Secretary, to which I was elected in May, 1877.

As I have already stated, the School funds were exhausted and yet to start teaching afresh and to carry out the agreement with the Hospital a large sum was needed. The Executive Council decided to appeal to the public for a sum of £5,000, payable in the five years the agreement ran. A meeting under the presidency of the Earl of Shaftesbury was held at St. George's Hall on the 25th of June, 1877, to inaugurate the appeal. Amongst the speakers were the Rt. Hon. W. Cowper-Temple, M.P., Lady Anna Gore Langton, Dr. Sophia Jex-Blake,

Mrs. Garrett Anderson, M.D., Dr. T. King Chambers, etc. The appeal was so successful that the whole sum was promised within a few months.

On January 16th, 1877, the Rev. Septimus Buss, LL.B., B.A., in the Convocation of the University of London, seconded by Mr. H. A. Nesbitt, M.A., moved the following resolution: "That it be referred to the annual Committee to consider a report upon the best means of carrying into effect the desire of Convocation that the degrees of the University should be open to women." The motion was carried by 22 to 16. In June, 1877, the University of London decided to admit women to its medical examinations.

In October, 1877, Dr. Cockle, Senior Physician to the Royal Free Hospital, gave an Introductory Lecture to the students in the Hospital, and nine new students entered under conditions much more favourable than those of 1874.

At this time the Staff of the Hospital consisted of two physicians, Dr. Cockle and Dr. O'Connor; and two surgeons, Mr. Gant and Mr. William Rose. The teaching was limited to attendance at the visits of the Staff and to the opportunities afforded by the clinical clerkships and dresserships. There were no special departments, no casualty department, no pathological teaching, no preparatory classes. Soon, however, an Assistant Physician, Dr. Allen Sturge, who also became Pathologist – the School paying expenses – and an Assistant Surgeon, Mr. James Shuter, were appointed, besides a Gynæcologist, Dr. Hayes, and an Opthalmic Surgeon, Mr., now Sir Anderson Critchett.

Much care and circumspection were necessary to make the new departure work satisfactorily. The officials naturally regarded it somewhat critically, but by tact and thoughtfulness on the part of the students and others, the arrangements were gradually fitted in and occasions of friction were avoided.

Between 1877 and 1882, the period covered by the first agreement with the Royal Free Hospital, the development of the School made substantial progress. Miss Prideaux, Miss Cock, Miss McCall, Mrs. Scharlieb, who had been a student in the classes organised in Madras by Surg.-General Furnell, Miss Tomlinson, Miss Webb, Miss Toms (Mrs. Stanley Boyd), Mrs. Ayrton and Miss Macdonald were among the students.

At the Intermediate Examination in Medicine, of the University of London, 1881, the Gold Medal and Exhibition in Anatomy were awarded to Miss Helen Prideaux, Mrs. Scharlieb took 1st class honours in Materia Medica and Pharmaceutical Chemistry, and Miss Tomlinson 2nd class honours in Organic Chemistry.

In November, 1882, Mrs. Scharlieb obtained the Gold Medal and Exhibition in Obstetric Medicine, with honours in Medicine and Forensic Medicine.

In 1880 two legacies were received: one from Miss Watts, of Thornhill Square, of £500, and one of shares in the Bank of Van Dieman's Land from Mrs. Oakes. At the time the bequest was made the shares were valued at £10,000, and Mrs. Oakes had expressed the wish that the income derived from them, which amounted to £500 a year, might prove a permanent help to the School. Mr. Oakes, one of the executors under the will (who took a great interest in the medical education of women) came to London from Australia to advocate the retention of the shares in accordance with his wife's desire; but, unfortunately, they carried an unlimited liability, which the trustees were advised would fall on them if the shares were accepted and the Bank failed. Such a heavy responsibility was therefore declined. Mr. Oakes kindly undertook to do the best he could for the School. Just then the failure of the City of Glasgow Bank, which ruined so many trustees, forcibly illustrated the risk of holding this class of property. For eighteen months the shares were unsaleable, but at length they were sold, and the proceeds, £4,051, remitted to the trustees. This legacy has been of the greatest service to the School ever since. It enabled the guarantee to the Hospital to be given with confidence; it was available for part of the cost when additions to the School buildings became necessary, and it recently enabled the Council to pay off the balance due on the second block of the new buildings, while part of it still appears among the School assets, represented by Midland Railway Preferred and Deferred Stock.

By the end of the five years' agreement twenty-three students had become registered practitioners. Thus the position that had so long been struggled for was gained, and the path cleared for other women.

During 1881 attention was drawn to the need of medical women for India, and a great impulse was given to this question by a message from the Maharani of Punna, brought to Her Majesty the Queen by Miss Bielby, who had been for a short time a student of the School. The Maharani wished the Great Queen of England to be informed "what the women in Indian zenanas suffer when they are sick." Her Majesty graciously sent a reply to the Maharani, expressing her interest and sympathy with every effort to relieve the suffering women of India.

The National Indian Association in London took up the subject of medical women for India, and Mr. G. A. Kittredge, of Bombay, started a fund for securing the services of women doctors for Indian women. With the aid of Mr. Sorabji Bengalli, a dispensary was opened at Bombay for the treatment of women and children by medical women. This institution was placed under the care of Dr. Edith Pechey, who when a student of the Edinburgh University had gained the marks entitling her to the Hope Scholarship.

Miss Bielby, who qualified in 1885, was appointed Senior Physician to the Lady Aitchison Hospital, Lahore, and Lecturer on Midwifery to its Medical School.

Soon after, Mrs. Scharlieb, M.B., B.S., had the honour of being received at Windsor by H.M. Queen Victoria, and at Marlborough House by T.R.H. the then Prince and Princess of Wales, before leaving for Madras in 1882, where she was appointed Lecturer on Forensic Medicine in the Madras Medical College and Examiner in Midwifery at the University of Madras.

Mr. Kama, another Parsee gentlemen of Bombay, built a fine hospital for the medical treatment of Indian women by women, and handed it over to the Indian Government. Dr. Edith Pechey was gazetted Physician to it in 1883.

Before the Countess of Dufferin proceeded to India in 1884, H.M. the Queen impressed upon her the importance of taking steps to carry out the wish for female medical help expressed by the Maharani of Punna. The Countess of Dufferin took energetic action to fulfil this command and the prospectus of the Association for supplying Female Medical Aid to the Women of India was issued at Simla in August, 1885, and met with a most cordial response from all classes, native and British.

Several of the Missionary Societies recognised the importance of their representatives having a complete medical training, and made special arrangements for their candidates to study at the School.

When a new agreement with the Royal Free Hospital for a further period of five years was under consideration in 1882, the subsidy of £315 which the School had paid since 1877 to the General Funds of the Hospital in compensation for possible loss was generously waived by the Committee, as the Hospital was found not to have suffered by its association with the School. The guarantee that at least £400 should be paid annually to the staff was augmented by £60 a year in order to provide fees for the Physician for the Diseases of Women and the Ophthalmic Surgeon.

In March, 1883, Mr. T. Barlow Kennett offered £100 on condition that £400 more were collected within two months. This was accomplished, and the Kennett Fund proved a great boon in helping to defray the general expenses of the School.

Early in 1883, Mr. A. T. Norton resigned the post of Dean, which he had held since 1874, during the most critical period of the movement, and during which he had rendered very valuable help to the struggling institution. Mrs. Garrett Anderson, M.D., was elected his successor.

In 1884 Mr. John Byron left the residue of his estate to the Trustees of the School, with instructions that it should be invested, and the annual interest used for the benefit of students needing pecuniary help for the prosecution of their studies. A sum of £692 9s. 6d. was realised, and the proceeds, about £23 a year, are applied according to the wishes of the testator. It may be interesting to the students to know that Miss Florence Nightingale was asked to become a Governor of the School in 1884. Ill-health prevented her complying with this request, but she wrote a most sympathetic reply, in which she said: "I could well rejoice that there is now an institution where women can obtain a complete medical education and I pray that you may go on and prosper, as you surely will."

Miss Helen Prideaux, who took the Gold Medal and Exhibition for Anatomy in 1881, passed the Final Examination for the M.B. Lond., in 1884 with Honours in Medicine, Obstetric Medicine and Forensic Medicine. She was then appointed House Surgeon to the Children's Hospital, Paddington. Unhappily in the discharge of her duties there she contracted diphtheria and died on the 29th November, 1885. Her character was a specially fine one, combining many sympathetic and tender qualities with a mind remarkable for its intellectual power and grasp of ideas. Her loss was deeply mourned, and at a meeting under the presidency of Sir William Gull, M.D., it was decided to found a Prize bearing her name to be competed for by graduates of the School.

Over £500 was subscribed and a prize of £50 was offered on certain conditions. The first Prideaux Scholar was Miss Florence Nightingale Toms, now Mrs. Stanley Boyd, M.D.

In 1884 a conversazione was held at the school to celebrate the tenth anniversary of its foundation in the modest way I have related. The supporters of the School had the satisfaction of feeling that they had rendered the thorough medical education of women possible. The three essentials wanting in 1874, namely:

1. A recognized course of medical training,
2. A clinical hospital,
3. A qualifying examination admitting to the Register, were now all supplied.

Dr. Buchanan Baxter, appointed Senior Physician to the Royal Free Hospital in 1881, was compelled by ill-health to retire in 1884. He died in 1885, much lamented, especially by the students, who greatly appreciated his admirable method of clinical teaching. Mrs. Buchanan Baxter kindly gave the principal contents of his library, about 200 volumes, to the Library of the School.

About this time the School lost some other good friends. The Rt. Hon. Henry Fawcett died in 1884. He initiated the admission of medical women into the higher ranks of the Civil Service by the appointment of Miss Edith Shove, M.B., as Medical Superintendent of the Female Staff at the General Post Office, London, and by making similar appointments at Liverpool and Manchester.

My husband, Mr. Joseph Thorne, always a very warm supporter of the School, who had been one of its Honorary Auditors for eleven years, died in 1885. The Rt. Hon. the Earl of Shaftesbury, one of the earliest and most influential friends of the medical education of women, also passed away the same year.

A distinguished student, Miss Tomlinson, M.B. Lond., became about this time incapacitated from continuing her most promising career by the after effects of a severe illness, causing loss of sight.

In 1885 it was found necessary to put up a lecture room in the garden, and to rearrange the Pavilion, as 30, Henrietta Street was then called. Considerable difficulties arose with the ground landlords, who again objected to the study of anatomy being carried on, on their premises. At length the alterations were sanctioned and carried out at a cost of £1,100, Mr. Stanley Boyd rendering great assistance with the plans. Early this year, 1885, Mr. Boyce Barrow, F.R.C.S., joined the Staff of the Royal Free Hospital.

The same year the Royal College of Surgeons, Ireland, threw open all its examinations, including the Fellowship, to women; the following year the Scotch Colleges admitted women to their Licentiate Examinations. It was not till 1888 that the Licence of the Society of Apothecaries, London, was re-opened to female candidates.

Up till 1886, the London School was the only one in Great Britain where women could obtain a qualifying training, and therefore all women medical students were concentrated at it. In that year a school was started in Edinburgh, which broke up the small number of such students. Considering the heavy expense of equipping and maintaining an efficient medical school and the need for providing it with all the appliances required for a modern medical education, it would, in my opinion, have been wiser to have consolidated and developed the original school before starting another.

The year 1886 was remarkable for the fact that all the nineteen students who went up from the School passed their respective examinations. An article appeared that year in *The Fortnightly Review*, entitled "Æsculapia Victrix," recounting the course of the movement for the Medical Education of Women. It was written by Mr. Robert Wilson, who had been a medical student at Edinburgh while we were attempting to study there and had watched all the phases of the struggle. He had shown us much sympathy, and I believe "The Song of the Neutral," "The Barrin' o' the Door," and other verses that appeared in the *Scotsman* were by him.

In 1887 Miss MacCall enlarged the work she had organised in the South of London by the foundation of a Maternity Hospital in Clapham. The Maternity established by the Sisters of St. John in Battersea was also placed under her care, and two dispensaries were opened. These institutions constitute a valuable extension of medical work by women.

The National Association for Supplying Female Medical Aid to the women of India placed two Scholarships of £25 a year each at the disposal of the Executive Council, one in commemoration of the Jubilee of 1887, and the other named after the Countess of Dufferin.

Mr. Bond, F.R.C.S., resigned the post of co-lecturer on Forensic Medicine in 1887. Mrs. Scharlieb, M.B., who had recently returned from Madras, where she had been lecturer on this subject in the Madras College, was appointed to succeed him, and thus began her teaching connection with the School, which has continued to the present time, though now she occupies another lectureship, that of Midwifery.

In 1887 the School and Hospital entered into another five years' agreement. With the approval of the Committee the guarantee of £460 a year to the Staff was not renewed, but all the clinical fees were, as before, handed over to them. The clinical fees have since considerably exceeded the guarantee, and several extra courses of instruction have been formed, for which additional payments are made by the School.

In 1888 the Metropolitan Board of Works changed the name of the street in which the School entrance was situated from Henrietta to Handel Street. The reasons for the change are obvious: there are two other Henrietta Streets within a short distance, and the name of Handel was chosen to connect the great composer with the locality, as several of his greatest works, including the Oratorio of the Messiah, were first produced at the Foundling Hospital, the Governors of which own much of the surrounding property, and are the ground landlords of the School premises.

In July, 1888, of the thirteen students who went up for the Intermediate Examination of the University of London, twelve passed: seven of these took honours; one in three subjects. Professor George Buchanan, referring to this fact in his opening address to the students of the Glasgow University of that year, said: "More than half of the honours of the University of London in Anatomy, Physiology, and

Materia Medica were taken by women as against all comers from all schools." All these women were students of this School.

Later in the year, Mrs. Scharlieb passed the M.D. Lond., the first woman to take this degree.

Several changes took place at the Royal Free Hospital in 1888. Mr. James Hopgood, who had been such a good friend to the School, resigned the Chairmanship of the General Committee, and Mr. Blyth, the Secretary, died after a short illness in April, 1888, and was succeeded by Mr. Thies. Mr. William Rose was appointed Professor of Surgery at King's College, and had therefore to resign his post as a surgeon at the Royal Free Hospital. Mr. James Berry, of St. Bartholomew's, and Mr. Battle, Surgical Registrar of St. Thomas's Hospital, were appointed Assistant Surgeons.

Miss Gray, L.R.C.P. and S.Ed., was appointed Clinical Assistant to the Homerton Fever Hospital, and was the first of the many women who have since received posts under the Metropolitan Asylums Board. Many other posts have been held by our students under the London School Board, the London County Council, and now the Central Midwives' Board. Mrs. Wright, then Miss I. G. Wilson, began her kind help to the School by starting a students' collection of books in 1888, and by presenting models to the Museum. Since then she has never relaxed her kind thought for the students, helping them in a variety of ways, giving comfortable chairs for the Common Room, etc., as well as providing £400 for the Mackay prizes and starting the Repayment of Debt fund.

When the National Association for the Promotion of the Medical Education of Women, which had its headquarters in Edinburgh, and the Ladies' Association, for the same purpose, at Birmingham, were dissolved in 1888, the accounts were closed by handing the balance of their funds, £44 9s. 7d., to the Bursary Fund of the School, from which help can occasionally be given to students.

Another scholarship was started from a small fund raised by Miss E. A. Manning, of the National Indian Association, and myself, for a student willing to practise in India under the Countess of Dufferin's Fund. By the request of the principal contributor, this was called the Stuart Mill Scholarship, and it is in the gift alternately of the United Kingdom Branch of the Countess of Dufferin Fund and of the Council of the School.

In 1890 Rukhmabai was amongst the new students. She is a Hindu lady whose refusal to carry out a marriage contract made for her in childhood caused considerable agitation on the question in Bombay. After a successful student career she qualified and returned to India, where she continues to do excellent work.

In April, 1890, one of our students, Miss E. L. Fleury, passed the Final Examination of the Royal University of Ireland with great distinction. She was declared First in order of merit in the 1st class of the Honours List and was awarded an Exhibition of £40. This fitly crowned an exceptionally brilliant student career, for Miss Fleury had gained the Exhibition of £20 at both the Second and Third Examinations in Medicine of the Royal University of Ireland. At the Intermediate Examination in Medicine of the University of London, Miss A. F. Piercy, now

Mrs. Willmott Evans, gained triple 1st class Honours, namely, the Gold Medal and Exhibition for Materia Medica and Pharmaceutical Chemistry, a Gold Medal for Anatomy, and 1st class Honours in Physiology and Histology.

A valuable donation of £100 was given in 1891 by Miss Sprigg, formerly a student of the School, now Mrs. Bennett, for the improvement of the Materia Medica Museum, and the collection was kindly arranged by Mr. Martindale. The same donor has also added to the collection all the drugs introduced into the British Pharmacopœia in 1894.

The sum of £500 was handed to the Council for the foundation of a Scholarship to commemorate Dr. Fanny Butler, one of the earliest students of the School, who died at Srinaghar, Kashmir, in 1889, while engaged there in very heavy work as a medical missionary. Miss Annie Butler wrote: "I do especially rejoice that by the foundation of this Scholarship my sister's name will be inalienably connected with the London School of Medicine for Women, for however much many students may have loved the School it would, I think, be simply impossible for any of them to have loved it more than she did. She would herself have deeply valued this remembrance and recognition in connection with her beloved Alma Mater." The Scholarship is awarded to a student approved by the Church of England Zenana Missionary Society.

Dr. Thomas King Chambers, one of the founders of the School and also one of its trustees, died in 1889. He took the liveliest interest in helping the School and aided it greatly in overcoming its numerous difficulties, and often spoke enthusiastically of "that grand work for women," carried on at the School. When he gave the opening address in 1879 he congratulated himself on having assisted actively in the development of two medical schools, that at the University of Oxford and ours. He was succeeded in his post of trustee by Sir Owen Roberts, M.A., one of the most constant and able friends of the School, whose support has been of so much value and to whom we practically owe the St. Dunstan's Scholarships.

The removal of the New Hospital for Women to a site near the School was a great advantage. The foundation stone of the new building at 144, Euston Road, was laid by H.R.H. the Princess of Wales, in 1889. The erection of this excellent hospital was principally due to the strenuous exertions of Mrs. Garrett Anderson, M.D., aided by other members of the Staff, and the final effort to pay for the building was a large Bazaar, opened by the late Marchioness of Salisbury. This institution, which grew from a few rooms in Seymour Place, with Miss Garrett, L.S.A., as the sole medical officer, to the present important hospital with its staff of physicians, and surgeons, fifty-four beds, operating theatre, cancer ward always full alas! and large outpatient department, is a striking object lesson, showing what excellent practical work, both medical and surgical, can be done by fully trained medical women. In March, 1900, Sir Thomas Smith, of St. Bartholomew's Hospital, bore most eloquent testimony to the value of the medical and surgical work carried on within its walls, and stated that after a prolonged and careful observation, he considers women are specially fitted for the surgical treatment of their own sex.

The Hospital provides posts of graduated responsibility for the younger qualified medical women under the Senior Staff. The Pathologists, Anæsthetists, Clinical Assistants, and Resident Medical Officers, etc., are nearly all former students of the School, as are also the members of the Senior Staff.

The New Hospital also accommodates the Medical Institute, the headquarters of the Association of Registered Medical Women, where women practitioners can consult works of reference and see current medical literature. It is also the meeting place where the Association assembles during the winter months, when valuable papers are read and discussed, and clinical evenings are held for the exhibition of special cases.

In 1890 the distance between the School and the Royal Free Hospital was lessened, and a pleasant walk made, by the conversion of St. George's Burial Ground into a public garden, with openings east and west. There is now an asphalt path under trees and between flower beds which renders the few minutes' walk both dry and pleasant. I wonder whether many students notice an old tomb about midway which marks the burial place of a granddaughter of Oliver Cromwell.

Early in 1891 the Council had to come to a decision in regard to the enlargement of the premises. The number of students had again outgrown the accommodation. The alterations in 1886 cost £1,100. The superior lease of the premises, which would expire in 1905, and the sub-lease of 7, Hunter Street, had been bought at a cost of £1,224. It was decided to connect the adjoining house, 7, Hunter Street, with 30, Henrietta Street, and on the 1st October, 1891, when Mrs. Stanley Boyd gave the opening address, the students and their friends found the School practically reconstructed, at a cost of about £1,800. The Council was in some perplexity as to this expense, although in receipt of liberal grants from several of the City Companies and others, when a kind friend, Mr. Matthew Whiting, after inspecting the improvements, placed a cheque for £1,000 in the hands of the Secretary, Miss Heaton.

In 1891, for the first time, a qualified medical woman, Miss E. E. Wood, M.B., now Mrs. Percy Flemming, M.D., was appointed demonstrator of Anatomy, and Miss Lucy Boole became demonstrator of Chemistry. A Maternity department was opened at the New Hospital for Women under the superintendence of Miss Frances Harris, M.B.

The resolution excluding medical women from the membership of the British Medical Association, which was passed in 1878, was rescinded by a large majority in 1892. During the intervening years Mrs. Garrett Anderson, M.D., was the only woman who was on the list of members, and the fact that the resolution was repealed is, I think, a great tribute to the impression she had made on her colleagues, and to the advance in the position of medical women in Great Britain.

In 1890 the Helen Prideaux Prize was awarded to Miss Adela Knight, M.B. Lond., a lady who came from Australia in 1885 to study at the School in consequence of an article on one of the Prize Givings she had seen in the *Queen* newspaper. After a distinguished student career she graduated in November, 1889. Her graduation excited much interest, as she was the first Australian woman to take the M.B. Lond., and in consequence she had the honour of a summons to Marlborough House, and of an interview with H.R.H. the Princess of Wales. Miss Knight was subsequently appointed Resident Medical Officer to the New Hospital for Women, where she superintended the transfer of the Hospital to its new home, and assisted in its reorganisation in the fine premises. Early in 1891 she went to Vienna for further medical and surgical study, before her return home later in the year. Unhappily she was taken ill and died, after a short illness, at Vienna, to the great grief of her friends and fellow students, who had looked forward to her doing much good work in Australia.

The International Congress of Hygiene met in London the same year. About sixty of its members visited the School. Prof. Baümler, of Freiburg, Dr. T. Barday, of Odessa, Dr. Möller, of Amsterdam, etc., were much interested in the arrangements for the medical education of women.

In 1892 the School was again enlarged, 8, Hunter Street being added to it. Mrs. Wright gave £400 to be used in Prizes in memory of her brother, McKay. The Executive Council decided to offer two prizes of £20 each on the results of the class examinations for the first two years' subjects. A calculation was made by the Accountant that the money would last twelve years. The first award was made in 1898. The Misses Naylor gave a herbarium of British plants collected by their sister, the late Mrs. Edward Wilkinson.

In 1893 the sum of £3,131 was transferred from the Pfeiffer Bequest to the Trustees of the School expressly for building purposes. The agreement with the Royal Free Hospital was renewed, the School undertaking to pay five per cent. to the General Funds of the Hospital on the School fees received from the students, in order to defray expenses consequent on their attendance at the Hospital.

Miss Aldrich-Blake, M.B., was appointed Assistant Anæsthetist to the Royal Free Hospital under Dr. Silk, and in 1894 she succeeded him to the higher post, which she has held ever since. Two Assistant Anæsthetists were also chosen from former students of the School to work under her, so that for the past twelve years the administration of anæsthetics has been in the hands of Alumnæ of the School. The death of Miss Jessie Hatch, who had been Clinical Assistant at the New Hospital for Women and subsequently Curator of the Royal Free Hospital Museum, and then Resident Medical Officer at the N.E. Fever Hospital, occurred in April, 1894. Her loss was deeply felt as the sterling worth of her character had made a great impression on her fellow students. It is interesting to recall the fact that one of them, Mrs. Percy Flemming, M.D., named her eldest daughter Jessie Hatch after her.

The sum of £400 was given by Mrs. Royce, of Leicester, as a memorial of the late Miss Mary Royce, L.S.A., a former student. The interest of the £400 furnishes a small honorarium to each of the Assistant Anæsthetists.

On July 22nd, 1895, their Royal Highnesses the Prince and Princess of Wales, with the Princesses Victoria and Maud, honoured the Royal Free Hospital by their presence in order to visit the part which had been recently rebuilt. The Princess of Wales graciously consented to receive contributions in aid of the Hospital

Building Fund. The students took an active part in the proceedings, and presented purses containing over £600 to Her Royal Highness, collected by themselves and their friends. The rebuilding of the front of the Hospital greatly improved the students' accommodation. Instead of being restricted to one small room, a larger one formerly reserved for the Medical Staff was assigned to them, and they were also allowed to use the large lecture room.

In the summer of 1895, that very good friend of the medical education of women, the Rt. Hon. Sir James Stansfield, M.P., retired from all public work, and had, therefore, to resign the Honorary Treasurership of the School, a post which he had held since its foundation. At the prize-giving, presided over by Her Grace the Duchess of Portland, an address expressing the value of the help he had rendered to the School in its early years, was presented to Sir James.

The School Magazine was started early in 1895, and it is agreed by all that it has justified its existence and realised the desire of its founders, that it should "promote fellow feeling among the different sections of the School, and link together past and present students." The motto, "Work is as it is done," a very appropriate one, was suggested by Dr. Helen Webb.

In 1895 petitions were presented to the Royal College of Physicians, London, and to the Royal College of Surgeons, England, praying them to admit women to their examinations. These petitions were signed by all the Staff of the Royal Free Hospital, and by a number of the heads of the profession, but the prayer was not granted, though the adverse majorities were small in each case, the numbers respectively being 100 for 109 against, and 96 for and 106 against the petitions being acceded to. Miss Aldrich-Blake took the M.S. degree of the University of London, being the first woman who had obtained this high surgical distinction. Miss K. M. Hunter, L.S.A., obtained the same year the D.P.H. Cantab, the first time this University had recognised medical work by a woman. Miss Hunter utilized the knowledge acquired for this degree in her subsequent work in combating plague in India.

Early in 1896 Mrs. Percy Flemming, M.D., was appointed Medical, and Miss Aldrich-Blake, M.D., M.S., Surgical Registrar of the Royal Free Hospital. A bacteriological department, under the superintendence of Dr. Andrewes and Mr. Roughton, was organised.

In 1896 a generous donation of £1,000 was given by Miss Payne-Townshend, who had taken some classes at the School in order to become acquainted with its working. The trust deed gave power to invest the money in School buildings, the interest at three per cent. to be used for the following objects: £5 a year to the Library, £5 to the improvement of the School Common Room, and the balance to the Bursary Fund.

Early in 1896 the Vice-Dean of the School, Miss Cock, M.D., was appointed a member of the Quarterly Committee of the Royal Free Hospital, and Miss Louisa Stevenson was elected one of the Managers of the Edinburgh Infirmary.

In 1896–97 the entry of students was so large that the rebuilding of the School, which had been under consideration for some years, became very pressing. The old building had become more and more dilapidated and inconvenient for the growing School. How it could be effected without stopping the work needed serious thought. Several new sites were suggested, but none possessed the advantages of the old one. At last it was decided that the building should be put up in separate blocks, and on Dr. May Thorne's suggestion, the first block was built on the lawn tennis court. Before anything could be done it was necessary to obtain from the ground landlords a lease long enough to justify the erection of a thoroughly equipped Medical School. A lease for eighty years was granted on condition that the rent should be £240 instead of £60 a year and that a building costing at least £16,000 should be erected. The Executive Council had only £9,400 in hand, strenuous efforts were therefore needed to make up the sum required. It was arranged that all surplus balances from the School funds should be given to the Building Fund, and the Medical Staff kindly agreed to pay for five years a percentage on the amount of the clinical fees received by them.

In order to simplify the business transactions and to relieve the trustees from the heavy personal liability of carrying out these conditions, it was considered advisable to incorporate the School under the Companies Act of 1862, omitting the word "limited," as the School is not carried on for profit, and on the 22nd December, 1896, the Governors passed a resolution sanctioning the proposed incorporation. Negotiations with the Board of Trade were then entered into, and occupied some time.

In order to mark the close association of the School and the Royal Free Hospital, which had lasted for twenty years and which had become more intimate as time went on, the Hospital authorities were asked to allow the name of the School to include that of the Hospital, a request which was granted.

In 1896 a Medical Society was started by the Hospital students, at which good work is done. A Hockey Club was organised in 1897.

In 1897 Mrs. Garrett Anderson, M.D., undertook the duties of President of the East Anglian Branch of the British Medical Association, to which she had been unanimously invited by the Council of the Branch. Her year of office proved very satisfactory. It marks the recognition of medical women as members of the profession in a special manner, for it shows that not only are women eligible as members of the chief professional Society of Great Britain, from which they had been excluded from 1878 till 1892, but that the principal position in a branch can be held by a woman with benefit to all concerned.

Miss Heaton, who had been Secretary to the School from its very inception, was compelled by ill-health to retire from the post in 1897, after twenty-three years of valuable service. The Council made a grant to her of £100 in recognition of her services during nearly a quarter of a century. She had mothered the students when they were only a small band, subject to many discouragements, and a strong affection existed between her and them. Their appreciation of her goodness was evidenced by the students, past and present, giving her a purse containing £300, and a silver teapot and stand to recall the many pleasant gatherings which had taken place in the garden and on the old verandah under her presidency. Miss Douie, M.A., Ed., now M.B., London, was appointed Miss Heaton's successor.

The Incorporation of the School took longer than was expected, owing to the Board of Trade requiring that not more than one member of the governing body should derive monetary benefit from the School. Hitherto there had been an Executive Council which included many of the Lecturers. To meet the Board of Trade's requirements the Executive Council was divided into two bodies, the School Committee, an advisory body, and the Council, the latter alone regulating the finances. The Council consists of the four honorary officials, two representatives of the Royal Free Hospital Committee, and four members elected at the Annual Meeting of the Association.

The Articles of Association were signed on the 3rd of August, 1898, when the Constitution passed in 1875 was abrogated in favour of the Articles sanctioned by the Board of Trade.

The plans for the new building were prepared while the negotiations with the Board of Trade were proceeding. It was decided to erect a block of laboratories, anatomical, physiological, chemical and physical, on the site of the lawn tennis court, which could be carried out without interfering with the existing buildings. These were commenced in the vacation of 1897, and were ready for use in May, 1898. The School Magazine of that month had an excellent paper on the abstruse subject of Electrotonus, by Miss A. H. Naylor. Their Royal Highnesses the Prince and Princess of Wales visited the premises on the 11th July, 1898, and declared the fine new Science Laboratories open. The ceremony was brilliantly successful. H.R.H. the Prince of Wales had kindly visited the premises a few days before, quite privately, and had seen the students, unconscious of his presence, engaged at work in the laboratories. He had afterwards been over the New Hospital for Women, and so was well prepared to speak at the ceremony of the 11th July. Her Grace the Duchess of Portland, Sir William and Lady Broadbent, Dr Creighton the late Bishop of London, Mrs. Westlake, Sir Alfred and Miss Garrod, Mr. and Mrs. Charles Burt, Lord and Lady Reay, etc., were present. Their Royal Highnesses took tea in the old Common Room, after visiting the Physiological Laboratory. It was thought well to try and build the second or Wakefield Street block as quickly as possible, and the Princess of Wales having kindly intimated her willingness to receive contributions, the sum of £4,500 was raised within five weeks. The students, as usual, entered heartily into the arrangements for decorating the School with flowers and flags, and the graduates enlivened the scene by wearing their academic robes, many of which looked very bright in the brilliant sunshine.

The autumn of 1898 was saddened by the sudden death of Miss Mabel Webb, M.B., Lond., Curator of the Royal Free Hospital Museum. Her health had not been good, but a long holiday seemed to have re-established it, and her death came as a great shock to all who knew her. Mrs. Webb, her mother, had recently given £1,000 to be invested in the School buildings, the interest at 3 per cent. to pay for a Research Scholarship in either Physiology, Chemistry or Pathology. It was decided to name this Scholarship after Mabel Webb. While Curator of the

Museum Miss Webb had drawn up a scheme to develop the bacteriological and pathological work in connection with it. Her fellow-students and co-workers felt that the best method of commemorating one so greatly beloved, and whose influence was so excellent, would be by carrying out her wishes in regard to this matter. A Committee was formed, subscriptions received, and estimates of the amount required obtained, when Mrs. Webb most generously offered to pay the entire cost of the building, the subscriptions to be used for the fittings. The plans were carried out, and this important department of the Hospital is now suitably equipped. The Museum was declared open by Lady Reay in March, 1900.

The Reid Trustees founded a Scholarship of £60 a year, tenable at the School, in memory of Miss Bostock, a former Reid Trustee, and an early friend and subscriber who always took a warm interest in its progress.

The instruction of students in Vaccination had become difficult in consequence of changes resulting from the new Act of Parliament. By the permission of the Committee and Staff of the New Hospital for Women a scheme was organised in connection with its Maternity. Miss May Thorne, M.D., was appointed Lecturer and Teacher of Vaccination by the Privy Council under the Local Government Board. The courses of study required for the Preliminary Scientific Examinations of the University of London were also arranged. Miss Edith Stoney was appointed Lecturer on Physics, and Mr. Mudge, A.R.A., Lecturer on Biology. Chemistry is taught by Miss de Brereton Evans, who has been Lecturer on that subject since 1898.

The Handel Street block of buildings was begun immediately after the opening of the science laboratories in Wakefield Street, and it was ready for use on October 1st, 1899. This block contains three lecture theatres, a biological department with excellent north light, Council room, Secretary's rooms, etc.

The Council had then to consider the serious responsibility of building the third and most expensive block, fronting Hunter Street, in order to complete the building. Every year labour and material were becoming dearer, and the inconvenience of the partially built premises increasing, so that it was necessary to face the difficulty at once, although the funds were exhausted. A General Meeting of the Association was called in July, 1899, when it was resolved to raise £8,000 by mortgage on the buildings already erected. It was decided that the upper part of the Hunter Street wing should be used as students' chambers, for which there was a considerable demand. The rent from these chambers replaces the rents of the old houses which, until their demolition, had been part of the income of the School. The block was finished by October, 1900. On the ground floor there is a fine common room and refectory for the students, and an anatomical museum. In the basement, housekeeper's rooms, kitchens, bicycle room, etc. On the first floor a large library and Materia Medica Museum.

At the Prize-Giving in July, 1900, Mr. Charles Burt, Chairman of the Weekly Board of the Royal Free Hospital, announced that the Board had decided to appoint two Resident Medical Officers from among students of the School. This announcement gave the greatest satisfaction, for to become a resident in one's own hospital is the laudable ambition of almost all medical students, and is a most desirable preliminary to responsible work elsewhere. Miss Garrett Anderson and Miss Woodcock, both holding the degrees of M.D., B.S. Lond., were appointed the following October.

Miss Aldrich-Blake, M.D., M.S., gave the opening address of the Winter Session, 1900. One of the visitors, Mr. J. F. Turle, a friend of Mrs. Garrett Anderson, heard that there was still a debt of £14,000 on the buildings, which with the fittings had cost over £35,000, and he most generously at once gave £5,000, on condition that no more debt was incurred till the whole of the existing liability was paid off. This generous donation gave immense relief to the Council, and they are very grateful to Mr. Turle for it.

The Council decided to name the Wakefield Street block the Pfeiffer Wing, the Handel Street block the Oakes Wing, and the Hunter Street block the Turle Wing, after the principal contributors to the Building Funds. The Council is also indebted to Mrs. Bennett Mrs. Ivory, Mrs. Durham, Mrs. Cox, etc., for contributions of furniture, and other gifts in equipping the School and adding to its comfort.

In the newly re-organized University of London the School is included in the statutory list of Medical Schools. Its lecturers are among the recognised teachers, and two women, Mrs. Scharlieb, M.D., M.S., and Miss Cock, M.D., are on the Faculty of Medicine of the University, as well as on other important committees.

The endowment, at Mrs. Garrett Anderson's suggestion, in September, 1901, of three hospital beds paid for by past and present students showed how much the appointments of female resident medical officers was appreciated, and a further important step was taken when, on the retirement of Dr. Hayes in October, 1902, Mrs. Scharlieb, M.S., M.D., and Miss Ethel Vaughan, M.D., B.S., were appointed respectively Physician and Assistant Physician for the Diseases of Women. This admission to the Medical Staff of the Hospital puts the climax to the association of the School and Hospital, and is particularly gratifying to those who can recall the early days when the School had to pay £315 a year to indemnify the Hospital from being injured by the connection. The Electrical Department, under Dr. Florence Stoney, was started in October, 1902. The important Maternity Department was begun in June, 1903, under Miss Turnbull, M.D., B.S., who has organised it most efficiently.

In July, 1902, I was invited to become a member of the Weekly Board, a position I willingly accepted.

The School owes very much to the authorities of the Hospital, both lay and medical, for the loyal manner in which the arrangements have been carried out during the long period of more than a quarter of a century.

On looking through the list of medical officers at the Royal Free Hospital, the names of many women are found holding responsible positions as Registrars, Clinical Assistants, Demonstrators, Anæsthetists, Electricians, Obstetric Assistants, etc., showing how much can be done by properly trained women. These posts also afford graduates of the School splendid opportunities for maturing and improving their powers.

Early in 1903 Mrs. Garrett Anderson, M.D., resigned the post of Dean, which she had held for twenty years. The Council at once offered Mrs. Anderson the post of President of the School, which she kindly accepted. The following quotation from the Magazine of June, 1903, expresses very well the sentiments felt by Mrs. Anderson's fellow workers: "Perhaps the School could never have arrived at its present position but for one mental characteristic which its Dean possessed in the most striking degree, the incapacity to tolerate the second-rate," and this was accompanied by a good sense and tact which overcame prejudice and inspired friends with the desire to help forward the essentials of a medical education for women. The foundation of the New Hospital for Women was due to her efforts, and also the re-building of the School. The School has much benefitted by her promotion of its interests. It is her friend, Mrs. Percy Sladen who has given each year since 1900 the sum of £700, without which there would have been a heavy deficit in the School accounts. Mrs. Anderson has also been good enough to promise £300 a year for 10 years to the School, the primary object being the payment of the heavy ground rent. Mr. J. G. S. Anderson's generous donation in 1902 of £1,000 was of great use.

Miss Julia Cock, M.D., who had for many years occupied the onerous position of Vice-Dean, was appointed Dean. In this capacity she has done and is doing very valuable work, specially in the important negotiations entailed by the association of the School with the University of London.

Happily the association of the School and the Royal Free Hospital has become more and more intimate as time went on, and the dinner which is held annually emphasizes the fact.

I think the contrast between the struggle for existence of the School in its early days with its present status shows the wonderful progress that has been made in regard to the practice of medicine by women.

The admirable work that has been done in many parts of the world by former students of the School, engaged in their most womanly mission, and the quiet energy that has characterised its existence, have been important factors in bringing about the great change in public opinion we now witness. For many years the London School was the only institution in Great Britain and Ireland where women received a full training, qualifying them to become registered medical practitioners. As it is, it is still the only one where its students can aspire not only to become Residents, but even, if specially distinguished, to obtain a post on the Staff.

In a sense the London School is the Mother School of all medical women in Great Britain and Ireland. I believe I am correct in thinking that had it not been proved by the work done at the London School and the New Hospital for Women that women can study and practice medicine and surgery successfully, other institutions in Great and Greater Britain would not have been opened to them.

The road has been cleared and the way made easy, but it remains for successive generations of students to carry on the traditions handed down to them; to follow in the footsteps of Helen Prideaux, Mabel Webb, Fanny Butler, Jessie Hatch, and many others, living as well as dead, who have shown that a medical woman can not only be skilful in the practice of her profession, but also an example to all other women for purity of mind and large-heartedness.

The School has had the able assistance of Mr. H. A. Henderson, first as a member of the legal firm of Shaen, Roscoe, & Massey, and subsequently as Honorary Treasurer who throughout has afforded the most valuable help by his wise advice and clear-headed counsel. Questions respecting Practical Anatomy and the School premises more than once threatened its existence, but Mr. Henderson's judicious treatment of the difficulty removed the obstacle and enabled the work to go forward.

The School has had a remarkable succession of teachers and demonstrators. As an example of what I mean a list of its Lecturers on Physiology may be given.

Professor E. A. Schäfer, Assistant Lecturer at University College, held the post from 1874 to 1883, subsequently was appointed Professor at the University of Edinburgh. Dr. Augustus Waller took his place from 1883 to 1884. He was succeeded at the School by Dr. MacWilliam, who became Professor at the University of Aberdeen in 1886. Dr. Halliburton was Lecturer from 1886 to 1897, when, to the regret of his students, he had to resign owing to the pressure of other work. Dr., now Professor E. A. Starling was his successor from 1897 to 1899. Dr. T. G. Brodie took the post in 1899, when he became Lecturer and Director of the Veterinary College. Miss Cullis, who for some time had been a demonstrator under him, was appointed his co-Lecturer in 1904.

Miss Boole's death in 1904 caused much regret. She had been a most conscientious and able teacher of Chemistry for many years.

Several tablets have been placed on the walls. On the mantelshelf of the Council Room the following sentence is inscribed: "The London School of Medicine for Women was established in August, 1874, through the efforts of Miss Sophia Jex Blake, M.D." On the wing containing the Laboratories appears: "In grateful memory of Emily Pfeiffer, whose bequest helped to build this wing, 1898." In the wing fronting on Wakefield Street: "This wing is named after J. R. Turle, Esq., to commemorate his gift of five thousand pounds to the Building Fund of the School," and in the Board Room there are the words "This wing is named after Mrs. George Oakes, of Paramatta, New South Wales, to commemorate her bequest of four thousand and fifty-one pounds." In the Common Room, so much used by the students, with its fine Turkey carpets, comfortable chairs and tables and bureau, are the words: "This room was furnished by a friend of the School in memory of her mother." This lady wishes to remain anonymous. I think we still want another tablet to preserve the memory of what Mrs. Garrett Anderson has done, although the whole School building is a monument to her. The fine large bookcase in the Common Room was the gift of Miss Lewin. The staircase has lists of donors lining the walls. In the Library the names of graduates who have gained honours and gold medals at the University of London and the Royal University of Ireland as well as these of the Prideaux Prize-holders appear.

A medical woman needs many important qualities. She should be wise and sympathetic with a clear, logical mind, much commonsense, good judgment, tact and acquaintance with human nature, able to inspire her patients with confidence. She is brought into close contact with so many of her fellow creatures, has so much varied experience of trying situations, that she requires not only a profound knowledge of medicine and surgery, but a firm grasp of the principles underlying them and the faculty of applying what she knows to suitable cases. She must be unselfish with a great capacity for taking pains. If she takes up surgery much practical skill is needed. She sees so much of the sorrows of life that her heart is often wrung by the griefs of her patients who depend upon her for counsel and comfort in their troubles. She must be able to face responsibilities, for the issues of life and death are often in her hands, and much depends upon her judgment; good health, too, is a most important condition. A medical woman should possess a combination of all that is best in womanhood. Her profession gives her a sphere of action for the exertion of the highest qualities. We look to present and future generations of medical students to justify the hard struggles of the pioneers of the movement and to show their appreciation of the efforts which have been made to secure to women liberty to be trained for the medical and surgical treatment of their own sex.

148, Harley Street, W.,
February, 1905.

Source Endnote

* Dr. Dupré remained Lecturer till 1901.

Editorial Headnote

Mary Scharlieb, *Seven Lamps of Medicine: Inaugural Address Delivered at the London School of Medicine for Women, October 1, 1887* (Oxford: Printed for Private Circulation by Horace Hart, 1888), and *A Woman's Words to Women On the Care of Their Health in England and in India* (London: Swan Sonnenschein & Co., Ltd, 1895), pp. 1–32

As one of the most prolific medical women writers, two of Mary Scharlieb's (1845–1930) earliest works appear in this volume. Although she published while actively practising at the New Hospital for Woman and later at the Royal Free Hospital, Scharlieb's contributions accelerated after she retired from her post in charge of the Diseases of Women section at the latter in 1908. Due to her own longevity, as well as her involvement in many causes from inebriety to eugenics over the years, Mary Scharlieb's writings covered over half a century of key developments in the lives and careers of medical women.

Scharlieb's background contributed to her eventual calling. Her own mother died ten days after her birth from puerperal fever, and she was brought up by her grandmother, then father and later stepmother. She was peripatetically, although well, educated, and married at the age of 20 to William Mason Scharlieb, a barrister completing his education before he returned to India to practise. The couple left for Madras in 1866, where they had three children by 1870. Scharlieb's experiences in India, where religion meant that women could not consult white male doctors, led her on the path to a medical education via initial training as a midwife at the Madras Medical College, where she received a diploma in 1874. Three years later, she left India to begin medical training as one of the earliest students at the newly-inaugurated London School of Medicine for Women, qualifying in 1882. Scharlieb became the first woman to receive an M.D. from London University in 1888 and M.S. in 1897. A successful career, initially in India and then in Britain from 1887 ensued; a CBE in 1917 and a DBE in 1926 cemented her public importance.[1]

Here she is represented as she was in day-to-day life: both a dispenser of advice to female medical students and as a professional support and guide for women negotiating the transition from girlhood, to wifedom, and onto motherhood. Although *Seven Lamps of Medicine* was published privately, it was mentioned in the usual abstracts of inaugural addresses in the medical papers,[2] but also considered in the *Englishwoman's Review*, where the writer joined the 'large assemblage' gathered to listen to Scharlieb.[3] For the *Hospital*, which concentrated on the style rather than the substance of the speech, the address was favourably received precisely because it was not usual and indeed had the effect of conveying 'the advantages which may arise to the profession by the admission of women to its ranks'. Far from the more typically unimaginative strain of the medical man's pronouncements, Scharlieb's thoughts were characterised by their abstraction from the 'figurative and the poetical' which should, argued the reviewer, be part of rather than disdained by 'the science and art of physic'. No medical man would have spoken like this, remarked the *Hospital*, but the expansiveness of the topic enhanced the medical woman's cause to bring a breath of fresh air to the staidness of professional behaviour.[4]

A Woman's Words to Women appeared at the end of October 1895 and was priced at six shillings.[5] In similar fashion to *Seven Lamps of Medicine*, it was received very positively both by the medical and lay press. The *Saturday Review* bemoaned the sheer number of scientific and medical books written by women in recent years, lamenting the conspicuous inferiority of their content in comparison to men's works. However, 'unreserved praise' could be heaped on Mrs Scharlieb's contribution, which inevitably trod a fine line due to topic, but successfully avoided both 'prurient reticence and prurient detail'. Wise and kind was the tone, decided the reviewer, and even Scharlieb's words could stimulate better physical and mental health in those addressed, especially if they lived in 'India and the tropics'.[6] The medical periodicals fell over themselves to admire the book; the *BMJ* even commended the 'highly' qualified author with 'highly' deserved praise all in one sentence. Clarity, wisdom, and practicality, traits not usually associated with women, medical or otherwise, characterised the volume and delighted the *Lancet*'s reviewer.[7]

A second, revised edition would appear nearly a decade after the first, cementing Scharlieb's reputation, before she had even published her most popular writings, as a medical woman who could speak both to her own sex and encourage the trust of the other.[8]

Notes

1 G. Jones, Scharlieb [née Bird], Dame Mary Anne Dacomb (1845–1930), Oxford Dictionary of National Biography, www.oxforddnb.com/view/10.1093/ref:odnb/9780198614128.001.0001/odnb-9780198614128-e-35968 (accessed 10 October 2023).

2 For example, 'Abstracts of Introductory Addresses Delivered at the Metropolitan Medical Schools: London School of Medicine for Women', *BMJ*, 2:1397 (8 October 1887), p. 770.

3 'Record of Events: London School of Medicine for Women', *Englishwoman's* Review, CLXXIII (15 October 1887), pp. 457–461; on p. 457.

4 *Hospital*, 3:54 (8 October 1887), p. 29.

5 'New Oriental Books Published in England', *Luzac's Oriental List*, VI:12 (December 1895), 232; 'Publications Today', *Times*, 30 October 1895, p. 12.

6 *Saturday Review*, 81:2099 (18 January 1896), p. 83.

7 *Lancet*, 146:3769 (23 November 1895), p. 1302; *BMJ*, 2:1864 (19 September 1896), p. 755.

8 'Autumn Announcements Supplement', *Academy and Literature*, 1691 (1 October 1904), 292; *A Woman's Words to Women. Second Edition, thoroughly revised* (London: George Routledge & Sons; New York: E.P. Dutton & Co., 1905).

12

THE SEVEN LAMPS OF MEDICINE: INAUGURAL ADDRESS DELIVERED AT THE LONDON SCHOOL OF MEDICINE FOR WOMEN, OCTOBER 1, 1887 AND A WOMAN'S WORDS TO WOMEN ON THE CARE OF THEIR HEALTH IN ENGLAND AND IN INDIA

Mary Scharlieb

Source: Mary Scharlieb, *The Seven Lamps of Medicine: Inaugural Address Delivered at the London School of Medicine for Women, October 1, 1887* (Oxford: Printed for Private Circulation by Horace Hart, 1888), and *A Woman's Words to Women On the Care of Their Health in England and in India* (London: Swan Sonnenschein & Co., Ltd, 1895), pp. 1–32

THE SEVEN LAMPS OF MEDICINE.

MANY years ago I chanced to read an eloquent and suggestive book entitled 'The Seven Lamps of Architecture,' written by one of the most simple-minded and earnest of men. The lamps with which Mr. Ruskin sought to illumine his stony path were those of Sacrifice, Truth, Power, Beauty, Life, Memory, and Obedience; and wonderful is the light they shed under his skilful management.

It has occurred to me that the path of the physician among the rocks and valleys, the swamps and thickets of his profession, is illumined by a radiant light shining more and more unto the perfect day; and that this light, like its prototype the sunlight, is separable into rays, each beautiful in itself and contributing to the perfection of the whole. These rays may be named Obedience, Thoroughness, Truth, Courage, Gentleness, Humility, Sacrifice. I do not pretend to see the whole spectrum, and to some of you it may be given to see the ultra-red and ultra-violet rays; but I will endeavour briefly to indicate to you their character and the sort of aid they offer by illuminating our onward and upward path.

DOI: 10.4324/9781003265238-12

Obedience first claims our attention; its flame must be fed with unremitting care, for only those who can cheerfully obey may safely command. 'Exactly in proportion to the majesty of things in the scale of being is the completeness of their obedience to the laws that are set over them.'

Many of you are this day commencing the preparation for your life-work; and in the name of the School Council, of your professors, and of your fellow-students, I bid you heartily welcome. It is fair to suppose that women enter the profession of medicine from love, not from compulsion; nor to fulfil, as do their brothers, a family tradition. Is it not likely, then, that the failings as well as the excellences of volunteers will be found among you? Far be it from me to damp your ardour and to daunt your courage, but forewarned is forearmed, and among the shortcomings of volunteers is a lack of obedience, an impatience of discipline. The young soldier reads with flashing eye and beating heart of the brave deeds of old. He longs to charge with the Six Hundred, to lead the forlorn hope, or to perish nobly, the regimental colours to be his shroud. So too you, as enthusiastic students, long for the day when you may stand between the living and the dead to stay the plague with your sanitary knowledge, when you shall be eyes to the blind and feet to the lame; but to the eager recruit come long weary days of training, of setting up drill, and of irksome obedience to orders he does not understand. To you come the prolonged scientific teaching, the dull formulae of Chemistry, the endless details of Anatomy, the mental gymnastics of Materia Medica; and, worst of all to some ardent but undisciplined spirits, the necessity for self-restraint and humble submission to rules which seem to have little or nothing to do with your future work. As medical students you are no longer children, and may not unnaturally think yourselves competent to arrange your work to your own liking, to attend this course of lectures and to omit that; to appear, or not to appear, at any given examination as seems best in your judgment. You must, however, remember that in entering any community, working to attain a special object, you can only work easily and well by conforming to the regulations of that community. Laws may be modified or abrogated, but so long as they are in force the individual cannot neglect them with impunity. According to Ruskin, 'Obedience is indeed founded on a kind of freedom, else it would become mere subjugation, but that freedom is only granted that obedience may be more perfect; and thus while a measure of licence is necessary to exhibit the individual energies of things, the fairness and pleasantness and perfection of them all consist in their restraint. How would it answer, think you, if in a hive some bees framed octagonal and others hexagonal cells? You have indeed the right of private judgment, but that is displayed in consenting, or refusing, to enter a community, not in trying to live an independent life within its pale. Nothing is perfect in the present stage of history: communities, like individuals, must ever seek a higher degree of development; but this growth is of necessity by slow degrees, by the body as a whole, and not by the aberrant action of individual members. Having placed yourselves *in statu pupillari* you will best consult your own interests by a cheerful and intelligent acquiesence in the arrangements made for your benefit.

Thoroughness. The second lamp is that of Thoroughness – a most essential quality for a doctor, and one more conducive to success than are the most brilliant endowments. Napoleon said 'La génie c'est la persévérance,' and a well-known English statesman defined genius as 'an infinite capacity for taking pains.' Epigrammatic sayings are seldom accurate, and few would be found to maintain that any amount of painstaking would enable an uncultured man to write like Milton or to paint like Raphael, but it is certain that nothing worth doing can be accomplished without diligence: 'What good gift have my brothers, but it came from search, and strife, and loving sacrifice?' asks Edwin Arnold; while Trousseau, in speaking to his class of the fame of the great doctors of France, demands of them, 'Do you suppose that they, and many others whose names are in the mouths of every one of you, could by the powerful gifts which nature bestowed on them have become princes of their art unless they had cultivated their natural powers at an early stage of their career? unless they had in early life greedily devoured the treasures of science which were spread out around them as they are spread out around you? unless, though wearied by, they had never been satiated with, labour; and had believed that they had no right to reserve for their own use the riches which they had acquired? Be this then your noble heritage. But, to secure it, toilsome exertions are required. Whilst you are yet young, and while you make your first essay in arms, let your fields be the Hospitals and Clinics; when your knowledge has increased, let the Hospitals and Clinics still be your fields; and let the Hospitals and Clinics still be your fields of industry after you have acquired all the scientific knowledge which we exact from you at the probationary examinations. By pursuing this plan you will attain expertness in the practice of your art, knowing what science teaches, and having within yourselves the power of originating.'

Trousseau said rightly that to secure our heritage toilsome exertions are required; and since the best work is done in a methodical manner, it is well to acquire habits of thoroughness early in your medical training, if they be not yours already. Each term studies should be carefully planned – each day and each hour arranged to the best advantage. Circumstances may force you to vary the details, but the general plan must be respected as far as possible. Here the variety of individual character and taste legitimately appear; and while one student learns most by careful reading, another succeeds only by making a précis, while a third arranges the fruits of study in a tabular form. The exact method matters less than the painstaking, conscientious carrying into effect of the plan selected. In hospital work a definite form of case-taking is essential. In vain does Trousseau exhort you to make the hospitals and clinics your fields of industry, unless you carefully note what you see and hear, and subsequently read the classical accounts of the diseases you have observed. Nor is it on student life alone that the lamp of

Thoroughness shines. Its ray illumines the stony path of the busy practitioner – without it success is impossible.

It is scarcely necessary to remind you that obtaining a qualification, far from marking the end of student days, is really the commencement of a higher education. To all practitioners, but especially to the newly-qualified, I would address the prayer, *Be students still!* Do not suppose that any magic is to be found in your final examination: for this ordeal, fiery though it be, is not the alchemist's crucible; it is but the assay of the mint!

> 'The rank is but the guines stamp,
> The man's the gold for all that.'

Do not dream that the letters appended to your names possess a charm whereby you will be endowed with wisdom and guided without trouble to success. Those of us who have worked hardest in our pregraduate days know best how small is our knowledge and how weak our strength. Probably the best work is done when the worry and anxiety of examinations are over; and, in the comparative leisure of commencing practice, each case furnishes us with materials for study, it may be for original research.

Patients and their anxious friends are keen observers. They quickly detect an unbusinesslike or inefficient discharge of our duties, while they fully appreciate a quiet methodical manner, an easy familiarity in the use of our instruments, and the value to themselves of the notes which ought to be taken of their cases. Always examine your patients on some well-known plan – organ by organ, system by system – else some important point will be omitted. Take careful notes of every point, enter the outline of your treatment; record its results, or apparent results, and gum in the charts and diagrams that will make your record valuable. In the evening, or the first leisure time, read up the subject in the text-books; consult the best monographs, and think over the whole matter. Subsequently, if possible, discuss the case (of course suppressing names) with a friend. It is wonderful how clear a previously obscure case sometimes becomes in the endeavour to bring it before another mind; wonderful, too, how much the formulating of our knowledge in words tends to show us both its strength and its weakness.

To be really thorough our profession must be to us a sort of religion; a golden band binding together all our faculties. For the thorough physician there are no such ideas as are conveyed by the words *trifling* and *insignificant*. Nothing can be small and of no consequence which concerns our patient's welfare or our own reputation. With this view we welcome art in our houses, and seek to make our waiting and consultation rooms as cheerful and attractive as our means permit. We cannot all have luxurious houses rich with rare china and valuable pictures; but we can all secure an agreeable modulation of temperature and light; we can charm the eye with flower and fern, and seek to enliven the tedium of the 'mauvais quart d'heure' by providing books and papers. May I suggest that because we are women more attention to these details is very properly expected of us; and that it is our duty to be as pleasant in our surroundings as possible. Our inmost selves find expression in our outward appearance; and an orderly, beautiful, and well-cultivated mind will be evidenced by suitable, pretty, and well-fitting attire. No one would now commit the follies ascribed by Molière to his learned ladies; but although the days of inky fingers are happily past, it is still well to remember that untidy hair and badly-fitting garments are signs of undesirable eccentricity, not of a superior mind. Pray do not suppose that I would urge the adoption by all ladies of the same model of clothing; but in these days of art-fabrics and cunning workmanship, with a choice of style from Redfern's latest to a flowing drapery of presumably Grecian descent, it is difficult to see why we should allow an easy victory to those who contend that women's minds are so badly developed as to be capable of but one set of ideas, and that when we cultivate what scientific capabilities we may possess, we have not left sufficient nerve-power to maintain our old reputation for love of the beautiful, and ready sense of the fitness of things.

Another result of the thoroughness I advocate is a keen sense of the value of time, an unfailing punctuality. Unpunctuality is really a form of dishonesty, for by it we rob others of their time, which is their most valuable possession. The person who rises late for breakfast breaks the first appointment of the day, and loses a quarter of an hour which frequently frets the temper and spoils the work. Doctors are so liable to be detained by accidents they cannot control, that they should avoid making precise appointments except under special circumstances, but an appointment once made is a promise, and must be kept as such.

Truth. No ray in our spectrum is fairer than is Truth. The necessity for it meets us at every point of our environment. The first essential is that we ourselves should be incarnations of Truth. According to Browning –

> 'Truth is within ourselves, it takes no rise
> From outward things. Whate'er you may believe
> There is an inmost centre in us all
> Where truth abides in fulness.'

No doubt we all have some natural perception of truth, as is shown by the ease with which we sometimes detect her divine form, even when obscured by the mists of ignorance and falsehood; but I rather believe that, as Ruskin says, 'Speaking truth is like writing fair, and comes only by practice. It is less a matter of will than of habit, and I doubt if any occasion can be called trivial which permits the practice and formation of this habit. To speak and act truth with constancy and precision is nearly as difficult, and perhaps as meritorious, as to speak it under intimidation and penalty; and it is a strange thought how *many* men there are, as I trust, who would hold to it at the cost of fortune and life for one who would hold to it at the cost of a little daily trouble.' We only do easily what we do habitually, and unless the habit of thinking, speaking, and acting truthfully is cultivated, we shall find ourselves untruthful against our will. It is not only that to be absolutely truthful demands a thoughtfulness and accuracy to which few accustom themselves, but we are all liable – and doctors more than most people – to be betrayed into an untruth. The demand for an opinion comes upon us so suddenly, the necessity for action is so urgent, that unless the path of the impulse towards truth is well worn it may not be followed. The difficulty comes to us in different guises, and affects each nature according to its own constitution.

To some doctors it is a most painful trial to tell a patient, or a patient's friends, the truth when it is unpleasant. The very tenderness of heart and ability to feel with, as well as for, others that in some respects enhance the value of a keen insight and an adequate knowledge, enhance also the difficulty of plain speaking. Thus: – we are called to see a little child, the parents complain only of a certain languor, a trifling irritability, and want of appetite, which they attribute to the state of the weather or to indigestion. They probably apologise for the trouble they are giving, and perhaps plead that the loss of other children has made them fanciful. How painful it is under these circumstances to toll, as it were, their darling's knell! what an effort it costs to warn them of suspected brain disease! Yet this must be done; and while we avoid undue alarm in cases where the issue is doubtful, and while performing our sad duty in the gentlest and most sympathetic manner, we must for our own sakes, as well as the parents', speak clearly.

Again: during the treatment of a case it may become evident that the patient's illness is caused, or aggravated, by alcoholism or some other error in the patient's self-management. Plain speaking is here the clearest duty: no doubt it is unpleasant; no doubt we must be prepared for the patient to seek another adviser; but the truth abiding in her inmost heart will acknowledge the justice of our accusation; and in many instances the doctor is more respected, and even beloved, for having discovered and declared the truth.

Another view of truth as our guiding lamp is the consideration of the perfect truth which must characterize our actions. Ruskin continues: 'It is surely becoming an honourable man to resolve that whatever semblances and fallacies the necessary course of his life may compel him to bear, or to believe, none shall disturb the serenity of his voluntary actions, nor diminish the reality of his chosen delights.'

Among the resemblances and fallacies we must avoid are those of appearing to do what we are not doing, and of seeming to know that of which we are ignorant. It is possible to continue a line of treatment after we are convinced that it is useless, and so to answer questions as to veil our ignorance under an assumption of knowledge. It is almost an insult for me to tell you that all deviations from the truth are wrong; and that, like all other sins, they bear within themselves the seeds of their own punishment.

Never be afraid to say 'I do not know.' No human being can be fairly expected to know everything. Omnipotence might as well be sought as omniscience. You will not be isolated in your honesty. Sir William Gull told me that he was always ready to confess his ignorance, and to patient and brother alike he frequently said 'I do not know.'

Apart from the ethical and moral view, a fearless truthfulness renders our work comparatively easy and painless. No one expects us to cure diseases that are by common consent incurable; but if from lack of courage we give our patients, or their friends, to understand that the ailment is slight, they will be justly aggrieved that we fail to cure the cancer or to restore the lost functions of an injured brain. Having carefully expressed, and in some cases explained, our opinions to the responsible member of the patient's household, our efforts at assuaging pain and prolonging life will be appreciated.

While on this subject permit me to warn you against dogmatically affirming that of which you are uncertain – a clear offence against truth, and against communicating an unnecessarily depressing opinion. We constantly see men and women who have been told that their days are numbered, or who have been warned against incurring this or that risk under penalty of death. In many instances these gloomy predictions have been happily falsified, and the patient naturally loses all faith in the prophet who has ventured beyond the bounds of knowledge and of common sense. To sum up all –

> 'To thine own self be true,
> And it must follow, as the night the day,
> Thou canst not then be false to any man.'

Courage. Without the warming cheering ray of this lamp we shall stumble over the boulders, sink in the morasses, and perhaps perish in the dark waters of despair. This is one of the qualities that the public greatly appreciate – the possession of which they desire in their doctor. There are two erroneous views prevalent: – first, that a doctor's courage is most tried in the performance of serious surgical operations, and second that women are deficient in this virtue. To me it seems that courage is most tried by the long continuance of adverse circumstances, by the failure of treatment, by the abnormal course a disease will sometimes run, and by the death of patients for whose recovery reasonable hopes had been entertained.

In the case of operations, as in all the concerns of life, knowledge is power; and the feeling of power contributes greatly to the calmness and dexterity with which it is performed. The nervousness from which all young operators suffer is to some extent an evidence of self-feeling, arising from an over-anxious desire to do well in the eyes of those around. The remedies are an accurate knowledge of what has to be done, of the accidents which may befall, and above all the custom of doing the operations. Our hands have to be specially trained to obey readily and easily the motor impulses; until, by long practice, the most delicate and complicated manipulations become almost automatic.

Courage is absolutely necessary in the moral treatment of our patients. We must have the heart to enforce the treatment and the discipline dictated by our reason. It cannot be a matter of indifference to the patient's welfare whether our orders are obeyed or disregarded. It is often necessary to treat patients as parents treat their children – first we must be quite sure what we want them to do, and then gently but firmly insist on their obedience. If the patient will not carry out our directions, it is better for our own reputation, for our peace of mind, and for the patient's safety, to decline further responsibility. This course demands in many cases no ordinary courage, but we must be prepared for such troubles, and have the strength to enforce our orders or to resign the case. In the long run it will be seen that we acted wisely, and the reputation for ability and courage thus gained will in time repay us for the temporary worry and disappointment.

The second error, that women have not courage, needs little comment, for it is daily refuted, and facts are stronger than argument. Women are generally admitted to possess the valuable form of courage known as endurance, and we are credited by the poet with

> 'The reason firm, the temperate will,
> Endurance, foresight, strength and skill.'

I hope this is true of many women, but it is impossible to insist too strongly on ample training and full qualification – impossible to reiterate too often that, since one only does well what one is accustomed to do, all women students, and women practitioners, should take every opportunity of turning theory into practice.

Courage is not only required in cases of great anxiety or sudden emergency, it is needed in everyday life. Other things being equal, the doctor with a pleasant face, bright manner, and cheerful word, will do the most good. Indeed, this quality of courage is, like that of mercy, twice blessed, and that which was at first an effort and cultivated for the sake of our patients, will, after a time, become the habit of the mind; and the bright cheerfulness, which becomes a doctor as the halo does a saint, will be an emanation from within not a mere outward appendage.

Gentleness. Remember, dear sisters, that because you are women, and because you have cultivated your minds, developed your higher natures, and renounced ease, luxury, and this world's pleasant days, much is expected of you.

The men of our profession have justly won the reputation of being the most tender, unselfish, and gentle of their sex. Should not we then be most womanly women, refined, gracious and sympathetic? for –

> 'Courteous we must be towards the lowly,
> To the weak and the sorrowful loving too.
> We must be courageous, refined, and holy,
> By nature exalted, and pure, and true.'

The profession of our choice brings us into contact with all that is most sorrowful, with all who most need sympathy; for –

'Sorrow is
Shadow to life, moving where life doth move,
Not to be laid aside until we lay
Living aside, with all its changing states,
Birth, growth, decay, love, hatred, pleasure, pain,
Being or doing.'

'Oh suffering world!
Oh known and unknown of my common flesh,
Caught in this common net of death and woe,
And life which binds to both – I see! I feel!
The vastness of the agony of earth!
The vainness of its joys. The mockery
Of all its best, the anguish of its worst.'

If we realise the truth of this, shall we not desire to lessen as far as possible the terrible load of human suffering?

'*The vastness of the agony of earth.*' Who has the sad privilege of knowing this as well as the doctor? In the hour of suffering; in the dismay and sorrow that fill the house of mourning, conventionalities are laid aside, human nature appears without its robe of pride, and stricken hearts turn to the earthly representative of that Good Physician to whom none ever appealed in vain. Then is it our high mission to comfort and console; we cannot indeed reverse the laws of nature, we cannot cause the shadow to return on the dial of life; too often it is our duty to bid the mother prepare to resign her babe, to interpret to anguished ears that would fain misunderstand the language of 'the beautiful angel Death'; to communicate to the dying the last divine message, to bid them be of good cheer, that –

'There is no Death! what seems so is transition.
This life of mortal breath,
Is but the suburb of the life Elysian
Whose portal we call death!'

Nor is it in silent chambers of the dead alone that our gentleness and quickness of sympathy are needed. We must always be ready with pleasant chat and cheering word to wile away long hours of suffering and suspense. We must be able to put aside our own anxieties, fatigues, and even actual illness, to meet our patients with an ever-active intelligence and keen appreciation of their condition. The intense fellow-feeling that we may acquire if we will, not only confers on us an improved power of diagnosis, but also so influences our patients as to facilitate all measures taken for their relief. It is no uncommon thing for patients to say, 'The very sight of my doctor does me good.'

We must then be gentle in manner, words, and tone of voice. No one would willingly be rough or brusque with the sick; but unless we remember how nervous and timid illness makes even the brave and resolute we have nothing whereby to measure and guide our conduct. We must not reserve our gentleness, courtesy, for those who seem very ill, and their friends. There are many conditions of mind and body in which the sufferer would fain have something definite the matter to account to himself and others for the vague weakness, the unrest and, above all, for the unnatural irritability. Half-frightened, and wholly ashamed by their want of strength and self-control, these patients are slow to seek advice and to tell the tale of their woes. They very truly need our help. Such states, undetected and unrelieved, are the frequent precursors of serious disease, but there is no task more difficult than to win the sufferer's confidence; and one rough word, nay, one unappreciative remark, suffices to check the half-made confidence. The tale cannot be told, and the last golden hope of bodily and mental health fades away into the darkness of despair.

Humility. – Do not shrink from walking in the light of this lamp. I am here to exhort you to the exercise of this lowly virtue whose name is derived from the earth itself. All things must descend deep if they are to ascend high. The awful but glorious iceberg, shining in the arctic sun, rears its cathedral-like form and heavenly brilliance but one third above the sapphire wave; two thirds are hidden, and what the splendid structure loses in height it gains in stability. The palm, waving its delicate fronds in the warm aether of the tropics, sends its stem as deep into mother earth as its slender column shoots towards the sun. For vast edifices men lay deep foundations. For all work worthy of the name there must be long and arduous preparation. Before honour is humility.

True learning is well aware of its own deficiencies. We all know in what estimation Newton and other great men held their own attainments; and whether we compare ourselves with the men of the past or of the present, with Harvey, Graves, and Trousseau, or with Burdon-Sanderson, Lister and Paget, we can but smile at our own tiny proportions. Humility well becomes us who know so little – and that little so imperfectly.

The vastness of the sciences upon the outskirts of which we are permitted to gaze confounds us. We stand like Moses on Pisgah's height, and enjoy but a fleeting vision of that glorious land.

> 'Fired at first sight with what the muse imparts,
> In early youth we tempt the height of arts,
> But more advanced, behold with strange surprise
> New boundless fields of endless science rise.'

We must not compare ourselves with ourselves, or we may be misled into the fatal belief that we may give thanks as did the Pharisee in the parable.

Consider for a moment how well this lamp can help us on our way. By walking in its light we shall avoid the censorious discourse, the self-complacency and conceit which strike us as spoiling the beauty of our neighbour's character. We shall be more ready to profit by the criticisms of others, and by our own failures and disappointments.

The prediction of the rejecting examiner, 'You will live to thank me for this,' will be assuredly fulfilled if failure leads us to a fairer valuation of ourselves as well as of our knowledge, to an earnest resolve to dig deep as well as to build high, above all to a life-long appreciation of the struggles of others and true sympathy with their failures.

Humility is an old-fashioned virtue, and people sometimes say, 'Ah well! I like a little proper pride!' So they do, in themselves, but in their fellow-man they prefer a sweet reasonableness, a quiet deference, and a forgetfulness of self. As those who announce themselves as the handmaids of science, and as sisters of sinful ignorant humanity, fling away, I pray you, your pride, and be clothed with humility.

Sacrifice. In conclusion, let me say a few words on the very crown and flower of our professional virtues, the secret spring of our actions, the brightest of our lamps. *Sacrifice.* – We are so strangely constituted that for anything to possess a high value in our eyes it must not only be valuable in itself but it must have been bought with a price. Labour, skill, love, nay even life itself, have been and are gladly given, by priest, physician, and missionary, in the service of the race; and the boons thus purchased are valued in proportion to the price paid. In all the relations of life we love people in proportion to what we suffer for them. Hence the devotion of nurse to nursling, of the strong to the weak, of doctor to patient. Does the child feel for its mother the intense and absorbing love she bears to it? The little child and the young adult do indeed feel a quiet, trustful love, which rises at times into gratitude; but to the mother, the child for whom she has faced the perils of maternity, for whom she has watched and prayed and fought the fight of life, is the object of a solicitude and a devotion that none but herself can understand.

What then is the sacrifice demanded of you? – While you are students you must not only give up many of the pleasures and enjoyments of youth, contenting yourselves with plain living and high thinking, but you must renounce your own ways, your own ideas, and submit yourself to those who are for the time your official superiors; the probation is long and tedious, five or six of the best years of your life must be thus surrendered, and after all it is valueless unless you are a cheerful giver. The gift even of your lives is valueless unless offered more than willingly – enthusiastically at the altar of suffering humanity.

Do not consider your profession this day from a practical point of view; do not regard it as a means of earning a livelihood; do not desire the wealth or the prestige that fate may have in store for you. Heap all the riches of your nature, your woman's heart, your cultivated mind, your high ideal of a noble life on this sacred altar. Think,

> 'If such a one, having so much to give,
> Gave all, laying it down for love of man,
> And henceforth spent himself to search for truth
> Wringing the secret of deliverance forth,
> Whether it lurk in bells, or hide in heavens,
> Or hover unrevealed nigh unto all.
> Surely at last! far off! sometime, somewhere
> The veil would lift for his deep searching eyes,
> The road would open for his painful feet,
> That should be won for which he lost the world,
> And death should find him conqueror of death.'

You owe this devotion to our pioneers, to those women who spent their money, their time, and their best energies to secure to their younger sisters a recognised position and an academic career. Gratitude, nay common justice, demands that you should show your appreciation of the benefits they purchased for you. Compare your well-ordered curriculum, your invaluable hospital training, and your absence of care, with the grudged teaching and painfully snatched clinical work of such women as Mrs. Anderson, Miss Jex Blake, and Mrs. Thorne. After all, your student days are but the preparation; you are now developing that knowledge and those qualities which will make your lives valuable to your fellow creatures, as Trousseau told his class: 'Then (with qualification) will you begin that priesthood which will honour you and to which you will do honour. Then too will commence that life of sacrifice in which your days and nights will be the patrimony of your patients. You must resign yourselves to sow in devotion that which you must often reap in ingratitude; you must renounce the sweet pleasures of the family, and that repose so grateful after the toil of laborious occupation. You must know how to confront loathsomeness, mortification of spirit and dangers. You must not retreat before the menaces of death itself.' The mortifications of spirit of which this great master spoke are sure to come. No doctor but was misunderstood, misinterpreted, and unjustly condemned. You will be calumniated by those you have served to the best of your ability, reproached by the ignorant, and perhaps – most trying of all – you may be misunderstood by members of your own profession. Well, you must learn that this is a part of your sacrifice, and remember that the dews of blessing heaviest fall where cares fall too. Be of good cheer, the best and noblest of your patients, of the public, and of your brethren, will bless you, appreciate you, and uphold you; only be true to yourselves, seek no earthly reward, seek to follow the leading of the Divine Light, and let the record of your professional life be one

'Of perfect service rendered, duties done
In charity, soft speech, and stainless days.
These riches shall not fade away in life,
Nor any death dispraise.'

A WOMAN'S WORDS TO WOMEN.

Chapter I.

THE YOUNG GIRL.

Her Education at Home and at School: Physical, Mental, and Moral

– Her Profession.

"Maiden with the meek brown eyes,
In whose depths a shadow lies,
Like the star in evening skies.

"Standing with reluctant feet,
Where the brook and river meet,
Womanhood and childhood fleet."

To the mind of a thoughtful person, there are few objects more interesting than the young girl. She stands, as Longfellow says, "where the brook and river meet," between the happy, careless days of childhood and the pressing duties and responsibilities of womanhood. The young girl is the mother of the future. She may be the destined helpmeet of man, and the mother to be of the men and women of the future, or she may be the spiritual and intellectual mother of children who will owe to her the development of the natures they took from another.

In these days it is impossible to believe that woman's only future is matrimony. The great excess in the number of women has led to their seeking other occupations and wider education. The whole status of woman has changed within the last twenty-five years, rendering the problem of their lives more complex, and demanding different advice, different self-management.

It is useless to ask whether women are better, stronger, nobler, and happier than they were. It may be that they are so; but even were they weaker, less good, and less happy, the times have changed, and they must change with them. Just as the over-stocking of the country in general has led to emigration, with its sorrows to the few, its advantages to the many, and its wonderful outcome in scores of "New Englands," so the overcrowding of what was once the only profession for women has led to their emigration into other professions, arts, and industries. As in the former case, individuals suffer. Some girls lose their health; some develop in undesirable ways; but the great majority have found the primal blessing – the true dignity and satisfaction that attend all honest work.

The present is a transition period, and one of rapid development; inevitably many mistakes are made, many imperfections exist, and the environment is scarcely as yet adapted to the new needs and altered relations of women. Never were the words more true, "Ye have need of patience," – patience with circumstances, with our fellow-creatures, and above all with ourselves. It has seemed to me that in a book professing to advise women on the care of their health, the first chapter should be devoted to the needs of the young girl, who now is often separated from her home and her mother, and who often desires advice that she cannot ask. It has also occurred to me that mothers, schoolmistresses, and others in charge of young girls, greatly need advice and assistance in their important duties. I am constantly asked questions by ladies who feel their responsibilities and their want of knowledge, and I am led to hope that the following pages may be useful to them. As a doctor and a mother, I make no apology for beginning with what too often comes last in consideration – the important subject of health.

Health really lies at the very root of a woman's usefulness; without it the highest intellectual gifts are not only useless – their development is impossible. Impossible, too, is the perfection of the moral nature. Many people think that sickness and suffering mature the character and increase its capacity for reflecting the Divine Image, but consideration will convince us that ill-health prevents the practice of the more active virtues, and renders the passive virtues of patience, submission, and unselfishness very difficult. As Jeremy Taylor quaintly puts it: "Few men mend with sickness as they are but few who with travel and a wandering life become devout." It is true that we all know instances of those who pass through the "cleansing fires," and like the three holy children of old, walk in their midst unscathed. But this involves a supernatural aid, the presence of the Fourth, whose atmosphere of peace alone can envelope and save them.

The exception does but prove the rule, and that, as is too well known to invalids, is that the highest development of which their natures are capable cannot be attained. Just as the eye is the organ of sight, and as sight is rendered imperfect by its accidents and diseases, so the brain is the organ of the mind, and on its structural integrity, on its due nutrition, depends the ease and perfection of its function. Call to your minds two pictures – one of the rosy, active schoolboy, a being brimming over with nervous energy, to whom lessons are easy, and who, with his tireless, ceaseless activity, brings back to all who know him bright memories of their youth. The other picture is of a young girl, slender, pale, with dilated pupils and languid step. She sits quietly gazing into vacancy. You ask her what she is doing, of what she is thinking, and she answers, "Nothing." This is only too true. The exhausted brain, badly supplied with impoverished blood, is always tired and incapable of exertion. Mr. Garret Anderson once said to me of such a patient: "She was born tired, and has been tired ever since. She often feels too tired to live, but she does not die."

If, then, our girls want to live happy, useful lives, if they wish to take the place in their homes, their colleges, and their professions, for which their original endowments ought to fit them, let them take jealous care of their physical health.

Every adult individual has his or her own standard of health, as each has an average weight and an average capacity for exertion. This standard may be gradually raised or gradually depreciated, but it is in the earlier years of life that the standard is fixed; afterwards the maintenance of the acquired level is all that is possible. Hence young people should be taught how best to attain to excellence in this respect.

The intelligent care of the health demands some acquaintance with the outlines of physiology and hygiene, for unless we know something of function in health we are unable to detect the variations of disease. As this is not a treatise on the laws of health, I can only offer a few brief suggestions, and advise my readers to study carefully such books as "Huxley's Elementary Physiology" and "Wilson's Hygiene."

Among the most important factors of health and usefulness is –

Food, and this is a subject on which very few young people think correctly. Too many girls have still the foolish idea that it is not lady-like to satisfy a healthy appetite, and since nothing is more a matter of habit they soon reduce their desires to what they consider the elegant standard. Others, again, believe that meat is likely to make them too robust; they therefore make such articles as pastry, cakes, and sweets their chief nourishment. If these young ladies were acquainted with the simplest rules of physiology they would know that the human body, like a housewife or a merchant, has a regular expenditure, to meet which a regular and adequate income is necessary. They would also know that to provide the requisite income of three hundred grains of nitrogen, and five thousand grains of carbon, in the best and most economical manner, a mixed diet of meat, fats, and farinaceous foods is desirable. It has been found by repeated experiments that to maintain normal weight a man requires daily three quarters of a pound of meat, two pounds of farinaceous food (as represented by bread, potatoes, rice, corn flour, etc.), and, at least, one ounce of butter. Besides this he needs some vegetable and mineral salts, that are found in vegetables and fruits, and about three pints of watery fluid, including tea and coffee. Here, too, the individual standard varies, and while some human beings seem able to thrive on little food, apparently using all they take to the best advantage, others are like badly constructed machines, and need much fuel. Women and girls do not need so much food as men and boys, but this difference is chiefly founded on the difference in employment, the occupations of women generally making less demand on their muscular system. When girls are doing the same work mentally and physically as their brothers, there is no more difference in their dietary needs than depends on their difference in size.

Another point of importance is the distribution of food in the working day. Too many girls and women suffer from a want of what they call their "breakfast appetite." When this is habitual it is a sure indication that there is something wrong – some organic disease or functional derangement that demands medical advice. A healthy girl, having three or four hours' work before her mid-day meal, needs a substantial breakfast of eggs, bacon, or fish, with plenty of bread and butter, and a pint of cocoa or coffee. To take such a breakfast in a comfortable fashion demands from twenty to thirty minutes, which too many busy girls consider a waste of time, and too many lazy girls find incompatible with the slothful habit of lying in bed after they are called. With the nourishment supplied by a proper breakfast, eaten about eight o'clock, nothing is needed until the mid-day meal. This may consist of bread and meat, or bread and cheese and fruit. It should not be too heavy, especially in the case of girls who have to attend afternoon lectures. Whatever organ is in active function makes a large demand both on the blood-supply and on nerve energy; if, therefore, the stomach has to dispose of a heavy meal, the brain will be relatively anæmic, and a painfully drowsy condition results. The afternoon tea, so dear to us working women, and so reprobated by some of our male friends, is always a welcome interlude, and a sufficient stimulus for the rest of the day's work. Unfortunately, few people understand the art of tea-making; few realise that all the refreshing and stimulating element (an alkaloid called *theine*) is readily soluble, and that after the first few minutes the only additions to the beverage are the bitter vegetable extractives, which seem to have a peculiarly bad effect on digestion. Dinner, the principal meal of the day, should, as a rule, be eaten about seven p.m. The early mid-day dinner of our forefathers may answer well for those who have no further work to do, but for all who need the afternoon for work, the late dinner is better. There is sense as well as custom in commencing the meal with a few spoonfuls of good soup. It stimulates the secretion of gastric juice, and sets in action the ferment needed to convert meat into a soluble form. To this should succeed fresh well-cooked meat, with several vegetables, and the meal may come to a close with fruit or light pudding. A dinner of many courses, including highly-seasoned dishes, and a large variety of pastry and sweets, is wholesome for no one, while for young people, and especially for those who eat in order to live and to work, it is an absurdity.

One word as to stimulants. These should be regarded by the young girl as medicines only. In many cases a wineglassful of sound claret with dinner may be useful, but it should be taken only under medical advice. This is specially true in India and other hot climates. The sense of exhaustion from the heat is very distressing, and may be relieved for a time by wine or other stimulants, but it soon returns, and unless the stimulant is regarded as medicine, and taken under proper precautions, the foundation of evil habits and of subsequent disease are rapidly laid.

Exercise and Rest. – In England, the working day usually begins about seven in the morning, when the early bath refreshes and braces both body and mind. An hour devoted to the intelligent care of the body, and to a careful mental survey of the day's work, is an hour well spent, and one that will result in the smoother and more agreeable despatch of business. To the devout, Jeremy Taylor's advice to employ the time in meditation, adapting the thoughts to the actions of the toilet, has a quaintness and originality that are refreshing. He says: "In your dressing, let there be ejaculations fitted to the several actions; as at washing your face and hands, pray God to cleanse your soul from sin; in putting on your clothes, pray Him to clothe your soul with the righteousness of your Saviour – and so on, in all the rest. For religion must not only be the garment of your soul to invest it all over, but it must also be as the fringes to every one of your actions, that something of religion appear in every one of them, besides the innocence of all of them."

Lectures, hospital work, and the daily routine of most offices commence at nine a.m., and thenceforward the earnest worker is fully employed. To those who are healthy and not over-burdened with work or responsibility, this fulness of work has a special and ever-recurring delight. There is the sense of "something attempted, something done," which is so satisfying. Some of us who are less strong in mind and body are apt to be discouraged, especially in the beginning of work. Let such remember Miss Proctor's advice:

"One by one thy duties wait thee,
 Let thy whole strength go to each;
Let no future dreams elate thee;
 Learn thou first what these can teach."

In this way, simply taking up each piece of work as it comes, resolutely refusing to fret about that which is beyond, we find energy and strength sufficient for the day. Many girls waste precious time, and still more precious nerve-power, in fearing that they will not be able to accomplish their tasks. We must bear our duties as children bear their pains, "with direct and gentle sufferance," without regrets for the past or fears for the future. If, with this sense of order in time we can combine order in space, and not work amidst untidiness, we shall do well. "Those who work in a mess get their minds in a muddle"; while external order and method insensibly affect our inmost selves, so tending to lucidity of thought and promptness of action. The mid-day meal should be a time of physical and mental rest, taken with pleasant companionship of chosen friend or beloved book.

If possible, the hour from one to two should be reserved for the light repast and needed repose. In the case of the young and healthy girl, a set of tennis or a quarter of an hour's walk will be refreshing, and restore the "equilibrium of forces." Work again from two to five will not then be found too exhausting, and after the refreshing tea, with its friendly converse and useful interchange of ideas, at least an hour should be devoted to exercise. By exercise I do not mean a dull, routine walk, nor a shopping expedition, but real exercise, that will throw every muscle into action, and make suitable demands on the respiratory and circulatory systems. All girls, but especially those who are studying, should belong to a tennis club, to a gymnasium, or to a swimming class. In the winter it is well to join a singing or dancing class, and gymnastics are then even more useful than in the summer. It is not to be supposed that every girl can attain to excellence in singing or dancing; but that is not the object. The fact is that such exercises, properly conducted, are means of health, and go far in the important matter of physical development. Besides this, it is to be remembered that the girls who distinguish themselves most in college or office are seldom those who excel in accomplishments and sports, so they may learn a useful humility, while those who are habitually beaten by them in graver pursuits may here enjoy an equally useful superiority.

It is very desirable that little or no work should be done after dinner, but in these days of hard work and keen competition it is often necessary to secure a quiet time in the evening for the preparation of the next day's work. Where this is the case no work should be permitted immediately after the meal. Music, singing, a hearty game with the younger children of the house, or a quiet stroll in the garden or square, should occupy an hour or at the very least half an hour, and then the evening work will be less injurious. Many girls, either from a form of indolence or from a want of good management, spend twice the necessary time over their preparation. It is difficult to understand this, but they certainly sit with books and papers before them and their minds far away. This is a bad habit, and one that saps the very foundations of intellectual and moral excellence. It is a sort of dishonesty, a mal-appropriation of time, and a useless waste of power.

Young people, and especially young girls, need plenty of sleep, and the more arduous their work in the day, the longer rest do they need. At least seven, and if possible eight hours sleep should be secured. They should retire at ten, so that they may be in bed and asleep by eleven.

Physiologists have watched the changes that occur in many glands. They tell us how their cells vary before, during, and after functional activity. The brain cells are not convenient for such observations, but there is no doubt that they also require intervals of rest, during which they may be built up and accumulate stores of potential energy. Such rest can be had only during sleep, for while we are awake we have no power to inhibit cerebral function. An overtaxed stomach may be emptied and kept at rest, tired limbs may repose on a comfortable couch, but the weary brain knows no rest save in sleep. If then, girls wish to do their work well and to attain to excellence, they must carefully secure the rest that their brains require.

The Toilet. – Every really womanly woman, every one who truly realises her mission, desires to "look nice," that is, to be a pleasant object of vision for her fellow-creatures. Nor does this quite exhaust the truth, for every womanly woman would wish to be pleasant in herself, and would be as nice in personal matters on a desert island as she would at the court of a great king.

The fundamental necessity of a good toilet is the care of the skin and its appendages, the hair and the nails. The days of imperfect ablutions are, I hope, the days of long ago with the girls for whom I write. Among the many students of my acquaintance there is scarcely one who does not take a bath once a day; but in some instances the bath is taken without any thought of adapting it to the individual, and it causes almost as much harm as good. In many books on Hygiene and Domestic Medicine the only form of bath recommended is the cold plunge or sponge bath. Nothing can be more invigorating and delightful to a healthy and robust girl, but its application is not of universal utility. If the little shock caused by the cold water is rapidly succeeded by a warm glow and sense of exhilaration, all is well; but in some instances there is no such reaction; the shock is prolonged, the fingers "go dead," the lips remain blue, goose skin appears, and perhaps a shivering fit. If this be the case the bath is injurious, and must be modified. One of the best modifications is that suggested by the late Dr. Baxter. He recommended delicate girls to stand in a foot-bath of warm water, to wrap around them a sheet wrung out of tepid or cold water, through which their limbs and bodies are to be vigorously rubbed for three minutes. The wet sheet should then be replaced by a warm, dry Turkish bath sheet, and the rubbing repeated, a small cup of hot milk or tea before completing the toilet securing the maintenance of reaction.

This bath may be made still more stimulating by substituting sea water, real or artificial, for ordinary water.

In some cases a warm bath is better borne, and where the system is feeble this may be accomplished with least fatigue at night. If so, a rapid sponging with a half dry sponge will suffice in the morning.

The clothes call for some degree of care and foresight. Few people reflect on the objects to be subserved by clothes. They should be so fashioned as to afford adequate covering and protection to the body without hampering its movements, and the materials selected should be as far as possible poor conductors of heat. All good ideas are liable to be exaggerated by those who originate or adopt them; and some, otherwise sensible people, appear to go crazy on the subject of the Jaeger sanitary system. Not only would they insist on all clothes being woollen, but they must also be of Jaeger's wool. Of course, the Jaeger materials are very delightful, warm, light, and unirritating, but their cost puts them out of the reach of many. It is a comfort to think that any lightly woven woollen material will suffice for all practical purposes. The clothes should be as light as is consistent with adequate warmth, and their weight should be fairly distributed, hanging as much as possible from the shoulders, and in no case constricting the waist.

It is no part of my design to advise the young girl upon the fashion of her dress, nor to criticise her good taste in selecting garments of tailor-made trimness or aesthetic looseness, I would only remind them that suitability of dress to occupation and occasion is the very essence of being well dressed. I would also have them remember that the orderliness and propriety of the mind is very generally reflected in the appearance and dress.

So many young women are now preparing for work in India, that I make no apology for saying a few words on dress in the tropics. It is well to realise at once that soft, light woollen underclothing is, if possible, more necessary there than it is in England. The great heat causes profuse perspiration, and renders chills, with consequent fever and dysentery, more frequent. Very fine cashmere or spun silk stockings should be worn, and during the day holland or canvas shoes. A fine woollen garment reaching from the neck to the knees is essential to those who hope to keep their health in India, and in many cases an additional safeguard in the form of an elastic Jaeger belt is desirable. At night, a fine thin woollen garment is necessary to protect from the sudden chills which often occur naturally towards morning, and still oftener from a sudden revival of energy in the man who pulls the punkah. As to head-gear, a pith or cork hat, trimmed with a silk or cotton scarf, called a *puggree*, is a necessary protection against the sun. It should be bought in England, as it is much needed on the steamer after leaving the Mediterranean. Spectacles of tinted glass are wanted to protect the eyes from dust and glare, and a light woollen or silk shawl to avert the ill consequences of the heavy dews and sudden variations of temperature.

Whether in India or in England, young girls cannot be too particular about the regular and adequate performance of physical duties. It is unfortunate that too many mothers shrink from the manifest duty of telling their young daughters the leading physiological facts which would often put them on their guard, and instruct them in what they should expect. Girls ought to be told that a neglect of the daily relief of the bowels is a physical sin, and one which is sure to entail its own punishment. They should also understand what simple dietetic remedies they may use – brown bread and butter – treacle, fruit and vegetables, a glass of water either hot or cold on first awakening, are all useful in promoting punctual and adequate relief. Girls should also be told by their mothers or other guardians of the development of organs, and the evolution of new functions which mark the transition from childhood to womanhood. Great alarm is caused by the unexpected occurrence of the first monthly period, and it is an absolute wrong and cruelty not to prepare the young girl for what, if unexplained, must appear to her in the light of an illness. The periodicity, the average duration, and other characters of the function should be mentioned, and certain simple rules as to the avoidance of cold, fatigue, and undue excitement should be given her. I am convinced that the terrible suffering so often borne by young girls and women in connection with what should be healthy and painless, most frequently arises from a want of intelligent care during the earliest years of womanhood. How can a girl know unless she be told that swimming, riding, rowing, tennis, and, indeed, all very active exercise, should be avoided for two or three days each month? Such restrictions may be inconvenient and irksome, but all doctors, and, unfortunately, most mothers, see too much of the misery which is caused by a want of knowledge in these matters.

Woman's sexual life commences at puberty. No doubt there are differences of structure from a very early stage of embryonic life, but the infant boy and girl have similar functions and similar physiological requirements.

Puberty, the process which transmutes the girl into the woman, occurs at very varying ages, and may be slow or rapid in its evolution. Its advent is announced by signs of development of the generative system, and by an analogous mental and moral change. The mammary glands become full, the nipples more deeply coloured and more erectile. These changes often cause a good deal of aching and discomfort too often neglected, and frequently aggravated by the dresses not being altered to suit the expanding figure. In connection with this mammary development should be mentioned the fact that the somewhat sudden addition to the weight of the upper part of the figure sometimes causes lateral curvature of the spine. The muscles of the back, which sufficed to balance the childish bust, are suddenly called upon to balance and to support womanly proportions, and unless they be strengthened by the natural calisthenics of an active country life, or by the artificial calisthenics of the gymnasium, they are likely to prove inadequate to their task. The muscles being easily fatigued, the girl is apt to seek relief in any lounging attitude that is comfortable, and the spine is dragged out of shape. Hence the necessity for frequently examining the spines of growing girls, and of seeking proper advice as to exercises and training before muscular defect has given place to bony deformity.

The clothing too often remains unsuited to the altered needs, and is both too short in the skirt to properly protect the limbs, and too tight in the chest to permit of proper muscular development or efficient respiration. A good test as to the fit of the clothes is that suggested by Mr. Bernard Roth. Let the girl stand with her clothes unfastened, her shoulders and heels pressed against a door or a wall. It will then usually be found that her clothes do not meet by a space varying from two to six inches. In many instances there is no conscious "tight lacing," the clothes do not feel very uncomfortable, and what discomfort there is is borne as a matter of course. Nature, however, is not so easily cheated, and the restrictions thus placed on healthy exertions bears fruit in feeble muscles and curved spines.

Mental Education. – Education is a word which is constantly on our lips, but the true meaning of which is apprehended by few. To many people it seems to imply simply a cramming in – an intellectual stuffing, of which the individual assimilates not much more than does the bird of St. Michael the sage and onions which fill his carcase; or perhaps, more truthfully, the profit is as real as that of the turkey who is daily gorged with a wasteful supply of food to fit him for his Christmas duties. It is only to some such process that we can liken the unintelligent way in which children, without regard to their individual capacity and tastes, are remorselessly pressed from standard to standard, their intellectual feeding being conducted on Procrustean principles. Instead of this, according to Herbert Spencer, "to prepare us for complete living is the function which education has to discharge; and the only rational mode of judging of an educational course is to judge in what degree it discharges such function." What then are the fractions which together make the unity we call life? Spencer has classified them thus: – "(1) Those activities which directly minister to self-preservation; (2) those activities which, by securing the necessaries of life, indirectly minister to self-preservation; (3) those activities which have for their end the rearing and discipline of offspring; (4) those activities which are involved in the maintenance of proper social and political relations; (5) those miscellaneous activities which fill up the leisure part of life devoted to the gratification of tastes and feelings."

As to the first necessity – that of self-preservation – that is to a great extent taught us by Nature, and amounts to an instinct; but, like most instincts, it not unfrequently fails us. We do generally avoid what we know to be bad for us; but we often do things that are very harmful through ignorance. We need to know far more than we do of the properties of those things by which we are surrounded, and yet how small a space does physical science occupy in most schemes of education. The second class of activities, "which, by securing the necessaries of life, indirectly minister to self-preservation" – in other words, the acquisition of knowledge, which confers the ability to earn a living – are sometimes left till formal education is at an end. It is extremely difficult to reconcile the conflicting claims of general culture and technical education; but, as a rule, it is well to remember that unless the foundation be broad and strong, the edifice cannot safely be high; and, medically, we know that a mind with all its faculties cultivated and developed is, other things being equal, more likely to remain healthy than one which has been trained in one direction only.

No knowledge is in itself worthless, and to an intelligent mind all information is interesting; but as facts accumulate and observations multiply, the difficulty of mastering many sciences has become greater, until it is now an impossibility, and a selection must be made among many interesting studies; and, indeed, as a rule, for those who wish to attain to excellence, a portion only of some one subject must be selected for the life work.

Of course, too early devotion to a certain study is much to be depreciated; such a course would tend to shut out many sources of training and of happiness. The individual would have but narrow interests, and would be unable to sympathise in the work and feelings of others. A broad and solid foundation of general knowledge should be laid, and then the acquisition of special knowledge will not have so injurious an effect.

The third class of activities, "those which have for their end the rearing and discipline of offspring," is the class for which absolutely no preparation has hitherto been deemed necessary. It is surely terrible to think that the parents of the nation are less well educated for their important duties than they are in any other respect. To judge by the usual curricula, a knowledge of Greek and Latin or a smattering of zoology and botany, is held more important than physiology and hygiene. Young men and women marry without any idea of the value of their health, without any means of recognising deviations from its standard, and without the knowledge necessary for its maintenance. When a child is born to them, neither parent knows how to feed it, how to clothe it, when it should cut its teeth, walk, talk, or pass through any of the various phases of development. The child is indeed a source of joy, but he is also the cause of many anxieties, the victim of ignorance and mismanagement. The loss of infant life is appalling, and the unsatisfactory health of children is scarcely less terrible. With all good intentions, and with unfeigned love for their little ones, parents too often are helpless through their ignorance. It is perhaps not generally practicable to have lectures to parents, and especially to mothers, on the rearing of children; but surely some acquaintance with simple physiology and hygiene should be acquired by all. In this respect we are worse off now than were our forefathers. In the olden days, girls were regularly taught by their mothers the simple knowledge they themselves possessed. All maidens knew something of cooking and something of leech-craft, as they called it. It is surely a step in the wrong direction which has excluded girls from these domestic mysteries, and has banished the still-room and herbarium. The laws of health are better understood now by the few; but while the doctor and the sanitary engineer have attained to some degree of knowledge, the many have relinquished all interest in the matter, and, in the intensity of their competition for academic honours or commercial prosperity, have practically abandoned all such subjects. This is greatly to be regretted, for no man can obey the laws of health for another, and no excellence of sanitary science in a medical adviser can ensure healthy conditions in his patient's home and nursery.

This is not the place in which to enlarge on this subject from the legislative point; it is more my duty in subsequent chapters to attempt to give a little simple instruction on the practical side.

The fourth and fifth classes of activities to fit us for duties to the State, and to develop artistic, literary and other tastes, need not detain us, as they do not primarily concern those for whom I write.

The Young Girl's Profession. – The time seems not far distant in which it will appear as natural and proper to train our girls for some definite work in life, as it has long been in the case of their brothers. There is no doubt that all human beings are happier and better for having a definite aim and object in life, in preparing for or being engaged in some work that is obligatory and cannot be set aside by the whim of the moment. The worst of the essentially feminine faults, such as vanity, slandering, unpunctuality, and excessive self-consciousness, have been developed during the generations in which the majority of us had no definite work. It is scarcely possible to imagine circumstances in which a woman determined to find work and interest should fail to satisfy herself, and, generally speaking, the nearest and most obvious work is the best. But there are, and have been, many women to whom the world seemed to offer no special work, and who lacked the power to set themselves to find out the exact work that suited them and to which they were suited. Now the tendency is for most girls to devote themselves to some definite and chosen work, and with the desire has come the increase of opportunity; new outlets for woman's energy, new spheres of industry have appeared since the commencement of the second half of the century; the professions of nursing, medicine, law, as well as that of education, also appointments as clerks in post and telegraph offices, book-keepers and accountants, are open to women. Education has been systematised, and the teacher's work has been raised from that of a badly paid servant to the dignity of a profession. To enjoy the dignity of work does not necessarily demand high intellectual gifts. There is room for clever fingers as well as for thoughtful brains, and the trades of house decorating, of millinery and dressmaking, are now freely entered by women of gentle birth.

Editorial Headnote

'Lady Doctors. Increasing Demand for Their Services. Some Objections. The Question of "Nerves"', *Observer*, 8 September 1907, p. 3

The *Observer* began publication in 1791, and was the first Sunday newspaper in the world. By the 1890s, it could also claim another pioneering achievement – the first global female editor. Rachel Beer (née Sassoon) (1858–1927) was born in India and grew up in Britain. She married into the *Observer* in 1887; the paper was owned by her husband, Frederick Arthur Beer (1859–1901), who had inherited it from his father. The marriage was soon dogged by ill health; syphilitic symptoms were experienced by Beer and later by his wife. Despite these significant problems, Rachel Beer wrote for and later edited the *Observer* from 1891. She would also buy and then edit the *Sunday Times* from 1893. After the death of her husband, Beer's own mental health declined significantly, and she was committed and both papers sold in 1904.[1] By the early twentieth century, and after the Beer reign, circulation had reached a very low point, just 5,000 copies when Alfred Harmsworth (1865–1922) bought the paper. Circulation began to increase and, by 1909, it had reached 40,000 with James Louis Garvin (1868–1947) as editor. In 1911, the paper was bought by William Waldorf Astor (1848–1919), who handed it to his son, Waldorf (1879–1952).[2]

From the 1880s, the paper covered 'the beginning of a vast social and moral revolution in India' through 'female medical advice and assistance',[3] but it also commented on the way in which medical women were presenting themselves. In October 1890, the *Observer* took issue with Mrs Stanley Boyd's inaugural address, accounting for the London School of Medicine for Women's progress, finding it 'partly, but not entirely satisfactory'. Forming part of the 'Review of the Week', the paper remarked that while lady doctors should work hard, for the benefit of their patients as well as their own careers, 'that they should work so hard as to endanger their health and forfeit all enjoyment of life is evidence of zeal rather than discretion'. In so doing, the article highlighted a key concern that medical women needed to prove themselves through the profession of constantly hard and superlative work. For the *Observer*: '[t]he lady, indeed, who first succeeds in showing that it is possible for ladies to be serious without being too serious will be an undoubted benefactress to her sex'.[4] The paper also complained about the attitude of Oxford University in 1890, whose House of Congregation had blocked women's admittance to medical degrees at the institution. It was a fact, sighed the *Observer*, that 'lady doctors at all events exist' and had found, especially in 'our Indian Empire – considerable opportunities of usefulness'. In similar fashion to the 1907 article reproduced here, however, support was tempered with doubts, however humorously expressed in this instance. It was necessary to ensure that female competence was evident '[o]therwise it may happen that they will mistake arsenic for Epsom salts, and so poison the Indian subjects of their Queen'.[5] A short piece from 1891 condemned the 'Ladies not admitted' attitude in Germany to women wanting to pursue professions, but depicted medical women as politically conservative and staid. 'English experience' had concluded that while shoemakers, far from learned, were the most socially and politically subversive element, the Germans had nothing to fear from lady doctors who 'exhibit as little desire to upset the pillars of the Constitution as our lady type-writers or our lady barbers'.[6]

The production of a mixture of assistance and detraction aside, however, as a key weekly paper, the *Observer* was utilised by medical women themselves. Strikingly, when the editorship was under Rachel Beer at the very start of the twentieth century, the New Hospital for Women pleaded very regularly for funds towards current expenses. 'The New Hospital for Women. Staffed by Medical Women' appeal could be found frequently throughout the years between 1901 and 1904.[7] Similarly, in July 1908, the paper marked a sea-change in attitudes to female doctors through an article on the 'very strong growth of feeling in the profession in favour of women', indicated by a positive vote regarding their admission as members or fellows of the Royal College of Surgeons.[8] That the *Observer* had called its article 'Women Surgeons' rather than the more usual 'Lady Doctors', used even a year before in the piece reproduced in this volume, suggested that the lay press was also treating medical women more favourably.

Notes

1 V. Curney, Beer [née Sassoon], Rachel (1858–1927), Oxford Dictionary of National Biography, https://oxforddnb.com/view/10.1093/ref:odnb/9780198614128.001.0001/odnb-9780198614128-e-48270 (accessed 9 October 2023).
2 'Key Moments in the *Observer*'s History – A Timeline', www.theguardian.com/gnm-archive/2002/jun/11/2 (accessed 9 October 2023).
3 'Notes', *Observer*, 16 December 1888, p. 5.
4 'Review of the Week', *Observer*, 5 October 1890, p. 5.
5 'Review of the Week', *Observer*, 23 November 1890, p. 6.
6 *Observer*, 15 March 1891, p. 6.
7 See, for example, *Observer*, 26 May 1901, p. 1; 24 August 1902, p. 8; 27 December 1903, p. 8; 11 September 1904, p. 1.
8 'Women Surgeons. Growth of Feeling in Their Favour', *Observer*, 12 July 1908, p. 3.

13

'LADY DOCTORS. INCREASING DEMAND FOR THEIR SERVICES. SOME OBJECTIONS. THE QUESTION OF "NERVES"', *OBSERVER*

Source: 'Lady Doctors. Increasing Demand for Their Services. Some Objections. The Question of "Nerves"', *Observer* (8 September 1907), p. 3

LADY DOCTORS.
INCREASING DEMAND FOR THEIR SERVICES.
SOME OBJECTIONS. THE QUESTION OF 'NERVES'.

The decision of the County Asylum authorities at Fulbourn, near Cambridge, to discontinue appointing lady doctors to their resident staff recalls attention to the long struggle on the part of women practitioners to share the medical profession on equal terms with their male rivals.

There is a widespread notion that women have so far failed to make much progress in invading the medical ranks, largely on account of professional jealousy. Such, however, according to an eminent authority of wide experience in the world of medicine, is far from being the case. He maintains that, as a rule, there is no such jealousy, nor any feeling that women are taking the bread out of the male doctors' mouths. Such instances are too few and insignificant to be taken into account.

The two great objections to the female resident doctors in hospital and asylums, it is said, are, firstly, the unsuitability of the domestic arrangements, and, secondly, the temperament of most women in the face of responsibility. As to the first objection, our institutions have been built on the supposition that the resident medical staff would be of one sex.

Then as to the question of temperament, there is, he urged, a tendency on the part of women either to cast about for someone to lean on or to take consequences much too seriously to heart. As an instance of this he quoted the sad case of Miss Hickman, the lady doctor at the Royal Free Hospital, who poisoned herself in Richmond Park.

'It all comes under the head of nerve', he said. 'In the case of a surgical operation the man is satisfied with doing his level best, and if the patient died he would

DOI: 10.4324/9781003265238-13

think it could not have been helped. But a woman would worry herself over it while operating, and even afterwards, and the consequence is that the next patient suffers also'.

GAINING GROUND

However, women doctors have in recent years made substantial progress, both in public estimation and in the numbers who have successfully entered the profession. It is true that, with the exception of the Royal Free Hospital in Gray's Inn-road, women practitioners are still precluded from the residents staffs of our London hospitals, but in all other directions they have given ample proof of their medical skill. The New Hospital for Women in Euston-road, now in its thirty-seventh year of existence, has been staffed entirely by women doctors from the start, and so much appreciated is the institution by women that applicants will wait patiently for months in order to obtain admission to this especial hospital rather than apply elsewhere. Reference to the last annual report shows that during the year there were no fewer than 208 major operations performed, and of this number 2023 recovered – a percentage of which the medical staff may well be proud.

At the Royal Free Hospital the resident medical staff has included two women doctors for many years past, the arrangement having been found to work with perfect smoothness. In addition to the above, there are medical institutions for women and children, officered wholly or partially by registered medical women, as Chelsea, Clapham and Plaistow, the Church Army Dispensary in Crawford-street, W., and in various parts of the provinces.

Altogether, according to returns made up to last autumn, there are 552 medical women practising in the United Kingdon, apportioned as follows: -

England and Wales	389
Scotland	122
Ireland	41

London, naturally, heads the list with a total of 172 lady practitioners, and the proportion in which the chief provincial towns are thus provided may be seen from the following table: -

Birmingham	7	London	172
Bristol	6	Manchester	9
Hull	9	Newcastle	3
Leeds	5	Nottingham	4
Liverpool	11	Sheffield	12

The above facts and figures show that women have at any rate made substantial progress within the forty years during which the movement has been in progress, and for this the chief credit is due to the London Royal Free Hospital London

School of Medicine for Women, which has granted no fewer than 476 medical degrees to women since it was started in 1874.

MASCULINE V. FEMININE 'NERVES'

Miss Douie, M.B., M.A., the secretary and warden of the school, informed a representative of THE OBSERVER that she considered the movement had been wonderfully successful. Like all other professions, there was an ebb and flow, but, on the whole, there was certainly an increasing number of women joining the medical ranks.

'The only thing which handicaps us', said Miss Douie, 'is that appointments are not as freely open to women as they are to men, but this is getting better than it used to be. When women do get appointed, you generally find people are very pleased with their work. It is a case of getting to know them. There seems to be an absurd misconception that women doctors are not trained in the same way as men, but the training is precisely the same, and they are under the same regulations. In all the schools, except this and Edinburgh and Glasgow, women share the work with the men. The cases of breakdown are few, and not more than you would get in any other profession'.

In answer to a question as to how women students' nerves stood the strain, Miss Douie said that they were in no way inferior to men. 'I have gone through the school myself, and I have never seen a woman shirk anything at the hospital. Ordinary operations do not require more physical strength than is possessed by the average woman. Our students go in a great deal for athletics, which, besides being an amusement, develops their muscles. They take life very much as other people take it, and are not morbid. I regard the criticisms of women surgeons as entirely unfounded, and anyone acquainted with surgery and the work our surgeons have done can disprove them. There are very few cases in which women have been displaced. Of course, in open competition a woman may be appointed and be out next time'.

'We always protest strongly against the idea that women are willing to work for less than men. Several students have refused appointments because they were offered less than the male doctors. We do not at all wish to undersell men in any way; we particularly object to it. The training is the same for both sexes, and the payment ought to be the same'.

'I think it is an early Victorian idea that women doctors do not marry', said Miss Douie, in answer to another question. 'In every department of life I think that men do not really prefer stupid women'.

PROSPECTS FOR LADY DOCTORS

As to how far medical women are successful in establishing themselves in private practice in England, another authority is of opinion that a woman has a better chance than a man. For if she settles in a good provincial town she usually has no competitor of her own sex to fear, and without buying a practice she is pretty sure, without exercising any extraordinary efforts, to earn about £200 a year after being in practice for two years. After that her income increases more rapidly, for it is in earning the first £200 in fees that the medical practitioner has the hardest struggle of his life.

This same authority is of opinion that the great majority of English medical women undoubtedly marry either before or soon after they complete their curriculum. 'In fact, one almost fancies that men either perversely seek as wives the very type of women whose intellectual tastes they pretend to detest, or prudently apply matrimony as a solvent of sexual competition'.

Editorial Headnote

F. Howard Marsh, 'Scarcity of Doctors', *Cambridge Review* (24 February 1915), pp. 221–222

When Howard Marsh (1839–1915) died in June 1915, he received a four-page obituary in the *British Medical Journal* and a two-page eulogy in the *Lancet*. Both added an enormous photograph of Marsh in his cap and gown, a distinguished figure who had died while Master of Downing College, Cambridge and Professor of Surgery in the same institution. This was an image which belied his 'breezy and unconventional' teaching style.[1] Marsh began as an apprentice to his uncle, and afterwards had a longstanding affiliation with St Bartholomew's Hospital, which he entered in the Autumn of 1858. *Plarr's Lives of the Fellows* remarked that he 'passed through his student career without distinction'.[2] Marsh became M.R.C.S. in 1861; F.R.C.S. in 1866. In the early 1860s, a variety of posts at Bart's were coupled with work at the Hospital for Sick Children in Great Ormond Street, where in 1862 he became House Surgeon; he would later become Consulting Surgeon there in 1889. At Bart's, Marsh became assistant surgeon in 1873, additionally held medical school appointments, such as demonstrator of anatomy, lecturer in surgery, became full surgeon in 1892, and consulting surgeon in 1904. From 1866 to 1903, he was Surgeon at the institution which was later known as the Alexandra Hospital for Children with Hip Disease; the other institution with which he would become perennially associated. In 1886, along with Agnes M. Bowditch, he founded the Children's Cottage Hospital in Berkshire. In 1903, Marsh was offered the Chair of Surgery at Cambridge, and four years later he was elected the Master of Downing College. He was also the first Commissioner of Scouts in Cambridge from 1912.

Although he published first on tracheotomies in children in 1867, Marsh specialised in diseases of the joints and advocated pioneering conservative surgical treatment for tuberculosis of the bones and joints, involving immobility and rest rather than risky, radical procedures such as excision of the hip, which too often resulted in death. In addition to numerous papers on the subject, he produced *Diseases of the Joints* in 1886, which had reached its third revised, enlarged edition by 1910 as *Diseases of the Joints and Spine*.

Howard Marsh was 'always on the side of broad views and generous ideas', a 'progressive'.[3] It is not surprising, therefore, that he was known as an active supporter and friend of medical women, promoting their admission to degrees and diplomas throughout his career.[4] His importance to the cause can be illustrated by the articles kept in their press cuttings and scrapbooks both by the London School of Medicine for Women and the South London Hospital for Women and Children which featured his encouraging words about women's medical and surgical capabilities in the lay press.[5] Marsh's comments must have been particularly treasured as these were some of the last writings penned before his death.

Notes

1 'Obituary', *Lancet*, 186:4792 (3 July 1915), pp. 39–40; on p. 40.
2 Marsh, Frederick Howard (1839–1915), Plarr's Lives of the Fellows, https://livesonline.rcseng.ac.uk/client/en_GB/lives [accessed 10 October 2023].
3 Sir Clifford Allbutt, in 'Obituary', *BMJ*, 2:2844 (3 July 1915), pp. 35–38; on p. 37.
4 *BMJ*, 3 July 1915, p. 36.
5 South London Hospital for Women Press Cuttings 1912–1917, H24/SLW/Y6/1 and London School of Medicine for Women and Royal Free Hospital Press Cuttings, Volume IV: January 1904 – August 1915, H72/SM/Y/02/004, London Metropolitan Archives.

14

'SCARCITY OF DOCTORS'

F. Howard Marsh

Source: F. Howard Marsh, 'Scarcity of Doctors', *Cambridge Review* (24 February 1915), pp. 221–222

SCARCITY OF DOCTORS

It is familiar to us all that when an important subject presents itself the air at once becomes thick with conflicting opinions, very strongly expressed, by people who are either quite unconsciously prejudiced, or who are mere gossips, speaking not according to knowledge, and never having given the question a quarter of an hour's serious thought. Both these groups forget that till they have mastered some, at least, of the main facts they are mere blind leaders of the blind.

We have a clear instance before us. People hear that, in the circumstances of the present war, there is a very serious shortage of Doctors, both for military service and for civil work at home. It is understood that about a million or two millions of men are shortly going to the front, and they must be fully supplied with Doctors. To secure this the service in our hospitals will be very seriously depleted; the same will be the case in every dept of public health; and a large proportion of the ablest general practitioners up and down the country have already obeyed their country's call, and have volunteered for active service. Here is a serious outlook, which no amount of loose talking will meet. The situation is governed by facts, and these facts are, that not only is there this shortage at the front and at home; but also that it must increase in an ever growing proportion as the war goes on, and further, that many men who, before the war, intended to make medicine their profession, have applied for commission as combatants.

In the search for some solution of this very real difficulty we are met by the question of women Doctors. Can they be turned to any useful purpose? Here again, before pronouncing any opinion, we must examine any facts that are available. We must ascertain what position women have, as a matter of fact, attained in the profession, and what their credentials are.

To being with, the London School of Medicine for Women, founded in 1874, and at the Royal Free Hospital, women undergo exactly the same training as that provided for men in the Medical Schools connected with the large Hospitals. The

DOI: 10.4324/9781003265238-14

curriculum extends over five years. The number of students is steadily increasing. In the present year the entries have reached 63, and the number of students in the School is now 220. When the time comes these students present themselves for the usual medical examinations. Until recently there was no provision for the examination of women at the conjoint board of the Royal College of Physicians and the Royal College of Surgeons, and women were obliged to submit themselves to the more severe ordeal of the University of London. The results have been remarkable. Not only have a very high percentage of women examined passed, but they have won, in open competition with men, the gold medal in each of the following subjects: Anatomy, Physiology, Midwifery (three times), Surgery, Medicine, Forensic Medicine (twice), and State Medicine. Since women have been admitted to the Conjoint Examination of the two Royal Colleges, one candidate has become a FRCS. Thus, so far as examinations go, women have attained very high distinctions. When it has fallen to my lot to examine women in Surgery I have found evidence that their work has been thorough and sound, that there has been no shirking, and that the note of the parrot or the jay (garrulus glandarius) was nowhere to be heard. I have had good opportunities of seeing women Doctors at work in many different positions. It is beyond doubt that, allowing for a percentage of failure, such as is certainly not absent on the men's side, women Doctors have achieved a very notable success, and very little has been seen of those defects and handicaps which, in the opinion of many, made failure a foregone conclusion. I know women who display every endowment and every qualification necessary for the higher levels of operative Surgery and whose results are as favourable as any obtained by men in similar groups of cases. I know others who from every point of view are well adapted for general practice, and who moreover have been notably successful. I do not think anyone who is acquainted with the facts of the case will deny that, in the various departments of public health, women have discharged their duties with complete efficiency. And why should anyone be astonished to hear these things said? Be it remembered that women doctors are a selected class, who have aspired to a high position, and who have won it in the face of great difficulties, by long and hard training in a suitable environment. What are the qualities women Doctors must possess? Are they not steadiness and fortitude, earnestness, conscientiousness, and a sense of duty and responsibility, tenacity and purpose, the power of taking pains and attention to detail. Are not these characteristics found in many a woman whom most of us are privileged to know in various other walks of life? And now that we are face to face with a national emergency may we not expect that it can be largely met by utilising the work which women have so fully shown themselves competent to undertake?

There are several depts in Medicine in which a well informed and candid observer must surely allow that women are qualified to play their part. To begin with, a great many more than half of the community are women and children, and there would seem to be, from many points of view, an inherent propriety and conveniency that women should attend them. I know that at present many women say they would not have a woman Doctor. If asked why, some give one reason and some another, and every one's feelings must be respected. A free choice is open to all. But when a little more time has elapsed and more is known of the quality and level of the work of which women Doctors are capable, a change of opinion may and, I venture to think, certainly will come.

Does not the fact that male patients are nursed by women sweep away considerations which might, at first sight, indicate a fundamental difficulty as to women Doctors for men? This is a matter, however, which will settle itself, for in an ample margin of cases women Doctors will decline to attend men, and men will decline to consult women Doctors.

The diagnosis and treatment of the affections of the chest, eye, ear, teeth and throat present nothing beyond the acquirements of a woman who has been through a general curriculum of five years, and who has subsequently worked at the theory and practice of the subject, under good teachers, in a special department, for two or three years. I cannot believe that women thus trained would be inferior to men who had worked on similar lines. The administration of anaesthetics might seem to be a test case. The answer is that in the Hospital for Women where critical internal operations are frequently performed the various anaesthetics are given entirely by women, with the remarkable result that in the last 3 years there have been only 6 fatalities in a total of 5856 cases.

In many other Hospitals and in private practice anaesthetics are largely given by women with a very satisfactory average of success.

In many of the provincial Hospitals women are acting as Resident Medical Officers. In these appointments they are intimately associated with the Matron and the Nurses, under the supervision of the Visiting Staff, and the general verdict is very much in their favour, especially as many of them are fully trained in clinical pathology and the use of the microscope.

Those in authority are making it a strong point to avoid underselling their male colleagues. Also it is fully understood that when men return from military Service women Doctors who have been temporary substitutes for them must retire in their favour. Justice cannot be done unless this is a binding compact. This should be no deterrent. Women who have done good work will readily find other openings.

Much depends on the women themselves. They suffer no restrictions in presenting themselves for pass and honours examinations; but undoubtedly the financial question is a very pressing difficulty. There is an urgent need for considerable enlargement of the Royal Free Hospital, for which a strong appeal is being made. Cannot the rich women of England make it a question of their own and supply the necessary funds? The sum required is £25,000.

I am informed that the War Office has offered to Medical women a Military Hospital of 500 beds in London, to be completely staffed and run by them. The Hospital will be provided, equipped, and maintained by the War Office. This shows the direction of the tide.

F. Howard Marsh.

Editorial Headnote

Beatrice Harraden, 'Women Doctors in the War', *Windsor Magazine*, XLIII (December 1915-May 1916), pp. 175–193

Beatrice Harraden (1864–1936) was a novelist, playwright, and short-story writer, as well as an ardent suffragist. She was educated at Cheltenham Ladies College and went on to receive a B.A. from Queen's College and Bedford College London, opened in 1848 to begin the higher education of women. She was a treasured former student.[1] Harraden's first novel was published in 1893 and entitled *Ships That Pass in the Night.* While the phrase has become one in standard English usage, the novel has been forgotten. However, it was described as one of the most popular works in the 1890s, replete with, as Harold Williams later sniffed when assessing modern English fiction, 'sentimental ethics and simple piety', the greatest of draws for the British middle class who preferred their tales to be wholesome and inoffensive.[2] In 1901, Harraden wrote to the *Bookman* to describe the circumstances of the publication of the novel. She remarked that it had been turned down by Messrs. Blackwood as too short and sad, so unlikely to sell, but it was promptly adopted by Messrs. Lawrence and Bullen, who provided the author with twenty guineas for the copyright. Inexperience and desire to publish forced Harraden's hand, and she accepted their terms. *Ships* was a phenomenal global success, massing editions throughout the year. It was pirated in America, ensuring that it appeared, without copyright, in every format from five cents to a dollar, likely to have sold, modestly, over half a million copies. Worldwide interest was generated from as far afield as New Zealand, Canada, South America, and India; a non-financial harvest that Harraden found 'priceless'.[3] Many other novels followed *Ships*. The 1903 work *Katherine Frensham*, for example, was described by G. Meredith in the medical periodical the *Hospital* (tellingly in its 'Nursing Section'), as 'so valued' due to its pathetic nature and 'rare charm' of the 'essentially feminine' combination of strength and sweetness.[4] It was this appealing nature which ensured Harraden's works would be translated, in her lifetime, into, for example, Danish, Dutch, French, German, Hungarian, Icelandic, Indonesian, Japanese, Russian, and Swedish. Beatrice Harraden's name, therefore, from the 1890s onwards, was a real draw for anyone lucky enough to secure her interest, and her works were read with genuine enthusiasm.

Alongside her fictional triumphs, Harraden devoted her life to women's rights, initially as a member of the Women's Social and Political Union, but later breaking away from the WSPU to join the Pethick-Lawrences' Votes for Women Fellowship.[5] She brought her two passions to bear when she was a proud marcher under the Scrivener's banner with Elizabeth Robins and Evelyn Sharpe, on 13 June 1908, for the famous procession of suffragists, which included a band of medical women.[6] In a letter to the *Times* in 1912, she explained why the moment was right for the development of the movement, which was akin to a religion. A 'deep force' was at work in the country, Harraden remarked, 'which impels women of all ages and conditions – women of 80, middle-aged mothers, young wives, and unmarried women of all professions and callings – to do, dare, risk, and sacrifice everything for the suffrage cause'.[7] The feeling was visceral for women, rather than one inspired by leaders, she argued.

The 1908 march was not the first time Harraden had combined with the medical profession. In 1896, she wrote, with the American physician, William A. Edwards M.D., a little volume called *Two Health Seekers in Southern California*. As a resident for over two years for her own ill health, Harraden was able to contribute the chapters on 'Southern California' and 'Out-Door Life for Women'. From 1915, another association was begun when Harraden acted as librarian at the woman-run Endell Street Hospital, presided over by Louisa Garrett Anderson and Flora Murray. She would later pen the preface to the latter's *Women as Army Surgeons: Being the History of the Women's Hospital Corps 1914–1919* in 1920.[8]

Notes

1 Mrs A. Tweedie (ed.), *The First College Open to Women Queen's College London: Memories and Records of Work Done 1848–1898* (London: Queen's College, 1898); 'Record of Events: London University. BA Examination Pass List', *Englishwoman's Review*, CXL (15 December 1884), p. 567.
2 Harold Williams, *Modern English Writers: Being a Study of Imaginative Literature 1890–1914* (New York: Alfred Knopf, 1919), p. 29; p. 439.
3 B. Harraden, 'Concerning "Ships that Pass in the Night"', *Bookman*, 20:115 (April 1901), pp. 10–11.
4 G. Meredith, 'Review of *Katherine Frensham*', *Hospital*, 35:900 (26 December 1903), p. 185.
5 E. Crawford, *The Women's Suffrage Movement: A Reference Guide 1866–1928* (London: UCL Press, 1999), p. 276.
6 E.S. Pankhurst, *The Suffragette: The History of the Women's Militant Suffrage Movement, 1905–1910* (New York: Sturgis Walton & Company, 1911), p. 243.
7 *Times*, 18 March 1912, p. 6.
8 W.A. Edwards, M.D. and B. Harraden, *Two Health-Seekers in Southern California* (Philadelphia: J.B. Lippincott Company, 1897); B. Harraden, 'Preface' to F. Murray, *Women as Army Surgeons: Being the History of the Women's Hospital Corps in Paris, Wimereux and Endell Street September 1914-October 1919* (London: Hodder and Stoughton, 1920), pp. vii-x.

15

'WOMEN DOCTORS IN THE WAR'

Beatrice Harraden

Source: Beatrice Harraden, 'Women Doctors in the War', *Windsor Magazine*, XLIII (December 1915-May 1916), pp. 175–193

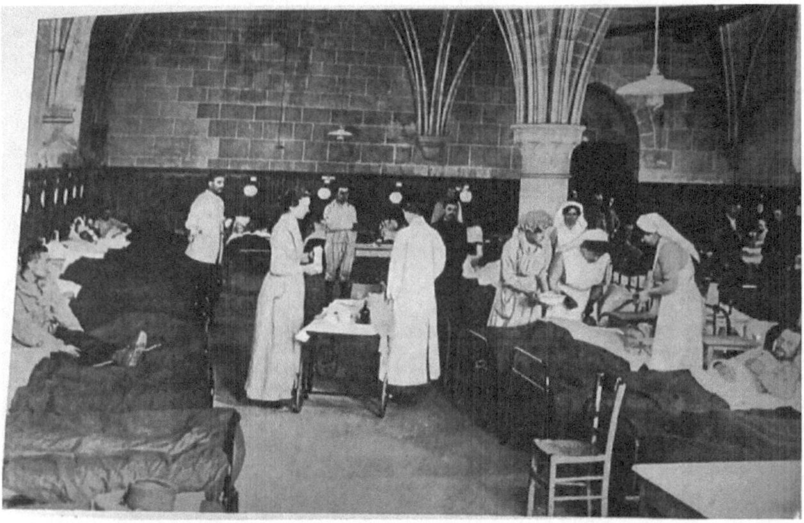

HOSPITAL AT THE MONASTERY AT ROYAUMONT, FRANCE, FOR SOME TIME DIRECTED BY SIR JOHN FRENCH'S SISTER, MRS. HARLEY.

WOMEN DOCTORS IN THE WAR

By Beatrice Harraden

IN the record of women's activities in the War, no chapter is more interesting and significant than the work achieved and the part played by the women doctors. To all those who have for long years laboured for free fields for woman's endeavour, and have had to wrestle with difficulties and tread down traditions, it must be a special source of pride and reassurance to witness the triumph of the women doctors all along the line – not only the triumph of fulfilment, but also the triumph of acceptance and recognition, and, more than that, the triumph of being wanted imperatively and of being ready for the call and opportunity. To the pioneers of the woman movement, therefore, the successful issue of the medical women's struggle would seem to be symbolic of the woman's cause as a whole, and all the more so because it entirely justifies the claim always put forward, but not always understood, that the co-operation of women is needed, not only for the good of their own sex, but for the good of the community.

It is a compelling instance of the eventual working out of the scheme of justice that medical women, who bore the heat and burden of the uprising of women in those distant days of forty years ago, should now have the satisfaction of heading the onward march through open country, with barriers broken down. And it must surely enhance their pleasure to know that all women, no matter what their own achievements in other directions, share in this pride, and add to it a deep admiration for the way in which these women have used all available opportunities for service, and created others by their splendid initiative, resourcefulness, and self-sacrifice. Forty years ago the first little band of women in Edinburgh who went up for a medical examination were surrounded by a crowd which hooted, yelled, menaced, threw mud, and would probably have resorted to violence, but that some of their more chivalrous class-mates formed themselves into a regular bodyguard for their protection.

"And encompassed by them," writes Dr. Sophia Jex Blake, who was one of the women, "we passed through the still howling crowds at the gate and reached

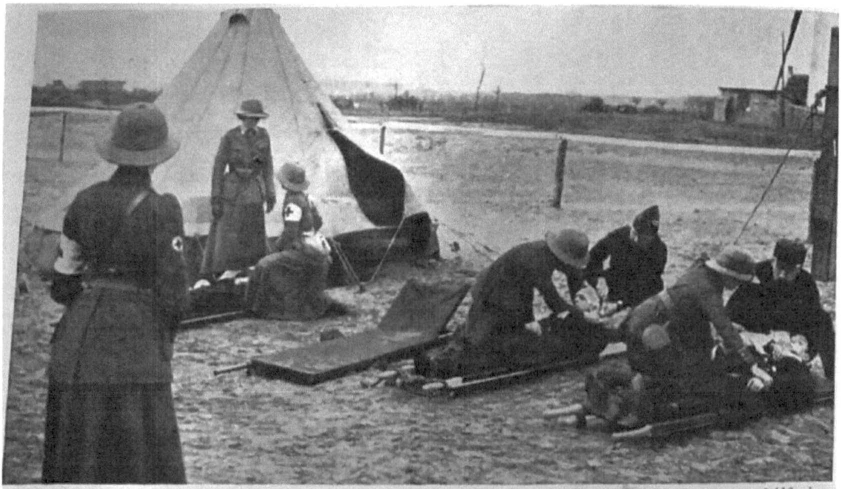

Photo by] [*Alfieri.*

MEMBERS OF THE FIRST-AID NURSING YEOMANRY CORPS AT WORK BEHIND THE TRENCHES.

home with no other injuries than those inflicted on our dresses by the mud hurled at us." That was forty years ago. And about four months ago the Prime Minister, Lord Curzon, and Mr. Balfour made an appeal in the Press for funds for the London School of Medicine for Women, thus emphasising the urgency of the country's need for more women doctors. No instance could be more illustrative than this of the complete change in conditions, outlook, and valuation.

To a suffragist, of course, the work done by the suffrage organisations is of special interest; but although the initiative has in most instances been theirs, and the administration in their hands, the support has by no means been confined to suffragist circles, and contributions have flowed in from the general public, from all sorts of people holding all sorts of political opinions, and from supporters not only throughout the British Empire, but in many other countries, too. Indeed, the story goes round that the first contribution received by the Scottish Federation of the National Union of Suffrage Societies towards the first Scottish unit was sent by an anti-suffragist, who said she was glad that they were at last doing something useful!

There are at this moment at least five military hospitals equipped, organised, and staffed entirely by women. In addition, there are two hospitals where more than half the doctors are women, and three others which have been equipped and organised by women.

The first unit of all the hospital units to be actually organised was that of Mrs. St. Clair Stobart, who was lay administrator, with Dr. Florence Stoney as head of the medical staff and in charge of the X-ray department; but they got to the Front a few days later than Dr. Louisa Garrett Anderson and Dr. Flora Murray, whose unit, with complete equipment, including X-ray apparatus, left for France on September 15, its offer of service having been accepted by the French Government.

Of these two units I would like to speak later, and will confine myself for the moment to the work of the National Union of Suffrage Societies, which has been responsible for no less than five units in France and Serbia, the Scottish Federation of the Union having initiated them and administered them under the splendid leadership of Dr. Elsie Inglis, who travelled up and down the country appealing for funds, and who has now gone to Serbia to help there.

The first hospital was started at Calais, with Dr. Alice Hutchinson and Dr. Phillips in charge, and with a staff of ten fully trained nurses. This work was undertaken at the request of Dr. Depage, the famous Belgian surgeon. In the typhoid annexe, of which they were given charge, they had the lowest death-rate of any typhoid hospital in Calais.

The next contingent to go abroad was a complete unit in charge of Dr. Frances Ivens, under the auspices of the French Red Cross, and it took up its quarters at the beautiful old Abbaye de Royaumont, seven miles from Chantilly and twelve from Creil, which is the principal distributing station for the wounded. The Abbaye, which dates from the twelfth century, and is said to have been founded by Blanche de Castile, had been disused for ten years or more – since the time when the French Government ejected the nuns – so it was found to be in a state of great

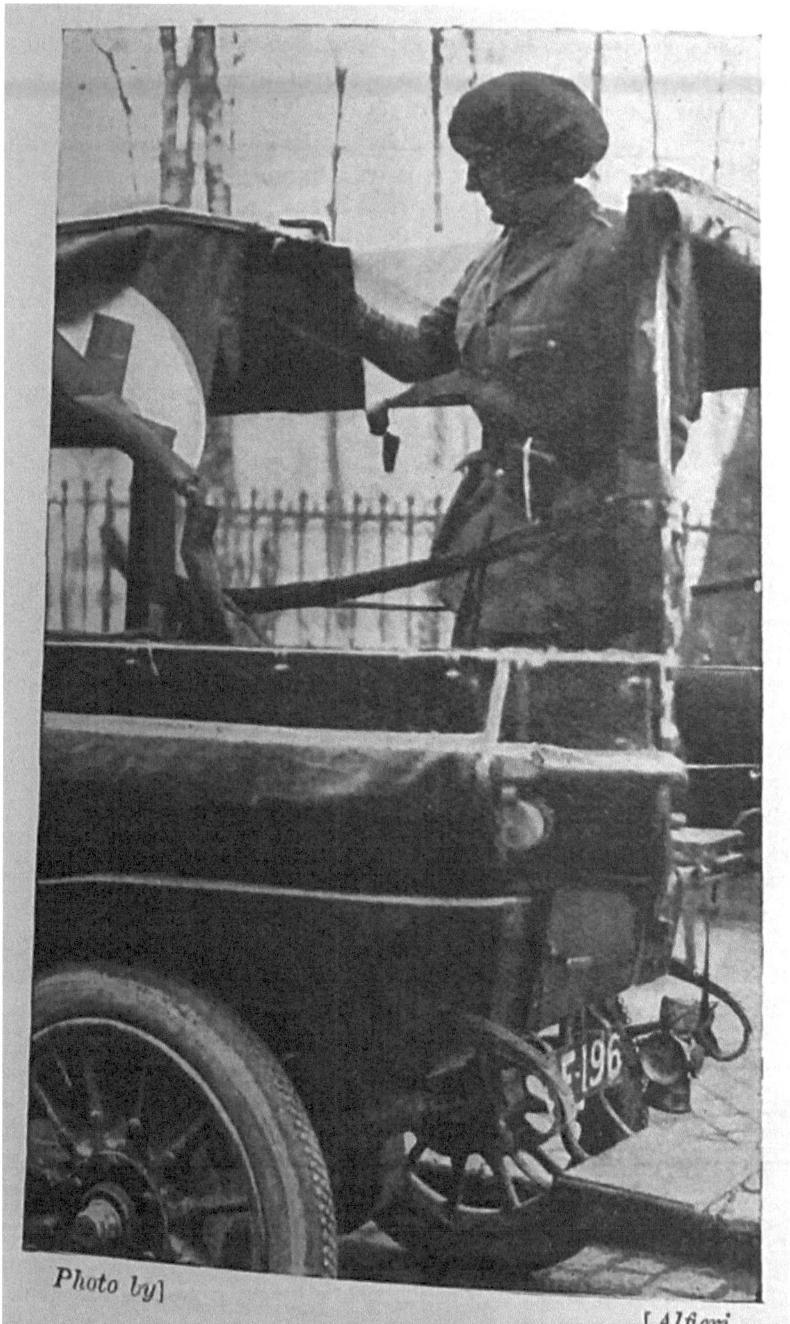

A RED CROSS CAR DRIVEN BY THE WOMEN'S NURSING YEOMANRY CORPS, AFTER A NARROW ESCAPE, A SHELL HAVING GONE RIGHT THROUGH IT, BUT WITHOUT EXPLODING.

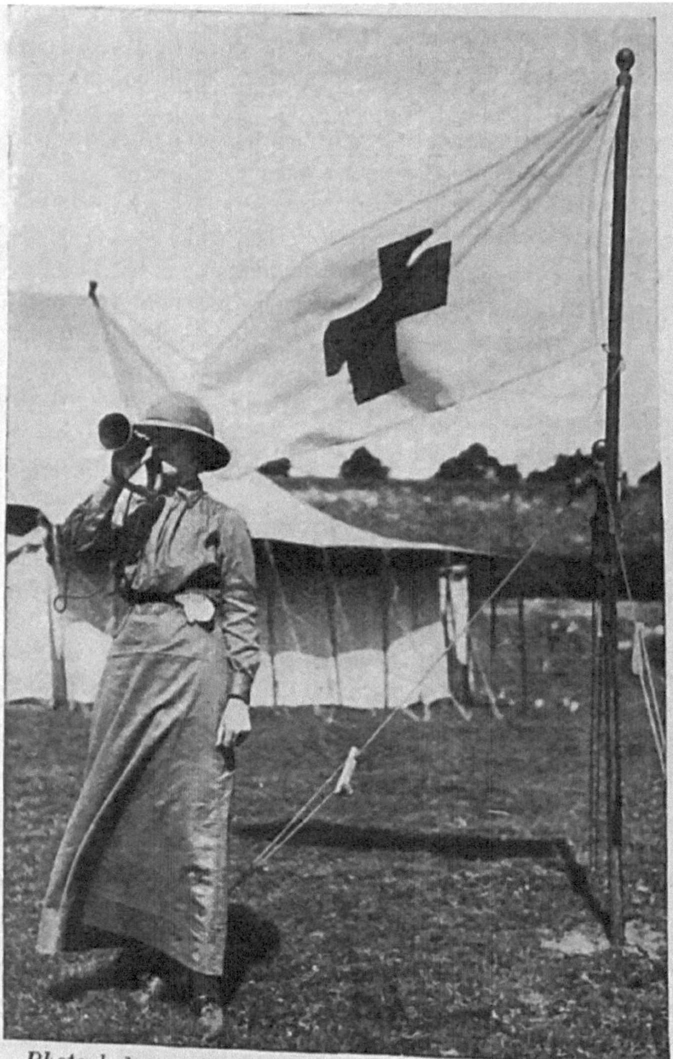

Photo by] [*Central News.*

SOUNDING THE REVEILLE IN THE CAMP OF THE WOMEN'S NURSING YEOMANRY CORPS IN FLANDERS.

disrepair. But, nothing daunted, the staff set to work, and in an amazingly short time grappled successfully with a whole host of difficulties. It was almost impossible to get outside help, and there were no stoves and no coals, and there was no hot water. The story of their experiences in getting the premises ready sounds something like what one might expect to happen in a disused ranch house in the wilds of the West. Finally the hospital was ready to be inspected by the French military hospital authorities, who gave their cordial approval, and recognised it as Hôpital Auxiliaire 301. It was equipped with an X-ray apparatus, and had attached to it a fleet of motor ambulances driven by women chauffeurs. It is the only hospital in the district fitted with an X-ray apparatus, and patients have been brought from all adjoining neighbourhoods to have their bullets extracted. The staff, over fifty in number, consists entirely of women, with the exception of the electrician. There were originally one hundred beds, but these have been increased to two hundred, and now a laboratory has been added. The work of this hospital has been greatly appreciated by the French military authorities, and a practical proof of the value of the unit lies in the fact that a special request has been sent down from the military authorities that Hôpital Auxiliaire 301 should take the most serious cases, and discharge them immediately they are convalescent.

The five wards are called after Blanche of Castile, Millicent Fawcett, Joan of Arc, Margaret of Scotland, and Queen Mary – in very truth representative women of all time. Mrs. Harley, sister of Sir John French, was for some months lay administrator at Royaumont, but she has now gone to Troyes to fill the same office in the second French unit. Miss Cicely Hamilton has been acting as clerk there since the beginning. Most interesting and delightful letters come from her, harbingers, let us hope, of a connected record and history of this fine undertaking, of which all women are so proud.

General Joffre has taken a personal interest in this hospital, and sent through his aide-de-camp a gift of three hundred francs for the men, out of a donation of one thousand francs entrusted to him for distribution in the neighbourhood.

The second French unit has been established at the Château Chanteloupe, Troyes, ninety miles south-east of Paris. It lies within forty miles of the firing-line, and its situation thus forms one of the principal stations for the reception of wounded from the seat of war. The hospital is a two-hundred-bed one, and is, with the exception of the operating theatre, entirely under canvas. The students of Girton and Newnham subscribed £1800, and it is known as the Girton and Newnham Unit. Dr. Louise McIlroy, of Glasgow, and Dr. Laura Sandeman, of Aberdeen, are in charge, and Mrs. Harley is lay administrator. It is directly under the French military authorities, at whose request it came into existence. It has an X-ray apparatus and a fleet of motor ambulances. A bacteriological laboratory, under the management of Dr. Ellen Porter, of Edinburgh, is an important feature of the hospital. It differs from the Royaumont and all other French hospitals in that it is the first hospital in which the French wounded have been nursed under canvas, and consequently it has aroused a great deal of attention everywhere. The Ministère de la Guerre has arranged with the Scottish Committee that this hospital should continue work for the duration of the War, and General Joffre's personal approval has been received that it should be a military hospital and under military control.

It is now proposed to open a clearing hospital, or *ambulance flottante*, near to the firing-line. The very bad cases would be first tended there, and afterwards sent on to Royaumont. The London Society of the National Union of Suffrage Societies has presented a travelling X-ray motor ambulance costing

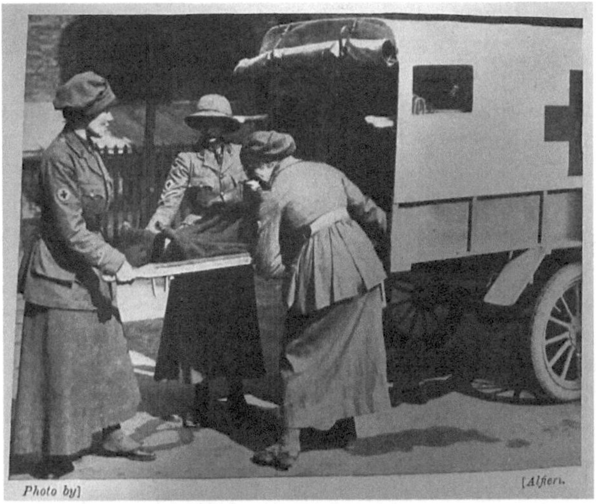

MEMBERS OF THE FIRST-AID NURSING YEOMANRY CORPS TAKING WOUNDED FROM BEHIND THE TRENCHES. MISS MURIEL THOMPSON (ON THE LEFT) HAS BEEN DECORATED BY KING ALBERT FOR BRAVERY IN THE FIELD.

over £1000, to be attached to this *ambulance flottante*, under the charge of Dr. Agnes Savile, of Harley Street, and has undertaken to maintain it for at least three months. I had the advantage of seeing this generous gift when it was shown recently in the grounds of that other pride of the woman movement,

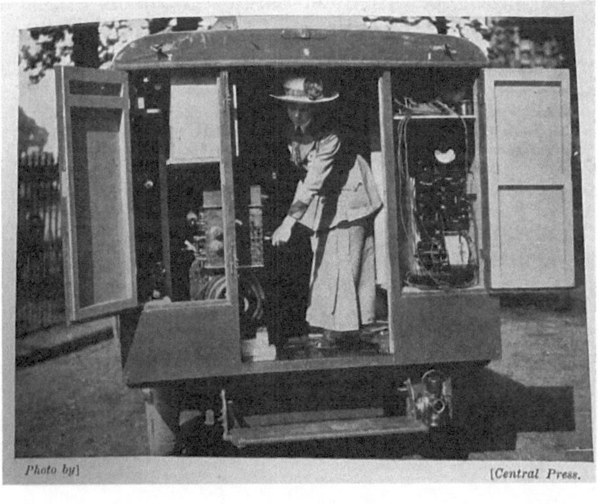

INTERIOR OF THE X-RAY MOTOR AMBULANCE PRESENTED BY THE SCOTTISH WOMEN'S HOSPITALS TO THE RED CROSS. IT CARRIES ITS OWN GASOLINE MOTORS FOR RADIOGRAPHY, WHICH IS UNDERTAKEN ENTIRELY BY WOMEN.

Bedford College, Regent's Park. The car carries a tent which can be packed into the rear, under which the table for taking photographs can be raised. There is a dark room in the car where photographs can be developed even while it is in motion. The car will be driven by a woman. It is very interesting to note the importance of radiography in this War, and the enthusiasm and natural aptitude of women for this department of service. Several women doctors have greatly distinguished themselves in it since the War began, and, in addition to others working in France and Serbia, Dr. Florence Stoney is in charge of this department at the military hospital, Fulham.

The sight of this wonderful car, and the realisation of the merciful purposes for which it was destined, held me for a long time. It was thrilling to think that it could just be telephoned for, and that it could speed from one field hospital to another, and thus be the means not only of sparing the wounded the suffering and physical strain of a long drive, but probably also of saving their lives and enhancing their chances of entire recovery.

In addition to these French units, the Scottish women's hospitals have sent two units to Serbia, and a third is in process of formation.

The first Serbian unit, in charge of Dr. Eleanor Soltau, and consisting of five women doctors, with nurses, dressers, and orderlies, arrived at Kragujevatz on January 6. Miss Douglas Irvine, the authoress, who accompanied the unit as clerk, writes: –

"It was welcomed by the authorities with eagerness, and found a need for its labours such as exceeded all that had been described in Western newspapers. The staff began work immediately in a hospital of one hundred and fifty beds, and soon, in order that these beds might be continuously devoted to only serious cases, they undertook also the supervision and surgical treatment of one hundred and fifty convalescent wounded. The X-ray apparatus of this hospital was in constant use, and our operator examined men who came not only from all the hospitals in Kragujevatz, but also from all the other towns – Belgrade, Nish, even distant Uskub. But, at the moment of writing, the need of Serbia is not for surgical, but for fever hospitals. There are still in the country very many wounded men whose ultimate recovery depends on the surgical treatment and nursing they receive, but they are less numerous than all the thousands who lie ill of typhus. When the staff of the first Serbian unit became aware of the seriousness of the typhus epidemic, they desired to help to fight it, and cabled to their Committee in Edinburgh for fever nurses. The Committee almost at once sent out the equipment of a fever hospital and two contingents, each of ten fully trained nurses, and also five doctors, asked for by the Serbian Government. The authorities in Serbia gave a building in Kragujevatz, which was disposed as a typhus hospital, and contains two hundred beds. This has now been transferred to Mlavadovatz, and is working under canvas."

Dr. Elsie Inglis, who has lately left for Serbia, reports that this unit has been responsible altogether for five hundred and seventy beds, and that General Soubititch, the Chief Medical Officer of the Serbian Army, said that "it was the best in Serbia, and that we did not expect impossibilities of the country, but made the best of what we could get."

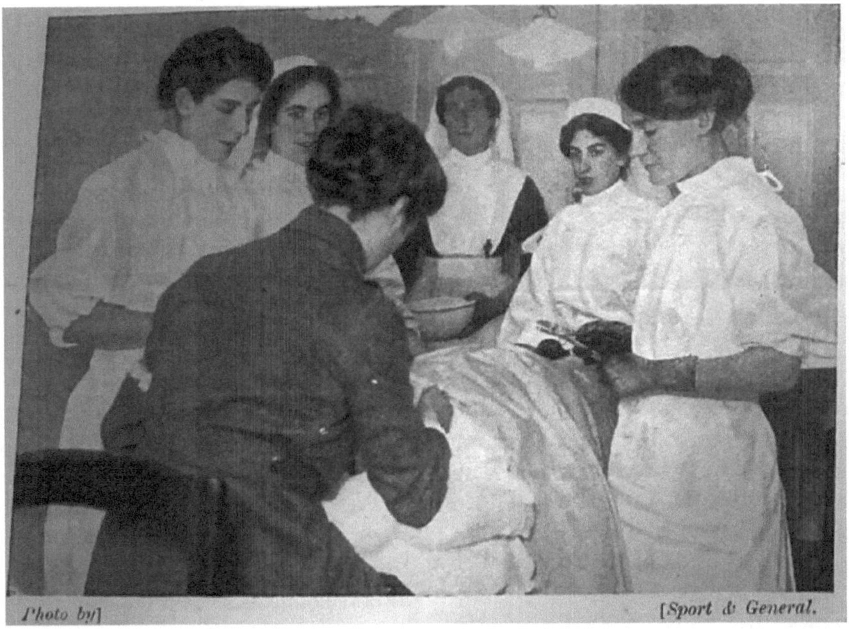

AN OPERATION IN THE ENGLISHWOMEN'S HOSPITAL IN PARIS.

Serbia's need, however, was so great that the Government asked for more help, and the second Serbian unit, in charge of Dr. Alice Hutchinson, was sent in April. It was staffed and equipped to nurse two hundred beds, to form a mobile base hospital, tents being the improved hygienic method of dealing with typhus and other epidemics and fevers. Dr. Alice Hutchinson's experience of military hospitals, in her work with the Women's Convoy Corps in the Balkan War, rendered her specially fitted for this work, and it is good to think that her valuable services were secured. This unit, on its arrival at Malta, was commandeered by the Governor to nurse our own wounded men from the Dardanelles, and when the unit left, Lord Methuen, the Governor, wrote: "It is not in my power to express my gratitude for this help given me by the Serbian unit. They leave here blessed by myself, surgeons, nurses, and patients alike, for they have proved themselves most capable and untiring workers. They never made the smallest difficulty, and would not have been sorry had I ordered them to remain another week."

This unit is now at Valjevo, on the north-west frontier of Serbia.

The third Serbian unit is shortly being dispatched. This is called the Wales and London Unit, the funds for its equipment having been subscribed by London and Wales, which has also sent a large motor ambulance to Serbia. It is staffed and equipped to nurse two hundred beds, and is entirely arranged with the idea of splitting up into a fever and a surgical staff, and its destination has been fixed for Ujitza.

All these units are working in touch with Colonel Hunter, of the R.A.M.C., who has been sent out by the War Office to take charge of the sanitary arrangements, and are sanctioned by Sir Ralph Paget, British Commissioner. They have posts of honour, being situated in the north-western district of Serbia, the area in which there has been the greatest amount of distress, and which, in the event of further hostilities, will again be seriously affected.

I have not dwelt on this distress, for it is well known by all of us that the sufferings of Serbia from one of the most disastrous epidemics of modern times have been appalling and heartrending. But here at least is one description of the conditions which the Scottish units found existing there at the beginning: –

"The most terrible sight I have seen here is the big fever hospital, a huge barracks, where there are said to be one thousand five hundred cases of fever, mostly enteric, typhus, and recurrent. Among their patients the acknowledged death-rate is ten a day, the fill of our hospital in a fortnight! With a fellow-member of the unit I went over the typhus wards one day. You really cannot imagine what it was like. There were only a few doctors for their hundreds of cases, and otherwise only orderlies, who are terrified for their own safety, poor wretches, and just crowd in corners, doing nothing unless driven to it. All along the corridors patients were packed together, and one of the corridors was so dark one could not see the patients' faces at first."

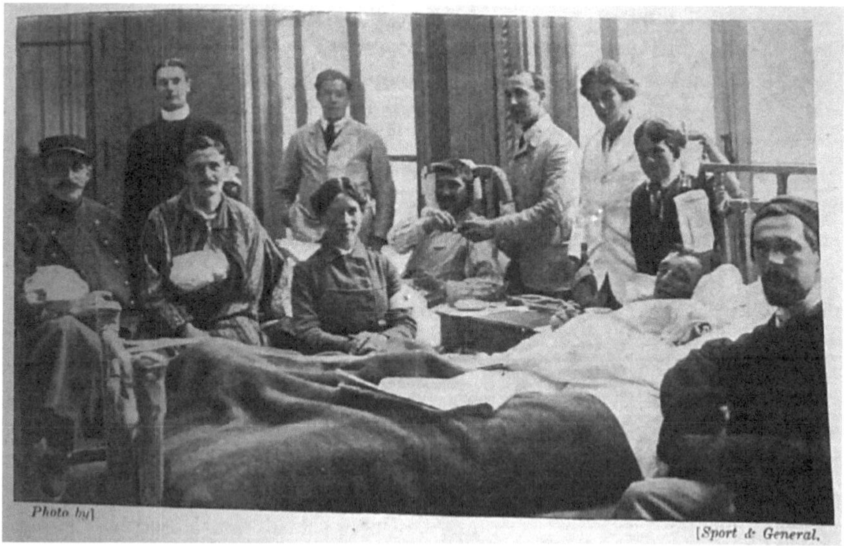

THE ENGLISH WOMEN DOCTORS' HOSPITAL, HEADED BY DR. GARRETT ANDERSON, IN PARIS.

It was to relieve conditions of this terrible nature that these heroic women, at great personal sacrifice and risk, undertook the work which they have so bravely and effectively carried out. Some have been very ill and have mercifully recovered. Some have died at their posts. Amongst the nurses and orderlies the death-roll has been excessive also, and the list of those who have given their lives includes the well-known name of that clever writer and most gifted woman Mrs. Percy Dearmer, and of Miss Neil Fraser, the famous golfer.

I cannot resist quoting, as a cheering instance of the improvement of conditions in Serbia, the following extract from one of Dr. Elsie Inglis's latest-letters. She writes:

> "The other day, Dr. Lilian Chesney got up a gymkhana for the patients in the hospital yard – a very simple affair, but it gave them the keenest enjoyment. In the middle of the sports I went into the wards to give tobacco to the men who were not able to come out and enjoy the fun, and whilst there I heard such laughter and cheers that I could not help thinking – there we all were, Turks and British and Serbs and Austrians, all playing together as happily as possible – perhaps if we played more together and knew one another better, such awful things as this War would not happen. At the end we gave some simple prizes – tobacco and cigarettes and knives."

A question frequently asked is why the Scottish women's hospitals are not working for their own country. The answer is, of course, that they wished to do so, but were given to understand that the needs of the British Army were fully met by established organisations. So they offered themselves to Belgium, France, and Serbia.

Since then, however, our own War Office has taken a different attitude towards the women doctors, and Dr. Louisa Garrett Anderson and Dr. Flora Murray now rank as majors in the British Army, and are in charge of the military hospital in Endell Street, for five hundred and fifty British soldiers.

These doctors organised a unit which they called the Women's Hospital Corps, and went to Paris on September 15, 1914, at the request of the Union des Femmes de France, one of the three constituent Societies of the Croix Rouge Française. The Corps consisted of seven doctors, three women orderlies, and an adequate staff of fully trained nurses.

Dr. Anderson kindly allows me to insert the following extract from one of her letters: –

"We were soon established in the Champs Elysées, in Claridge's Hotel, a magnificent new building with marble halls and painted ceilings. 'Never thought as I'd sleep in a marble 'all, I didn't, and so I laid awake and looked around me all night, I did,' as one of the patients said. It was to have opened in the autumn, and was built to attract millionaires, but the War came and brought stretcher-loads of wounded instead.

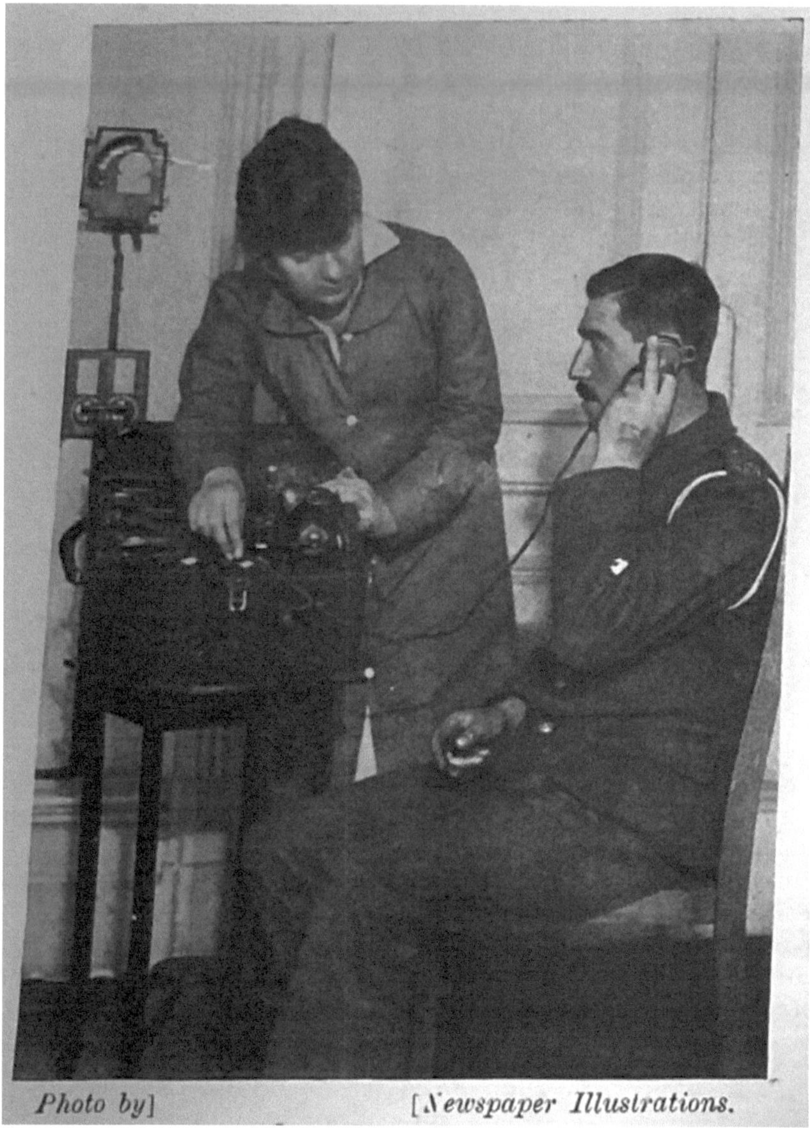

WOMAN DOCTOR TREATING A CASE OF SHELL DEAFNESS WITH AN ELECTRIC KEYBOARD.

"Friends gave us a magnificent equipment, which included an X-ray apparatus, instruments, and operating table and surgical dressings measured by the ton in weight.

"Claridge's Hotel provided the shell of a beautiful hospital. In less than a week, with the assistance of a carpenter and lathes and calico, the hotel was transformed into a hospital. The ladies' cloak-room, with tiled floor and walls, made the operating theatre, the hairdressing saloon was fitted as the X-ray room, and a large room with a beautiful ceiling light made the mortuary chapel.

"During the first weeks in Paris we were very busy. Most of the men were badly wounded. Transport arrangements were still defective, and the patients suffered greatly before they reached us.

"We will not forget the beauty of Paris in the early autumn mornings, and the processions from the hospital. The Champs Elysées was bathed in soft lights; the Arc de Triomphe looked ethereal; the trees were golden, and the distances faded into misty blue. All the beauty and poetry of Paris did honour to the dead. The firing picket drew up before the gate, the coffin, covered by the flag, was saluted by men in the streets, while the women crossed themselves and ran to put flowers upon it. A wreath, with '*France Reconnaissante*' upon it, was carried on the hearse, and members of the corps walked with it. Poor people in the streets used to stop us to give money *pour les blessés*."

Their hospital was a great success. The perfection of their equipment and organisation, and the quiet, methodical way in which both doctors went about their work, aroused warm admiration amongst the Parisians, and later amongst the many British military who came to inspect the hospital. They had British as well as French wounded, and it was to arrange about the British that one of the highly-placed officials of the Army originally came to the hospital.

Another visit from him followed on the first. He did not, however, seem to want to remove the British, but, on the contrary, asked if the work could be extended, so that more patients could be taken in if necessary. After this our militant doctors appear to have run the gauntlet of innumerable British military officials and Army and civilian medical men, and the upshot of the whole matter was that the British War Office got to know definitely that here was valuable work being done under the French Red Cross, and that there was no reason why it should not be done for the British Army. So when later the battle-line had moved further north, and fewer wounded were being brought to Paris, and the Women's Hospital Corps opened another hospital at Wimereux, near Boulogne, in the Château Mauricien, this is what happened: –

"On Monday afternoon," says the Journal, "we went into Boulogne and called at the headquarters. We walked into a bare room, where two officials were sitting at different ends of a table, presented our cards and our letter of introduction. Colonel – looked up at us and said: 'Oh, yes, I know all about you. You are the Women's Hospital Corps. You are extremely welcome here. We are delighted to hear you are going to establish yourselves' – and more of the same kind. The other Colonel said: 'How many beds will you have?' We told them we were established, that we would have up to a hundred beds, and asked them whether we should be used. He said: 'Yes, you shall be used to the fullest extent.' We asked whether we should be working under them, and he said: 'Certainly; you will be working

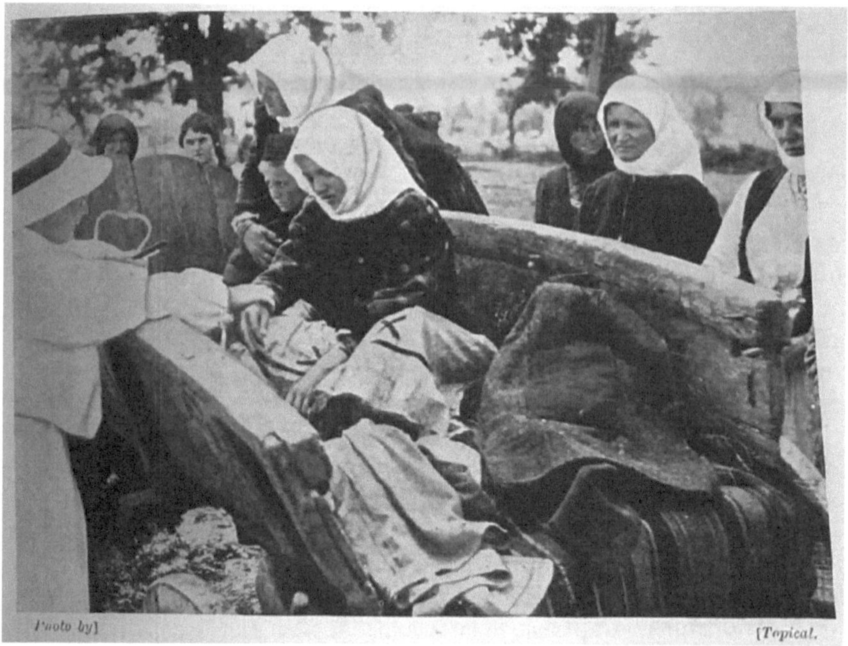

NURSES OF MRS. ST. CLAIR STOBART'S STAFF ATTENDING TO PATIENTS AT A WAYSIDE DISPENSARY AT KRAGUJEVATZ, IN SERBIA.

directly under me.' He then began to give me instructions as to what books to wire for, what forms and statistics to keep, and how to classify cases, while Dr. Anderson broached the question of rations. He said at once: 'Yes, you must have rations, certainly. And have you a quartermaster?' We had never thought about a quartermaster, but we said: 'Oh, yes, we have a quartermaster' – simultaneously, in our minds, appointing Orderly Campbell!"

This hospital, then, has been the first of those organised and staffed by women to be given official recognition by the War Office. They lived on Army rations, and indented for stores, clothing, and coal. It is interesting also to learn that two of the younger doctors of the staff were at once borrowed by the R.A.M.C., and were employed at one of the stationary hospitals, where they rendered invaluable service.

But notwithstanding these new developments of the work, the Women's Hospital Corps continued to keep on the Paris hospital as well; but as both fewer French and British wounded were being sent to Paris, and as, in addition, there were increasing difficulties connected with the heating of it, they finally retired from the French Red Cross, and transferred all their staff and equipments to Wimereux. They evidently left the scene of their early successes regretting and regretted.

"You have set a standard," said one of the military officials to them, "which is quite unknown, even amongst the auxiliary hospitals. It is a fine thing to have you here. It would be a misfortune if you were to leave, because you are such a good example of what a hospital ought to be."

They appear to have finished up with a real Christmas party and two plays. Here is the delightful description from the Journal: –

"Christmas preparations beginning. Got a lot of coloured paper and started the men on their decorations. This occupation kept them happy for the whole week and very busy, all vying with each other as to which should have the prize. Elaborate skill in most wards!

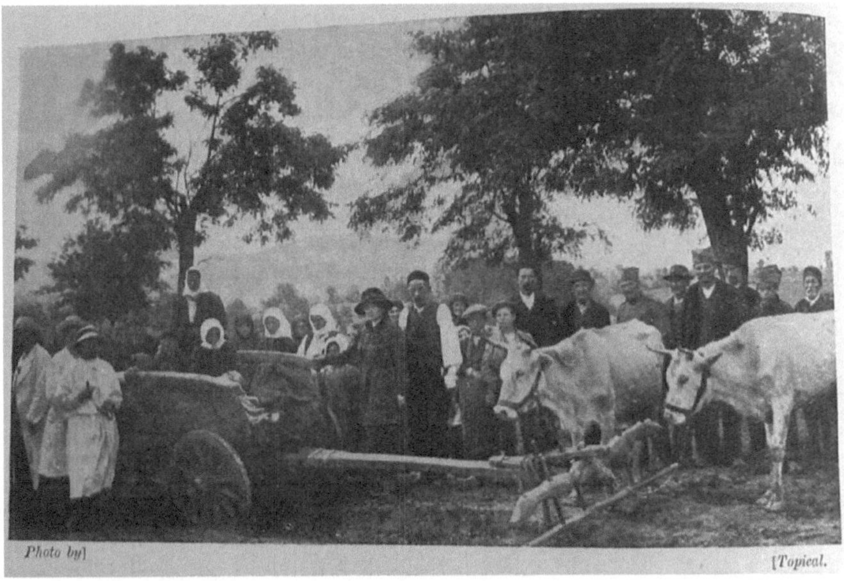

Photo by] [Topical.

A WAYSIDE CONSULTATION BY SOME OF MRS. STOBART'S NURSING STAFF IN SERBIA.

"We had a real Christmas atmosphere on Christmas Eve, when, in the half-dark, by the light of the braseros, the men and the night-nurses were seen hanging stockings all round the beds. At five o'clock I was wakened by roars of laughter, shouts of joy, reminiscent of nursery life, which continued on for the rest of the day.

"Our programme was to get the dressings over early, and then we collected all the tables in twos – seating accommodation for eighty-six – had all the beds conveyed in, and we had a grand dinner. We had excellent turkey, plum puddings, port wine, and so on. They enjoyed themselves tremendously. Then, when the puddings came up, we had a procession of myself and six nurses, each bearing a lighted pudding round, and they cheered and cheered the puddings again and again.

"After that we got arranged in the front ward, and the performance began.

" 'The Deserter' was an excellent play. They gave us a recruiting station, a scene at the Front, a desertion, and a court-martial, with the sentence carried out, the whole thing done with the greatest composure and steadiness, which made it very realistic. But what delighted us most of all was the way they took the officers off. The colonel, shuffling his papers and throwing a brief word at the unfortunate delinquent; the lieutenant, trying to bully the sergeant – they had got them absolutely, gesture, voice, manner, and appearance. In the middle of the performance Colonel – arrived and inquired what we were all doing here. One realised that his presence in the front would make the men feel extremely uncomfortable, so I did my best to get him out of the place as quickly as possible.

"The ward at the other end was quite jealous of the success of this ward, and announced that it would give an entertainment the following night. So we were given a story of a burglary and a scene in court. I missed most of it myself, but arrived on the scene in time to see a judge, in red flannel, with a cotton-wool wig, who every now and then himself roared: 'Silence in court!' "

The following interesting passage from the Journal throws a light on the French soldier, of whom we over here know so little: –

> "We have been very much struck by the mental shock from which the French soldiers are suffering. Our own men are of a less spiritual fibre. They have a stronger physique, and though the older ones are most obviously affected by the horrors of what they have gone through, and come out of the trenches nauseated, disgusted, and overwhelmed by the sights which they have seen, and which they will never forget, the French have, in addition, to bear the fearful anxiety of an invasion. In their delirium, and under an anæsthetic, they talk about France, and their beautiful country, and their homes, and the horror of the Germans coming round Paris. We ourselves in England have no conception of what it means to have that additional anxiety when one is fighting. All this increases the nervous shock and distress, and lessens the vitality."

Equal success and appreciation awaited the Women's Hospital Corps at Wimereux, and so admirable was their work there that, at the beginning of March, the War Office offered them the organisation of a general hospital of five hundred and twenty beds in or near London, and they accepted the offer and returned home. Their hospital is the military hospital, Endell Street, W.C. Their staff consists of fourteen doctors, amongst whom are a pathologist, an ophthalmic surgeon, and a dental surgeon. There are thirty-six nursing sisters and eighty orderlies, and that same quartermaster appointed by telepathy on that auspicious occasion at Wimereux continues her work here on this enlarged scale.

For some mysterious reason it would seem to be a law of the Medes and Persians that military hospitals should not be written about, but it is well known that the men are looked after by the Women's Hospital Corps with the greatest skill and devotion, that everything is done by the whole staff to make them happy, and to maintain a homelike and cheery atmosphere, which greatly helps in their recuperation.

Dr. Louisa Garrett Anderson and Dr. Flora Murray have made, by the vision which prompted them to go to France, and by the success of their work, and the recognition they have won from the War Office, a contribution of unspeakable value to the woman movement all the world over, while there is no doubt that their initiative, alertness, and attainment have stimulated and encouraged further activities amongst the French medical women themselves.

It is singularly fitting that one of these new pioneer medical women should be the daughter of Dr. Elizabeth Garrett Anderson, whose own pioneer work in the past helped to win for women their entry into the medical profession. And it is delightful to learn that when she heard that they intended to go to France to undertake this work, she said: "If you go, you will put forward your cause by a hundred years." And when she saw them off at the station, her parting words were: "If I had been twenty years younger, I should have taken them myself."

That is the spirit which won the battlefield for women in the past.

Mrs. St. Clair Stobart, who did admirable work for the wounded in the Balkans, was among the first to take the field on the outbreak of war. She began work in Brussels, but was arrested by the Germans as a spy. She and the others with her were, however, released, and escaped to England, and, nothing daunted, at once set about organising a hospital unit, staffed by women, to help in Belgium. She invited Dr. Florence Stoney to be head of the medical staff and to take charge of the X-ray department, the apparatus of which had been generously given by Lady Cowdray. The following is part of Dr. Stoney's account: –

"We started for Antwerp, at the invitation of the Belgian Croix Rouge, on September 20, 1914. There we had a hospital with one hundred beds, the number of which was increased later to one hundred and thirty-five. Our staff consisted of six women doctors, ten trained nurses, as well as several women orderlies. We were working there just over a fortnight, during which time we had more than two hundred cases, most of them straight from the trenches. They were Belgians and a few British. In the latter days surgery was rendered difficult because the water-supply was cut off, and for this reason, water for the whole hospital had to be fetched from a well. On October 8 the bombardment took place. We were eighteen hours under shell-fire before we could place our patients in comparative safety. During this time not a single one of our party was hit, though the ground was littered with shell, and houses round were burning.

"We ourselves finally got away across the bridge of boats on London motor buses, sitting on British ammunition cases. The road out of Antwerp was one sad procession of fleeing peasants, troops, cattle, guns, wagons, children, carts, all moving in the same direction as rapidly as possible. As we left Antwerp, the city was blazing in over twenty places, the oil reservoirs by the river being a pillar of fire one hundred feet high; but nothing else seemed to matter once we got away from the whiz of the shells, and for two nights we were thankful to get a wooden floor to sleep on. The bridge of boats across the Scheldt was blown up by the Belgians twenty minutes after we crossed.

"Our hospital unit was next invited by the French Croix Rouge to go to Cherbourg, and there we established ourselves, on November 6, in Château Tourlaville, as the Anglo-French Hospital No. 2, under the sanction of the British Red Cross and St. John Ambulance."

Here they worked, looking after very seriously wounded French, Belgians, and Africans, and gaining golden opinions from the authorities, and working under the Port doctor. Dr. Conteaud, Médecin Général de la Marine, wrote of the Women's Hospital at Cherbourg: –

> "J'ai admiré le sangfroid, le calme, et l'habilité des doctoresses, qui ne laissent rien à envier aux qualités professionelles des hommes médecins."

And General Gaffiot, Commandant of the Fifth and Eighth Sub-divisions, wrote: –

> "J'ai emporté de la visite à Tourlaville un sentiment de grande admiration pour la superbe installation de cet hôpital, et pour les soins si dévoués donnés aux blessés français."

The good work done there makes one regret all the more that the hospital was so far from the Front that it had finally to be given up. Mrs. St. Clair Stobart organised another unit for Serbia, and Dr. Florence Stoney, as already stated, returned home, and is in charge of the X-ray department at the military hospital, Fulham, a hospital of over nine hundred beds. The history of the whole of this enterprise is particularly interesting, because it is an admirable illustration not only of the ability and initiative of women, but also of their courage, cool-headedness, and endurance. The picture often rises before me of those doctors and nurses carrying down to the cellars their helpless patients when the bombardment of Antwerp began. Miss Macnaughtan, the authoress, accompanied Mrs. Stobart's unit to Antwerp, and stayed on afterwards, giving devoted service in many directions.

Special mention should be made of the Australian Women's Hospital, in one of the quietest parts in Auteuil, which was founded by Mrs. William Smith, of Melbourne, and her two daughters, Dr. Helen Sexton and Mrs. R. Blackwood. The latest news of this hospital is that it has now been recognised as a military hospital.

The space at my disposal prevents me from dwelling at length on many of the other undertakings carried through, and still being carried through, by women doctors, in groups or singly. But I must not omit to mention Dr. Agnes Bennett, who was in Egypt when medical workers were badly needed, and was taken into the New Zealand Army Medical Corps with the rank and pay of captain. She at once went on duty at the Egyptian Army Hospital, which has been lent to the New Zealand Government. There she found Dr. Grace Russell, who is a medical officer in the employ of the Egyptian Government, engaged in all sorts of public health work, and who had been lent to New Zealand. Dr. Russell was called away owing to an outbreak of typhus among the natives. Nor must I omit the name of Dr. Isabel Ormiston, who was decorated by the King of the Belgians for the splendid services to the Belgian wounded at Ostend, and later at the Queen of the Belgians' hospital at La Panne. She is now one of the staff of the hospital that was sent by the Wounded Allies' Relief Committee to Montenegro.

This account cannot in any way aim at being comprehensive, because of the difficulty of getting details, owing to the absence of the workers themselves, and the vastness of the area over which the activities are spread. There are several hospitals which have been equipped by English, Canadian, and American women, or both equipped and organised by women only, but not staffed by them, and of these, Lady Paget's in Serbia ranks as one of the very best. And a field ambulance, organised by Dr. Hector Munro, had on its staff four women, whose pluck in the firing-line has met with wide recognition. Miss May Sinclair accompanied this unit in the beginning, and gives a wonderful account of her experiences in her volume called "A Journal of Impressions in Belgium."

A British field hospital for Belgium, consisting of four women and three men doctors, also worked at Antwerp, Ghent, Bruges, Ostend, and on a hospital ship. One member, Dr. Maude, was then asked by the War Office to go as anæsthetist to an R.A.M.C. unit in Calais. Later she took charge of a rest-house near Dunkirk, where convoys could call for medical assistance, and leave cases which could not stand the whole journey in one day. This was in the danger zone, and her wounded were very often the victims of bomb attacks. The Women's First-Aid Nursing Yeomanry, some members of which are attached to the Fifth Division of the Belgian Army, is doing splendid service, often in the actual firing-line.

Imperfect though this record is, it will at least give some idea of the activities of the medical women in this War, and of the efficiency of their work. As Surgeon-General Sir Alfred Keogh said recently: "The idea that the medical education of women is an experiment must pass away. It has proved its worth, and nobody can doubt that it has come to stay – and to stay for the public good."

BIBLIOGRAPHY

ARCHIVAL MATERIAL

Album of Newspaper Cuttings Relating to the New Hospital for Women, H13/EGA/144, London Metropolitan Archives.

Papers Relating to Miss A.J. Beatty (1897–1908), DD/815/192, Administrative Records of the West London Hospital, London Metropolitan Archives.

Elizabeth Garrett Anderson Letters and Papers, HA436, Ipswich Record Office, Suffolk Archives.

London School of Medicine for Women and Royal Free Hospital Press Cuttings, Volume IV: January 1904–August 1915, H72/SM/Y/02/004, London Metropolitan Archives.

London School of Medicine for Women and Royal Free Hospital Press Cuttings, Volume V: Sept 1915–Oct 1920, H72/SM/Y/02/005, London Metropolitan Archives.

London (Royal Free Hospital) School of Medicine for Women Magazine (1895–1918)

South London Hospital for Women Press Cuttings 1912–1917, H24/SLW/Y6/1, London Metropolitan Archives.

Minutes of the Managing Committee of the New Hospital for Women, Book II: May 1882-March 1895; 4 July 1883, H13/EGA/020, London Metropolitan Archives.

Minute Books of the Managing Committee of the New Hospital for Women. Book IV: April 1906-November 1915, H13/EGA/022, London Metropolitan Archives.

Scottish Women's Hospitals Royaumont, Copies of Letters Received at Headquarters from July 1915 to October 1916', Mitchell Library, Glasgow.

American Medical Women's Association: https://livesonline.rcseng.ac.uk/client/en_GB/lives

At the Circulating Library: A Database of Victorian Fiction, 1837–1901: https://www.victorianresearch.org/atcl/

Census – 1851–1911

Changing the Face of Medicine: Celebrating America's Women Physicians: https://cfmedicine.nlm.nih.gov/physicians/

Church of England Births and Baptisms, 1813–1919

Medical Dictionary

Medical Register

New South Wales, Australia: Index to Deceased Estate Files, 1859–1958; Probate Calendar (Index of Wills and Administrations), 1858–1995

Oxford Dictionary of National Biography: https://www.oxforddnb.com/

Plarr's Lives of the Fellows: https://livesonline.rcseng.ac.uk/client/en_GB/lives

England and Wales Probate Calendar (Index of Wills and Administrations), 1858–1995
UK Midwives Roll, 1904–1959
University of London Student Records, 1836–1945: https://www.london.ac.uk/senate-house-library/our-collections/special-collections/archives-manuscripts/university-london-students-1836–1939
The Waterloo Directory of English Newspapers and Periodicals: 1800 to 1900. Series Two: https://www.victorianperiodicals.com/series2/

PRIMARY SOURCES

Newspapers and Periodicals

Aberdeen Journal
Academy
Academy Fiction Supplement
Academy and Literature
American Publishers' Circular and Literary Gazette
American Journal of Dental Science
Annals of Surgery
Archives of Medicine
Association Monthly
Athenaeum
Atlanta Medical and Surgical Journal
Atlantic Monthly
Australasian
Blackwood's Edinburgh Magazine
Book Buyer
Bookseller, Newsdealer and Stationer
Boston Daily Advertiser
Boston Sunday Globe
British Architect
British Medical Journal (*BMJ*)
Canadian Journal of Medicine and Surgery
California Medical Journal
California and Western Medicine
Chambers's Journal
Chap-Book
Chicago Medical Examiner
Church: A Journal of American Churchmanship
Common Cause
Congregationalist
Contemporary Review
Cosmopolis
Critic
Current Issue
Current Literature: A Magazine of Contemporary Record
Daily Evening Bulletin

Daily Mail
Daily News
Daily Telegraph
Derby Daily Telegraph
Dublin Journal of Medical Science
Eclectic Magazine
Edinburgh Medical Journal
English Review
Englishwoman's Review of Social and Industrial Questions
Equal Rights
Everybody's Magazine
Examiner
Friend of India
Girl's Own Paper
Glasgow Herald
Glasgow Medical Journal
Godey's Lady's Book and Magazine
Graphic
Guy's Hospital Gazette
Harper's Weekly: A Journal of Civilisation
Home Mission Monthly
Hospital
Hospital Gazette and Archives of Clinical Surgery
Indian Medical Gazette
Insurance and Commercial Magazine
Journal of the American Medical Association (*JAMA*)
Journal of National Medical Association
Journal of South Carolina Medical Association
Journal of the Women's Education Union
Lancet
La Revue
La Semaine Littéraire
Leicester Chronicle
Liberator
Literature
Literary Era: A Monthly Repository of Literary and Miscellaneous Information
Literary Digest
Living Age
London Journal
London Quarterly Review
Luzac's Oriental List
Manchester Courier and Lancashire General Advertiser
Manchester Guardian
Manchester Times
McGill Fortnightly: A Fortnightly Journal of Literature, University Thought and Event
Medical Critic and Psychological Journal

Medical and Surgical Reporter
Medical Times and Gazette
Michigan Alumnus Quarterly Review
Military Surgeon
Missionary Review of the World
Morning Post
Musical Standard
Musical World
Nation
Naturalists' Leisure Hour and Monthly Bulletin
New England Farmer: Devoted to Agriculture and All Its Kindred Arts and Sciences
New Orleans Medical and Surgical Journal
New York Age
New York Medical Journal
New Yorker Medicinische Monatsschrift
New York Times
New York World
North American
Observer
Our Young Folk's Weekly Budget
Outlook
Outlook of Missions
Pall Mall Gazette
Penny Illustrated Paper
Practitioner: A Journal of Practical Medicine
Publishers' Circular
Publishers' Weekly
Punch
Punch's Almanack
Review of Reviews
Saturday Review
Southern Workman
Spectator
Speaker
Standard
Temple Bar
Theologische Literaturblatt
Times
Wesleyan-Methodist Magazine
Western Daily Press
Westminster Review
Woman at Home: Annie S. Swan's Magazine
Woman's Medical Journal
Woman Worker
Women's Penny Paper
Women's Suffrage Journal

Books and Pamphlets

Annual Report of the New Hospital for Women (London: Alexander and Shepheard, 1872–1918)

Anon., 'Officers of the Eclectic Medical Society', *Transactions of the National Eclectic Medical Association of the United States of America, for the Years 1891–92*, XIX (Orange, NJ: The Chronicle Press, 1892).

Caldwell, A.B. (ed.), *History of the American Negro. South Carolina Edition, Volume III* (Atlanta, GA: A.B. Caldwell Publishing Co., 1919).

Catalogue of Copyright Entries, Part I: Books; Dramatic Compositions Maps and Charts (Washington: Government Printing Office Library Division, 1908).

Croly, J., *Sorosis: Its Origin and History* (New York: J.J. Little & Co., 1886).

Crosby, A.H., 'Orthodoxy and Heterodoxy in Medicine', in *Transactions of the New Hampshire Medical Society (eighty-Seventh Anniversary) Held at Concord, June 19 and 20, 1877* (Concord, NH: Republican Press Association, 1877), pp. 77–92.

Dall, C.H., *'Woman's Right to Labor'; or, Low Wages and Hard Work: In Three Lectures, Delivered in Boston, November, 1859* (Boston: Walker, Wise, and Company, 1860).

Diver, M., *The Englishwoman in India* (Edinburgh and London: William Blackwood & Sons, 1909).

Education and Professions: The Woman's Library, Volume I (London: Chapman & Hall, 1903).

Efforts for Social Betterment Among Negro Americans. A Social Study Made by Atlanta University, under the Patronage of the Trustees of the John F. Slater Fund (Atlanta, GA: Atlanta University Press, 1909).

Encyclopedia of American Biography (New York: The American Historical Society, Inc., 1936).

The English Catalogue of Books for 1895 (London: Sampson Low, Marston & Company, 1896).

Evans, M.A., *Martha Schofield. Pioneer Negro Educator. Historical and Philosophical Review of Reconstruction Period of South Carolina* (Columbia, SC: DuPre Printing Company, 1916).

Faithfull, E., *Three Visits to America* (Edinburgh: David Douglas, 1884).

Forty-Seventh to Sixty-Ninth Annual Announcements of the Woman's Medical College of Pennsylvania 1896–1897 to 1918–1919)

General List of Books, in Various Branches of Literature, Published and For Sale by Longman's, Green, & Co. (New York: Longman's, Green, & Co., 1906).

Handbook of South Carolina. Resources, Institutions and Industries of the State (Columbia, SC: The State Company, 1907).

Hildebrand, B. (ed.), *Uebersicht über die neuesten Publikationen Deutschlands und des Auslandes: Gewerbe und Industrie, Jahrbücher für Nationalökonomie und Statistik* (Jena: Gustav Fischer, 1895).

Hurd-Mead, K.C., *Medical Women of America: A Short History of the Pioneer Medical Women of America and a Few of Their Colleagues in England* (New York: Froben Press, 1933).

The Indian Law Reports. Bombay Series, IX (Calcutta: Thacker, Spink, and Co., 1885).

Jex-Blake, S., *Medical Women: Two Essays* (Edinburgh: William Oliphant & C., and London: Hamilton, Adams, & Co., 1872).

King, W.H. (ed.), *History of Homeopathy and its Instituions in America, Volume III* (New York and Chicago: Lewis Publishing Company, 1905).

Leonard, J.W. (ed), *Woman's Who's Who of America: A Biographical Dictionary of Contemporary Women of the United States and Canada* (New York: The American Commonwealth Company, 1914).

Lovejoy, E.P., *Certain Samaritans* (New York: The Macmillan Company, 1927).

Marshall, C., *The Woman's Medical College of Pennsylvania. An Historical Outline* (Philadelphia: P. Blakiston, Son & Co., 1897).

Memories of Jane Cunningham Croly 'Jenny June' (New York: G.P. Putnam's Sons and London: The Knickerbocker Press, 1904).

Miller, K., and Gay, J.R., *Progress and Achievements of the Colored People. A Beacon Light for the Coming Generations* (Washington DC: Austin Jenkins Co., 1917).

Nevins, A., *The Emergence of Modern America, 1865–1878, Volume VIII of A History of American Life in Twelve Volumes* (New York: Macmillan, 1927).

Fifty-Third Annual Report of the New England Hospital for Women and Children for the Year Ending September 30, 1915 (Boston: Geo. H. Ellis Co., 1916).

Pankhurst, E.S., *The Suffragette: the History of the Women's Militant Suffrage Movement, 1905–1910* (New York: Sturgis Walton & Company, 1911).

Polk's Medical Register and Directory of North America. Index to the Physicians of the United States, 9th revised edition (Detroit, Baltimore and Chicago: R.L. Polk & Co., 1906).

Repplier, A., *J. William White, MD. A Biography* (Boston and New York: Houghton Mifflin Company, 1919).

Robinson, L.A., *The Health of our Children in the Colonies: A Book for Mothers* (London: Longmans, Green, and Co., 1906).

Savill, A., *Music, Health and Character* (New York: Frederick A. Stokes Company, 1924).

Scawen Blunt, W., *My Diaries. Being A Personal Narrative of Events, 1888–1914: Part One 1888 to 1900* (London: Martin Secker, 1919).

Scharlieb, M., *A Woman's Words to Women. Second Edition, thoroughly revised* (London: George Routledge & Sons; New York: E.P. Dutton & Co., 1905).

Sorabji, C., *India Calling: The Memories of Cornelia Sorabji* (London: Nisbet & Co. Ltd, 1934).

Souchon, E., *Original Contributions of America to Medical Sciences* (n.p.: Transactions of the American Surgical Association, 1917).

Steward, S. M., *Woman in Medicine: A Paper Read Before the National Association of Colored Women's Clubs at Wilberforce, Ohio, August 6, 1914* (Wilberforce, Ohio: n.p., 1914).

Stanton, T., (ed.), *The Woman Question in Europe: A Series of Original Essays* (London: Sampson Low, Marston, Searle, and Rivington, 1884).

Strachey, L., (trans.), *The Memoirs of an Arabian Princess* (New York: Doubleday, Page & Company, 1907).

Tweedie, A., (ed.), *The First College Open to Women Queen's College London: Memories and Records of Work Done 1848–1898* (London: Queen's College, 1898).

Union of South Africa. Report of the Under Secretary for Education for the Year ended 31st December, 1918. Part I Child Welfare (Cape Town: Cape Times Limited, 1919).

University of Washington Territory. Seattle, WT. Annual Register for 1879–80 (Seattle, WT: Stewart & Ebersold, 1880).

Vietor, A.C., *A Woman's Quest: the Life of Marie E. Zakrzewska, MD* (New York and London: D. Appleton and Company, 1924).

Washington, B.T., *The Story of the Negro: The Rise of the Race from Slavery, Volume II* (New York: Doubleday, Page Company, 1909).

Wilde, O., *Reviews* (London: Methuen and Co., 1908).

Williams, H., *Modern English Writers: Being a Study of Imaginative Literature 1890–1914* (New York: Alfred Knopf, 1919).

Secondary Sources

Beetham, M., *A Magazine of Her Own? Domesticity and Desire in the Woman's Magazine, 1880–1914* (London and New York: Routledge, 1996).

Bellafaire, J., and Graf, M.H., *Women Doctors in War* (College Station: Texas A&M University Press, 2009).

Bennett, J.D.C., 'Princess Vera Gedroits: military surgeon, poet, and author', *BMJ*, 305:6868 (19 December 1992), pp. 1532–1534.

———, 'Abdominal Surgery in War – The Early Story', *Journal of the Royal Society of Medicine*, 84 (September 1991), pp. 554–557.

Bonner, T. N., *To the Ends of the Earth: Women's Search for Education in Medicine* (Cambridge, MA and London: Harvard University Press, 1992).

Brock, C., "Women in Surgery after the Great War', in C.G. Jones, A.E. Martin, A. Wolf (eds), *The Palgrave Handbook of Women and Science: History, Cultures and Practice since 1660* (Cham: Palgrave Macmillan, 2022), pp. 593–610.

———, 'The Disappearance of Sophia Frances Hickman', *History Workshop Journal*, 80:1 (Autumn 2015), pp. 161–182.

Condrau, F., 'The Patient's View Meets the Clinical Gaze', *Social History of Medicine*, 20:3 (December 2007), pp. 525–540.

Crawford, E., *The Women's Suffrage Movement: A Reference Guide 1866–1928* (London: UCL Press, 1999).

Crowther, M.A., and Dupree, M.W., *Medical Lives in the Age of Surgical Revolution* (Cambridge: Cambridge University Press, 2007).

Farkas, C-A., 'Fictional Medical Women and Moral Therapy in the Late-Nineteenth Century: Daughters of Aesculapius, Mothers to All', *English Literature in Transition, 1880–1920*, 54.2 (2011), pp. 139–164.

Harris, S.M., *Dr Mary Walker: An American Radical* (New Brunswick, NJ and London: Rutgers University Press, 2009).

Hunt, C., *The National Federation of Women Workers, 1906–1921* (Basingstoke and New York: Palgrave Macmillan, 2014),

———, 'Binding Women Together in Friendship and Unity?', *Media History*, 19.2 (2013), pp. 139–152.

Hunt, K., *Equivocal Feminists: The Social Democratic Federation and the woman question, 1884–1914* (Cambridge: Cambridge University Press, 1996).

Klifto, K.M, Quan, A., and Dellon L., 'Mary Edwards Walker (1832–1919): Approach to limb salvage therapy', *Wound Repair and Regeneration*, 27 (2019), pp. 285–287.

Lutzker, E., 'Edith Pechey-Philpson, MD: Untold Story', *Medical History*, 11:1 (January 1967), pp. 41–45.

McIntyre, N., *How British Women Became Doctors: The Story of the Royal Free Hospital and its Medical School* (n.p.: Wenrowave Press, 2014).

McIntyre, N., 'Britain's first medical marriage: Frances Morgan (1843–1927), George Hoggan (1837–1891) and the mysterious "Elsie"', *Journal of Medical Biography*, 12:2 (May 2004), pp. 105–114.

Nakayama, D.K. (ed.), *Black Surgeons and Surgery in America* (Chicago, IL: American College of Surgeons, 2021).

Raban, S., (ed.), *Examining the World: A History of the University of Cambridge Local Examinations Syndicate* (Cambridge: Cambridge University Press, 2008).

Schuller, K., *The Biopolitics of Feeling: Race, Sex, and Science in the Nineteenth Century* (Durham, NC: Duke University Press, 2018).

Sparks, T., *The Doctor in the Victorian Novel: Family Practices* (Farnham and Burlington, VT: Ashgate, 2009).

Swenson, K., *Medical Women and Victorian Fiction* (Columbia, MI: University of Missouri Press, 2005).

Whiteley, G., '*The Tree of Knowledge*: New Insights on Katherine Mansfield, Oscar Wilde and "A Woman"', in G. Diment, G. Kimber and M.W. Todd (eds), *Katherine Mansfield and Russia* (Edinburgh: Edinburgh University Press, 2017), pp.175–189.

Williams, L., *No Easy Path: The Life and Times of Lilian Violet Cooper, MD, FRACS [1861–1947], Australia's First Woman Surgeon* (Brisbane: Amphion Press, 1991).

Wilson, B.J., 'Relearning in Military Surgery: The Contributions of Princess Vera Gedroits', *Clinical and Investigative Medicine*, 30:4 (August 2007), pp. 159–167.

Young, A., 'Ladies and Professionalism: The Evolution of the Idea of Work in the *Queen*, 1861–1900, *Victorian Periodicals Review*, 40:3 (Fall 2007), pp. 189–215.

INDEX

Note: Numbers in *italics* indicate a figure.